AF880709

AMELOGENINS: MULTIFACETED PROTEINS FOR DENTAL AND BONE FORMATION AND REPAIR

Michel Goldberg (Editor).

Professor Michel Goldberg U747- Laboratoire Différenciation de Cellules Souches et Prions, U747, Université Paris Descartes, 45 rue des Saints Pères, 75006 Paris, France; Tel: 33 6 62 67 67 09; E-mails: mgoldberg.goldberg004@gmail.com or michel.goldberg@parisdescartes.fr

CONTENT

CHAPTERS

PART 1: GENE AND CELL REGULATIONS

PREFACE

Now at the end of my task as editor of this book, I would like to share the two criteria by which I selected my co-workers. Firstly they were chosen because they are among the best in the field that they were asked to cover. Of course, I could have selected a few others who are also excellent research scientists, but this would duplicate the talents and introduce redundancies. I beg the indulgence of these colleagues and apologize for those who were not included in the final short list of contributors. The second reason is the friendship that we have developed during all these years, meeting after meeting, during conferences, workshops, exchanging information, discussions, molecules, ideas, and in many cases drinking or dinning together. Obviously, any choice is questionable and spoilt by any bias of selection, but at the endpoint, it was a good one and I could not have dreamt a better team.

This mutual friendship meant that most authors instantaneously accepted my request and agreed to participate in this stimulating project. The exceptional list of authors who immediately and enthusiastically agreed to contribute, meant that I had little extra to do to convince the very few who had too much work, to accept this additional task. This then meant that this initial task of inviting authors was quite easy.

Later, I had to put some pressure on the shoulders of some of them to receive the chapters in due time. Finally this also was overcome. I have so much enjoyed receiving each manuscript, reading it and realizing that each excellent contribution was exactly at the level of excellence and insight that I was expecting. I hope that you as readers of this book will have this same experience, especially the PhD students who are willing to learn something about these molecules, and for the experts, scientists or clinicians, who are looking for a strong basis for their knowledge and/or support for everyday clinical practice.

In 1942, Deakins found that immature enamel contains 19%, by weight organic matter, and after maturation only 1.8% [1]. This later value was further revised and it is now accepted that the enamel matrix does not contain over 0.6% organic matter by weight. In the early 1960s, it was shown that the transitory enamel proteins displayed a very special amino acid composition, including high proline content (approximately one quarter of all the amino acid residues), with glutamic acid, leucine and histidine being the other major amino acids. For these findings, tribute should be given to John Eastoe for his analysis of enamel proteins [2, 3]. The amino acid composition of the developing enamel matrix differs from either collagens or keratins. During maturation, these unusual proline-containing proteins preferentially disappear, whereas others disappear less rapidly and are partly retained in the mature enamel. Eastoe suggested that these transitory hydrophobic proline-rich proteins be called amelogenins (AMEL) [4]. They are substantially different from the acidic matrix proteins found in mature enamel, termed "enamelins" (ENAM) by Mechanics in 1971 [5]. This category of enamelin proteins was more recently termed "nonamelogenins", and including more recently identified matrix proteins; ameloblastin (AMBN) [6], enamelin (ENAM), tuftelin, and amelotin.

For years, amelogenin was only implicated in the formation of dental enamel, both in the nucleation of crystallites, and as a molecule exclusively expressed by ameloblasts. However during the last decade, it was found that amelogenins are multifaceted proteins. Though they play an important role during enamel formation, they must also be removed from the mineralizing matrix and are degraded immediately after secretion and later during maturation by two specific proteases MMP20 and KLK4 (see chapters 4 and 9). These degradation products include specific domains of the original amelogenins which may be refolded or otherwise form fragments that may also have a role in enamel formation. If these degradation processes are altered, defective enamel will be formed, leading to some forms of *amelogenesis imperfecta* (AI). Being a link between the extracellular matrix and the cell membrane surface, amelogenin may contribute to biological events as a member of the matricellular family. Amelogenins are also signaling molecules, acting on dental tissues formation during odontogenesis [7], primarily on secretory ameloblasts, but also on differentiating and mature odontoblasts [8, 9]. Moreover, it was discovered that amelogenin also interacts with bone cells, osteoblasts and osteoclasts [10]. The concept that amelogenin is not entirely tissue specific is supported by the identification of this protein in non dental and non mineralized tissues.

Therefore our views on the functions played by amelogenins have been substantially modified during the last few years. As a consequence there was a need to review these new functions and aspects of amelogenins. New concepts have also arisen from studies on the role of amelogenins in biomineralization, and are still a matter of debate. Finally, amelogenins have been used experimentally for pulp therapy, periodontal healing and regeneration, and this third aspect also needs to be critically analyzed and evaluated.

The first part of this book opens with a chapter devoted to the knowledge provided by lessons from evolution. From an evolutionary viewpoint, *AMEL* was created after an *AMBN* duplication, itself resulting from a copy of *ENAM.* The N- and C- regions were unchanged during evolution, whereas others were susceptible to mutation, which in mammals lead to different forms of X-linked *amelogenesis imperfecta*. These different aspects are analyzed by Jean-Yves Sire in (chapter 1).

The next eight chapters focus on the gene coding the amelogenin molecule, on cellular aspects in developmental biology, membrane receptors, and intracellular regulation pathways. This then leads to a review of amelogenin degradation and the consequences on enamel defects, namely AI.

High levels of amelogenins are produced during the secretory stage of amelogenesis. The amelogenin genes have 7 exons, except in some rodents where 2 additional exons are found. Reports are made on regulatory regions of the gene and on alternative splicing of the primary RNA transcripts. In many species, the amelogenin gene is nested within an intron of the *Arhgap6* gene, generally in the opposite orientation (antisens). In addition, it has recently been shown that amelogenin mRNA and the coded protein are also detectable in several non-dental tissues. Megan Pugach and Carolyn Gibson summarized all these findings (see chapter 2), whereas Wu Li, Pamela DenBesten and their group reported on the role of exons 8 and 9 in rodents (chapter 13). This chapter could have been chapter 3, but since the chapter describes the functions of exons 8,9, focusing mainly on basic rather than clinical applications, I decided to place this chapter as Chapter 13.

The potential role of *AMEL* was evaluated experimentally by producing amelogenin knock-out mice, invalidating either the full length molecule or the leucine rich amelogenin peptide (LRAP). Ashok Kulkarni and his collaborators have covered this part (Chapter 3). They show that severe alterations in the enamel were formed when amelogenins were absent, but still some disorganized enamel structures were formed, suggesting that other matrix proteins also modulate enamel formation. Going from the gene to the mRNA and from the mRNA to the protein, ameloblasts are implicated in the synthesis, secretion, intra- and extra-cellular proteolysis of amelogenins and non-amelogenin proteins. These molecules are obviously crucial in enamel formation, and also have the capacity to influence osteogenic events.

The part, devoted to cell functions, is written (and beautifully illustrated) by Rima Waren, Sylvia Zalzal and Antonio Nanci (Chapter 4).

Among the enamel non- amelogenin proteins, ameloblastin and enamelin are critical for the formation of enamel mineral ribbons. Yong-He Chun, Jan Hu and Jim Simmer brilliantly review the properties of these molecules and their interactions with amelogenin in chapter 5.

The enamel matrix proteins bind a class of proteins called lysosomal associated membrane proteins (LAMP1, Lamp2 and CD/LAMP3). These molecules interact with the AP-3 complex to initiate receptor-mediated endocytosis. AP-3 dysfunctions lead to enamel abnormalities, described here by Michael Paine and his collaborators (Chapter 6).

For years, we have taught our students that amelogenin was a protein specifically expressed by ameloblasts, characteristic of the phenotype of these cells, and involved as a transitory molecule in enamel formation. Deutsch and his co-workers [11-13] tell us now that amelogenin is also present in many other tissues. Amelogenins do not only play a major role in enamel formation but also display other functions during the development of the embryonic craniofacial complex. They are recognized to act as signaling molecules. These additional properties lead to the exploration of the possible role on regeneration of tooth supporting tissues. Dan Deutsch and his collaborators review these biological aspects (Chapter 7).

Establishing a link between normal and pathologic enamel structures, Timothy Wright has examined the consequences of amelogenin mutations on AI (Chapter 8). Finally, amelogenins and non-amelogenin enamel matrix proteins are degraded by two proteinases. MMP20 and/or KLK4 are implicated in the extracellular cleavage of enamel matrix molecules. Severe enamel alterations termed *amelogenesis imperfecta* are due to gene mutations of these proteinases (reviewed in chapter 9) by John Bartlett and his co-workers.

The two chapters of the second part of the book are devoted to enamel mineralization, as a model for biomineralization. From the numerous published data, the potential role of amelogenin is still far from yet being clearly elucidated. Dental enamel matrix proteins display a complex distribution within the matrix. Amelogenins seem to be widely distributed among the forming enamel crystals, whereas the non-amelogenins immediately surround the enamel crystal surface. The respective chemical properties of each of these molecules provide some evidence for functional specificities. For example, non-amelogenins (previously referred to as enamelins), are more effective than the amelogenins in retarding seeded growth of enamel apatite crystals [14]. The role of amelogenin in promoting mineralization requires additional clarifications and perhaps implicates new concepts and technological approaches, as reported in this part of the book. Mineralization is concentration dependant, and amelogenin promotes in vitro nucleation at concentrations up to 6.5μg/ml but not at higher protein concentrations, whereas the amount of calcium phosphate is seen to decrease [15]. Others have developed the concept that the hydrophobic portion of amelogenin plays a role as inhibitor of crystal growth [16]. Despite numerous studies, data related to the function(s) of the leucine-rich amelogenin peptide (LRAP) in enamel biomineralization are conflicting. Some reports conclude LRAP does not control apatite crystal growth [17], whereas others suggested amelogenins regulate the nucleation, growth and organization of forming enamel [18].

Janet Moradian-Oldak and Rajamani Lakshminarayanan, using very recent concepts, demonstrate that amelogenin belongs to the class of Intrinsically Disordered Proteins. They describe and characterize the conformational plasticity, the multi-functionality, the self-assembly properties and the specific interactions with other targets (Chapter 10).

The implication of amelogenins in biomineralization is not yet fully understood. The role of the full-length amelogenin in organizing the formation of amorphous calcium phosphate, how the molecule guide the organization of linear needle-like structure that subsequently fuse are clarified by Henry Margolis and Elia Beniash (Chapter 11).

The third part of the book is focusing on the potential role of amelogenins [or enamel organic derivative (EMD)] as tools for dental and periodontal regenerative therapies. When Lars Hammarström collaborated with the Biora Company, he used purified porcine enamel matrix proteins in a product called Emdogain [19]. The mixture contained mostly amelogenin but also a series of other molecules, including proteases. When this mixture of proteins was put on the market, the evidences for the presence of amelogenin in the Hertwig's root sheath were weak and controversial, with conflicting reports among species, and therefore, the clinical application of amelogenin or EMD to periodontal regeneration was empirical and perhaps premature. Though these issues raised valuable questions, the product was found to work. We now have the answer to some of the questions related to the function of Emdogain in periodontal regeneration.

While using recombinant spliced molecules such as A+4 or A-4, very similar to LRAP, or LRAP + the amino acids expressed by exons 8, 9, we were able to run *in vivo* and *in vitro* studies and shed some light on the actual effects of amelogenins, on cells of the dental pulp. These studies give answers to questions related to how adult STEM cells or progenitors are recruited, and how they proliferate and differentiate. The cell differentiation processes or the expression of extracellular matrix molecules that play a role in dentin formation are implicated in dentin repair and pulp regeneration/mineralization. This strategy is applied to the dental pulp, bone and to the treatment of periodontal diseases.

Studying the mechanisms regulating these processes, Arthur Veis and his collaborators draw attention to the fact that small spliced isoforms of AMEL participate in the development of dental tooth germs. During embryogenesis, they are also found in non-dental organs. Chapter 12 shed lights on cell signaling, membrane receptors, and on intracellular trafficking between the surface of the cells and the nucleus where after A+4 or A-4 stimulation, molecules implicated in biomineralization are synthesized.

Additional data are brought by studies on exons 8 and 9, only found in rodents, that shed light on these therapies (see Pamela DenBesten et al., chapter 13). Altogether, these molecules are also tools for the repair of mineralized tissue (dentin, pulp, and cementum) and periodontal tissues.

Most studies were carried out on *in vitro* models. *In vivo* some experimental approaches were performed by our group, with the active collaboration of Art Veis's and Pam DenBesten's groups, providing insights on the cascade of events and the cellular mechanisms that are involved on pulp repair (Chapter 14). I would like to thank them for their warm friendship, for sharing molecules and science, and their help in editing our chapter written in Frenglish rather than pure English.

Additional chapters focus on the use of an artificial matrix created by nanotechnology in which amphiphilic peptides undergo self-assembly into nanofibers presenting biological signals to support cell proliferation and signaling properties to direct ameloblast differentiation. Such alternatives to traditional dental materials are extremely promising (see Malcolm Snead et al., chapter 15).

Other projects have implicated LRAP and its signaling effects on osteogenic differentiation along the canonical Wnt signaling pathway. This approach allows bone regeneration as shown by a rat femoral critical size defect model (see Yan Zhou et al., Chapter 16).

Finally, Anton Sculean and his collaborators (Chapter 17) present a critical and fair evaluation of the clinical effects of enamel matrix protein derivative (EMD) on periodontal defects in acute and chronic animal models, and from human case reports. Well-controlled studies demonstrate the improvements which may be obtained and underline the limits of the clinical applications of EMD.

Answering these numerous points was the aim of this book, written to transfer and establish strong links between the basic scientific knowledge and the clinical approach. I believe that we have covered most of the burning scientific points, and this will be useful in future.

REFERENCES

[1] Deakins, M.: Changes in the ash, water, and organic content of pig enamel during calcification. J Dent Res 1942; 21:429-35.

[2] Eastoe J. E. Organic matrix of tooth enamel. Nature 1960; 187:411- 2.

[3] Eastoe J. E.: The amino acid composition of proteins from the oral tissues - II The matrix proteins in dentine and enamel from developing human deciduous teeth Archs Oral Biol 1963; 8; 633-52.

[4] Eastoe JE. The chemical composition of bone and tooth. Advance Fluorine Res Dent Caries Prev 1965; 3: 5-17.

[5] Mechanic G. The multicomponent, re-equilibrating, protein system of bovine embryonic enamelin (dental enamel protein): chromatography in desaggregating solvents. in Tooth Enamel II, its composition, properties, and fundamental structure. Fearnhead RW & Stack MV, Eds., Bristol, John Wright, 1971 pp 88-94.

[6] Krebsbach PH, Lee SK , Matsuki Y, *et al.* Full-length Sequence, Localization, and Chromosomal Mapping of

Ameloblastin- a novel tooth specific gene. J Biol Chem 1996; 271 : 4431–5.

[7] Bourd-Boittin K, Fridman R, Fanchon S, *et al.* Matrix metalloproteinase inhibition impairs processing formation and mineralization of dental tissues during mouse molar development. Experimental Cell Research 2005; 304: 493-505.

[8] Bourd-Boittin K, Septier D, Hall R, *et al.* Immunolocalization of enamelysin (Matrix Metalloproteinase-20) in the forming rat incisor J Histochem Cytochem 2004; 52 : 437-45

[9] Veis A, Tompkins K, Alvares K, *et al.* Specific amelogenin gene splice products have signaling effects on cell in culture and implant in vivo. J Biol Chem 2000, 275: 41263-72.

[10] J. Hatakeyama J, D. Philp D, Hatakeyama Y, *et al.* Amelogenin-mediated Regulation of Osteoclastogenesis, and Periodontal Cell Proliferation and Migration J Dent Res, 2006; 85 : 144-9.

[11] Deutsch D, Haze-Filderman A, Blumenfeld A, *et al.* Amelogenin, a major structural protein in mineralizing enamel, is also expressed in soft tissues: brain and cells of the hematopoietic system. Eur J Oral Sci 2006;114 Suppl 1:183-9.

[12] Haze A, Taylor AL, Blumenfeld A, *et al.* Amelogenin expression in long bone and cartilage cells and in bone marrow progenitor cells. Anat Rec 2007; 290:455-60.

[13] Gruenbaum-Cohen Y, Tucker AS, Haze A, *et al.* Amelogenin in cranio-facial development: the tooth as a model to study the role of amelogenin during embryogenesis. J Exp Zool B Mol Dev Evol 2009; 15, 312B(5):445-57.

[14] Doi Y, Eanes ED, Shimokawa H, *et al.* Inhibition of seeded growth of enamel apatite crystals by amelogenin and enamelin proteins *in vitro*. J Dent Res 1984; 63 : 98-105.

[15] Tarasevich B, Howard CJ, Larson JL, *et al.* The nucleation and growth of calcium phosphate by amelogenin. J Crist Growth 2007; 304: 407-15.

[16] Beniash E, Simmer JP, Margolis HC. The effect of recombinant mouse amelogenins on the formation and organization of hydroxyapatite crystals in vitro. J Struct Biol 2005;149:182-90.

[17] Habelitz S, DenBesten PK, Marshall SJ, *et al.* Self-assembly and effect on crystal growth of the leucine-rich amelogenin peptide. Eur J Oral Sci 2006; 114 Suppl 1:315-9.

[18] Margolis HC, Beniash E, Fowler CE. Role of macromolecular assembly of enamel matrix proteins in enamel formation. J Dent Res 2006; 85:775-93.

[19] Nakamura Y, Hammarström L, Lundberg E, *et al.* Enamel matrix derivative promotes reparative processes in the dental pulp. Adv Dent Res 2001; 15:105-7.

CONTRIBUTORS

Tabitha A. Abrazinski	Laboratory Assistant, BS Forsyth Institute
Jerry Antone	Laboratory Assistant, BS Forsyth Institute
John D. Bartlett	Senior Member of Staff, PhD Forsyth Institute
Elia Beniash	Associate Professor University of Pittsburgh School of Dental Medicine 589 Salk Hall, 3501 Terrace Street Pittsburgh, Pennsylvania 15261 USA
Anat Blumenfeld	Ph.D., Hebrew University, Jerusalem, Israel
Dieter Bosshardt	Department of Periodontology, University of Bern, Bern, Switzerland
Michel Brecx	Department of Conservative Dentistry and Periodontology, University of Tübingen, Tübingen, Germany
Steven J. Brookes	Senior Lecturer, University of Leeds
Dan Deutsch	Professor, Hebrew University, Jerusalem, Israel
Yong-Hee P. Chun	Assistant Professor, Department of Periodontics, University of Texas Health Science Center at San Antonio, San Antonio, Texas 78229-3900
Pamela DenBesten	Professor, University of California, San Francisco, CA, 94110
Sasha Dimitrova-Nakov	Assistant Professor, Oral Biology, PhD student, Paris Descartes, U747, France
Carolyn W. Gibson	Professor, Department of Anatomy and Cell Biology, University of Pennsylvania School of Dental Medicine 240 S. 40th Street, Philadelphia, PA, 19104 USA
Michel Goldberg	Professor emeritus, University Paris Descartes, U747 Biomedicale St Pères, France
Yael Gruenbaum-Cohen	D.M.D. Ph.D., Hebrew University, Jerusalem, Israel
Yassine Harichane	Assistant Professor, Oral Biology, PhD student, Paris Descartes, U747, France
Naoto Haruyama	Global Center of Excellence Program, International Research Center for Molecular Science in Tooth and Bone Diseases, [2]Maxillofacial Orthodontics, Department of Maxillofacial Reconstruction and Function, Division of Maxillofacial/Neck Reconstruction, Graduate School, Tokyo Medical and Dental University, Tokyo, Japan
Junko Hatakeyama	Global Center of Excellence Program, International Research Center for Molecular Science in Tooth and Bone Diseases,, Tokyo

	Medical and Dental University, Tokyo, Japan
Yuji Hatakeyama	Global Center of Excellence Program, International Research Center for Molecular Science in Tooth and Bone Diseases,, Tokyo Medical and Dental University, Tokyo, Japan
Amir Haze	M.D. Ph.D., Hebrew University, Jerusalem, Israel
Jan C-C Hu	Professor, Dept. of Biologic and Materials Sciences, University of Michigan School of Dentistry, Ann Arbor, MI, USA, 48108
Z Huang	Research Associate, The University of Southern California, Center for Craniofacial Molecular Biology, 2250 Alcazar Street Clinical Science Annex 107 Los Angeles, CA 90033
Stanca Iacob	Instructor, Department of Biochemistry, Rush University Medical Center 1735 W. Harrison Street, 5th Fl-CRB, Chicago, IL 60612, USA
Odile Kellermann	Professor, University Paris Descartes U747 France
Ashok B.Kulkarni	Functional Genomics Section, Laboratory of Cell and Developmental Biology, National Institute of Dental and Craniofacial Research, National Institutes of Health, Department of Health and Human Services, Bethesda, MD, USA
Rodrigo S. Lacruz	Research Associate, The University of Southern California, Center for Craniofacial Molecular Biology, 2250 Alcazar Street, Clinical Science Annex 107, Los Angeles, CA 90033
Rajamani Lakshminarayanan	Senior Research Scientist, Singapore Eye Research Institute, Singapore 169611
Grace F. Lopez	Laboratory Assistant, BA Forsyth Institute
Wu Li	Associate Professor, University of California, San Francisco, CA, USA
S. Peter Lyngstadaas	Professor, University of Oslo
Mary Mac Dougall	Associate Dean for Research and Director, Institute of Oral Health Research, Birmingham, Alabama, USA
Henry C. Margolis	Senior Member of the Staff The Forsyth Institute 140 The Fenway Boston, Massachusetts 02115 USA
Antonio Nanci	Professor, Laboratory for the Study of Calcified Tissues and Biomaterials, Faculty of Dentistry, Université de Montréal, Montréal, Québec, Canada
Christina J. Newcomb	Graduate Student, Department of Materials Science and Engineering, Institute for BioNanotechnology in Medicine, Northwestern University, Chicago
Michael L. Paine	Associate Professor, University of Southern California

Anne Poliard	Professor, University Paris Descartes EA2496, France
Megan K. Pugach	Department of Anatomy and Cell Biology University of Pennsylvania School of Dental Medicine, 240 S. 40th Street, Philadelphia, PA, 19104 USA
Anton Sculean	Professor Dr Med Dent. Chairman, Department of Periodontology, University of Bern, Freiburgstrasse 7, Bern, Switzerland.
Jason L. Shapiro	Graduate Student, University of Southern California
Ramaswamy Sharma	Postdoctoral Fellow, PhD Forsyth Institute
Shay Sharon	Ph.D. and D.M.D. student, Hebrew University, Jerusalem, Israel
Dekel Shilo	Ph.D. and D.M.D. student, Hebrew University, Jerusalem, Israel
Nechama C. Silverstein	Ph.D. student, Hebrew University, Jerusalem, Israel
James P. Simmer	Professor, Dept. of Biologic and Materials Sciences, University of Michigan School of Dentistry, Ann Arbor, MI, USA, 48108
Jean-Yves Sire	Directeur de Recherche CNRS, Equipe "Evolution et développement du squelette", Université Pierre et Marie Curie, UMR 7138, 7 quai Saint Bernard, 75005 Paris, France
Malcolm Snead	Professor, The University of Southern California, Center for Craniofacial Molecular Biology, 2250 Alcazar Street, Clinical Science Annex 107, Los Angeles, CA 90033
Samuel I. Stupp	Professor, Department of Materials Science and Engineering, Institute for BioNanotechnology in Medicine and the Department of Chemistry, and the Department of Medicine, Northwestern University, Chicago, IL.
Yoshiro Takano	Professor, Tokyo Medical and Dental University Graduate School, Tokyo. Japan
Kevin A. Thompkins	Assistant Prof., Departments of Oral Biology and Implantology, Faculty of Dentistry, Chulalongkorn University, Bangkok, Thailand
Coralee E. Tye	Postdoctoral Fellow, PhD Forsyth Institute
Arthur Veis	Professor emeritus, Feinberg school of Medicine, Department of Cell and Molecular Biology, Northwestern University, Chicago, IL 60611, USA
Rima Waren	Research Assistant, Laboratory for the Study of Calcified Tissues and Biomaterials, Faculty of Dentistry, Université de Montréal, Montréal, Québec, Canada
Rungnapa Warotayanont	Resident, Department of Orofacial Sciences, University of California, San Francisco, School of Dentistry, 513 Parnassus Ave S-704, San Francisco CA 94143-0422

Shane N. White	Professor, University of California, School of Dentistry, Los Angeles, CA
J. Timothy Wright	Bawden Distinguished Professor and Chair, Department of Pediatric Dentistry, School of Dentistry, The University of North Carolina, Chapel Hill, NC, USA
Yucheng Xu, **Investigations performed at USC, CCMB** ***Present Address:***	Senior Scientist, Molecular Biology and Genomics, GlaxoSmithKline, R&D China 2F,Building 3, 998 Halei Road, Zhangjiang Hi-Tech Park, Pudong, Shanghai 201203, China
Sylvia Francis Zalzal	Laboratory Coordinator, Laboratory for the Study of Calcified Tissues and Biomaterials, Faculty of Dentistry, Université de Montréal, Montréal, Québec, Canada
Yan Zhou	Research Assistant Professor, The University of Southern California, Center for Craniofacial Molecular Biology, 2250 Alcazar Street, Clinical Science Annex 107 Los Angeles, CA 90033

CHAPTER 1

Origin and Relationships of Amelogenin, and the Evolutionary Analysis of its Conserved and Variable Regions in Tetrapods

Jean-Yves Sire

UMR 7138, Université Pierre et Marie Curie, 7 quai St-Bernard, 75005 Paris, France; E-mail: jean-yves.sire@upmc.fr

Abstract: Hypermineralized tissues related to enamel are identified in early vertebrates, 450 millions years ago (Ma). The enamel matrix proteins (EMPs), amelogenin (AMEL), ameloblastin (AMBN) and enamelin (ENAM) being enamel specific, we can deduce that they were recruited early in vertebrate evolution. Molecular analyses support their presence by the end of Precambrian period (>600 Ma), i.e., prior vertebrates differentiated a mineralized skeleton. However, our knowledge of EMPs is currently limited to tetrapods, i.e., 360 Ma. *AMEL* was created from *AMBN*, itself resulting from a duplication of *ENAM*. EMP genes are therefore paralogs. The evolutionary analysis of AMEL highlights conserved and variable regions. The N- and C-terminal regions contain numerous residues that were unchanged during 360 Ma, which supports important functions. Only a few positions are known to play a role. Other positions are considered as being crucial because they are unchanged. Five of them are known to lead to a genetic disease, X-linked amelogenesis imperfecta (AIH1) when substituted. The largest AMEL region, encoded by exon 6, is less variable in mammals than in sauropsids and amphibians, but it accumulates numerous indels in all lineages. It was created through the repeat of PXQ triplets. Similar repeats occurred independently at the same locus in mammalian species, but their meaning is still obscure. The evolutionary analysis of AMEL allowed to validate functional residues and positions known to lead to AIH1 when changed. It also highlighted residues that could have interesting functions and predicts these conserved positions will lead to AIH1 when substituted.

Key Words: Amelogenin, EMP, Enamel, Tetrapods, Evolutionary Analysis, Conserved Positions, Amelogenesis Imperfecta.

INTRODUCTION

These last years, the evolutionary analysis of genes encoding proteins involved in various functions proved to be an efficient method in order to identify specific regions that undoubtedly play structural and/or functional roles [1, 2]. These findings are supported by the conservation of amino acids, either unchanged or substituted only by chemically similar residues, during hundreds of millions years (Ma). This method takes advantage of the increasing number of sequenced genomes available in databases. The datasets of sequences are expanding rapidly, and in particular in mammals, in which the genome of 36 species[1], representative of the main lineages, can be now explored. Most placental lineages have differentiated approximately 100 Ma [3, 4]. When including sequences representative of the two basalmost lineages, monotremes (e.g., platypus) and marsupials (e.g., opossum, wallaby), the evolutionary analysis of any mammalian gene covers more than 200 Ma of evolution [5]. A period of 100-200 Ma is long enough for accumulating numerous nucleotide substitutions at random. In mammals, the substitution rate (neutral sites) is estimated between 1 and $8x10^{-9}$ substitutions/nucleotide site/year, depending on generation time in the lineage [6] (molecular and life history evolution are closely interlinked [7]). This means that virtually all nucleotide sites can be substituted during 200 Ma of evolution. Most of these mutations that accumulate over time due to genetic drift are

[1] Keep in mind that there are circa 5,000 mammalian species [8].

either silent (do not change the amino acid) or neutral (the residue is substituted but this change does not influence the structure and/or function of the protein). Advantageous mutations can be favored through positive selection, while purifying selection acts to eliminate deleterious mutations. Therefore, when a residue is kept unchanged during mammalian evolution, one can assess that this position is certainly important because it has been subjected to purifying selection. In order to obtain more information, the evolutionary analysis can be extended to amniote (310 Ma), tetrapod (350 Ma), or even gnathostome (450 Ma) level [4]. However, in this case the encoded protein must be subjected to the same selective pressures in these lineages as in mammals.

The aim of this chapter is to review the results that have been obtained these last years when applying this method to amelogenin (AMEL), the major and best known enamel matrix protein (EMP). For several years, in my lab we are particularly interested in the origin and evolution of EMPs, a family composed of three constitutive proteins involved in enamel formation and mineralization: AMEL, ameloblastin (AMBN) and enamelin (ENAM) [9-11]. Our major objective is to trace back these proteins in vertebrate evolution in order to understand how the current diversity of hypermineralized tissues, as observed in all lineages, was acquired during evolution [12]. We perform evolutionary analysis in order to identify conserved regions of these proteins that could help to find their genes in all, non mammalian vertebrate lineages. In addition, these investigations allow to (i) highlight conserved regions and residues that certainly play important functions, and (ii) accurately predict positions that would lead to genetic defaults in humans if they were modified [13,14].

In the following, I will first summarize the current knowledge on the origin and relationships of AMEL, then I will focus on the evolutionary analysis of this protein, with particular attention to regions that were identified as being structurally and/or functionally important for the molecule. Eventually, I will show how the evolutionary analysis of AMEL helps in validating and predicting mutations leading to X-linked amelogenesis imperfecta.

ORIGIN AND RELATIONSHIPS OF AMEL

AMEL was Probably Created Prior Enamel/Enameloid Appeared in Vertebrates

In amniotes, the three EMPs are enamel specific (see section 4) and, as such, one can expect that their recruitment in early vertebrates and their subsequent evolution in the various lineages were closely related to those of enamel and enamel-like (hypermineralized) tissues. The earliest hypermineralized tissues (enameloids and enamel-like tissues), covered the odontodes[2] ornamenting the dermal bony plates located on the body surface of jawless vertebrates that lived from the Early Ordovician (480 Ma) to Late Devonian (380 Ma) periods (Figure 1).

Enameloid is currently defined as a kind of hypermineralized dentin, the formation of which includes a contribution from both the odontoblasts (mostly collagen) and the ameloblasts (collagen, and probably EMPs and proteases) [15,16]. The ameloblasts participate in the maturation process leading to an highly mineralized tissue. During evolution, enameloid appeared probably first [12] then was either replaced with enamel in various lineages (e.g., in most amphibians, reptiles and mammals), or retained in cartilaginous fish, teleost fish, and in caudate larvae (salamanders and newts). The two tissues, enameloid and enamel, were present in ancestral osteichthyans, and enamel-derived tissues still cover the scale surface of various living species, mostly ray-finned fish [12,17].

In living vertebrates, the formation of these hypermineralized tissues is certainly related to the presence of EMPs and one can speculate that these proteins were already present when the first vertebrates acquired these hard, protecting tissues (i.e., > 500 Ma). EMP recruitment probably post-dates the two genome duplications that occurred in the Precambrian period (> 600 Ma) [18], but it undoubtedly benefitted from tandem gene duplications that played a major role in enamel and enameloid evolution (Figure 1).

[2] Tooth-like elements that are considered the ancestors of teeth [12,19]

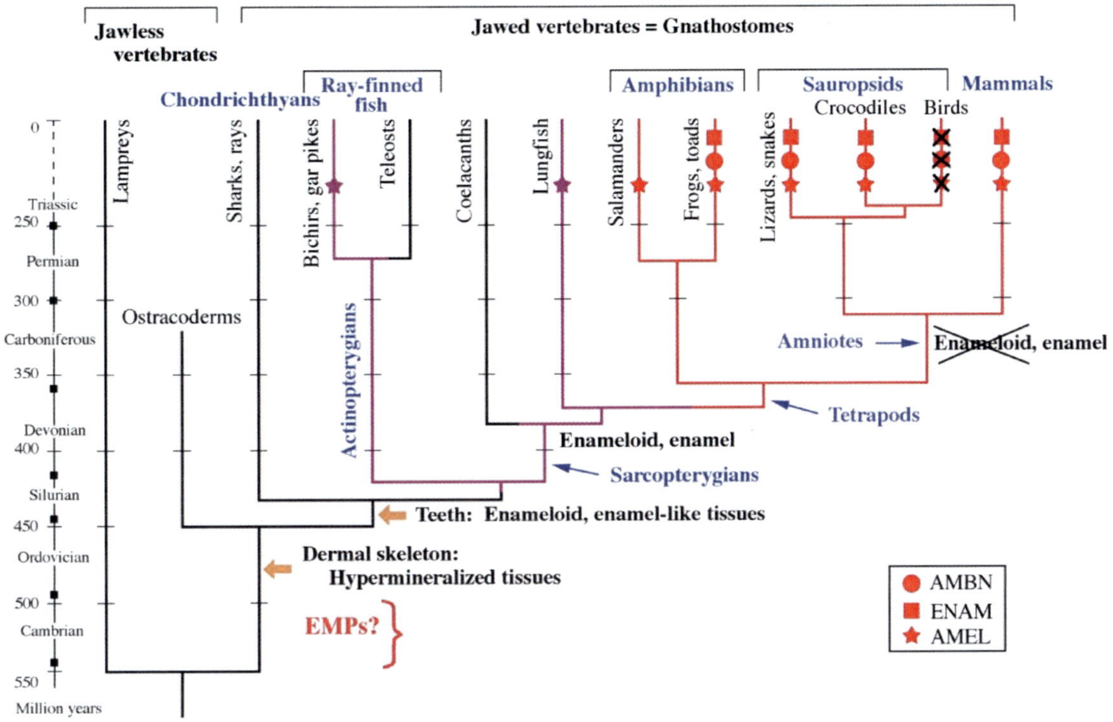

Figure 1: Origin and evolution of the hypermineralized tissues in vertebrates and current data on the identification of enamel matrix proteins (EMPs). Hypermineralized tissues related to enameloids and enamels were identified in the dermal skeleton of early, jawless vertebrates, 500-450 millions years ago (Ma), which suggests the presence of EMPs. Enameloid- and/or enamel-like tissues were present in the teeth that were recruited in early gnathostomes and their dermal skeleton. Enameloid is conserved in cartilaginous fish, ray-finned fish and tetrapods, in which it is still present in larval salamanders. EMP genes are known in representatives of all tetrapodan lineages, which indicates that they were already present in their last common ancestor (red lines). EMP genes are present but invalidated in lineages that have lost the ability to form teeth (e.g. birds). In addition, data from structural and immunohistochemical studies strongly suggest that the amelogenin was present earlier in vertebrate evolution (pink lines).

Gene duplications are generally consecutive to unequal crossings over (i.e., errors in homologous chromosomal recombination) and this did occur for the EMP genes. While one of the two copies of the ancestor of the EMP genes conserved its function, the other copy was free from selective pressure. It mutated faster than the other copy as these mutations had no deleterious effects for the organism. During millions years this ancestral EMP gene accumulated mutations that led to various changes providing new function and/or structure for the protein. These changes improved the fitness of the tissue in which the protein was secreted and the later was therefore conserved. However, are the three EMPs evolutionary related, i.e., do they derive from a common ancestral EMP gene? Two evidences indicate they could be paralogous genes: they are involved in enamel formation and mineralization, and their coding genes have a similar structure. In silico analyses of AMEL relationships have shown that EMPs are old proteins which are encoded by paralogous genes.

AMEL is known for nearly 30 years and numerous biochemical and in vitro studies have been performed to understand its function during enamel formation and mineralization. Several research groups are still working routinely on AMEL (see reviews in this book). This long lasting interest can be explained as AMEL is the most abundant protein in forming enamel (90% of the organic matrix of forming enamel in bovine). A large collection of *AMEL* sequences has progressively accumulated not only in mammals but also in various tetrapod species [20-22]. This dataset allowed to perform a series of evolutionary analyses. The first study aimed to estimate the period when amelogenin was recruited in the ancestral vertebrate genome [23].

Databases were searched for similarities between the five coding exons of *AMEL* and other sequences. The only significant result was found between *AMEL* exon 2 and the exon 2 of *SPARC* (osteonectin), a gene known in protostomians and deuterostomians. In *AMEL* and *SPARC*, most of exon 2 sequence encodes the signal peptide, an important region of the protein that allows the functional protein to be secreted in the extracellular matrix. This finding suggested a common origin for these exons and further analyses indicated that *AMEL* was probably acquired through a duplication of an ancestral *SPARC* in the deuterostomian lineage. This duplication was dated > 600 Ma, i.e., prior the so-called "Cambrian explosion" (around 530 Ma), a contemporary period with the origin of vertebrates (530 Ma) [24], and hence, prior the first hypermineralized tissues attributed to early vertebrates were found in the fossil record. This datation was confirmed later using another method (see section 2.2).

EMP Genes are Paralogs, and AMEL was Created from AMBN

In 2003, when the first human genome was available (DNA sequences and genes annotated on chromosomes), Kawasaki and Weiss [25] elegantly demonstrated the existence of the secretory calcium-binding phosphoprotein (SCPP) family. This family comprises currently more than twenty genes in humans, all encoding proteins involved in calcium phosphate regulation: mineralization of bone and dentin (the so-called SIBLINGs) and enamel (EMPs), binding calcium in milk and saliva, etc. These proteins were regrouped in a "family" not only because they share similar functions, but also because they have a common ancestor, from which they derive through tandem duplication. Their chromosomal location on a same chromosome (with the exception of *AMEL* that is elsewhere), their common gene structure and their similar protein characteristics of the N-terminal region, strongly witness for such a relationship. The key stone of the theory of a common origin of the SCPP genes is *SPARC-L1* a relative of *SPARC*. Indeed, this gene (i) is located on the same chromosome as the SCPPs, (ii) is adjacent to the SIBLING genes and (iii) shares a similar structure in the 5' region [26]. Therefore, the SCPP genes (including the EMP genes) do not derive from *SPARC* as proposed by our research group [23], but probably from its relative, *SPARC-L1* [26].

Because they belong to the SCPPs, EMPs have strong relationships with other members of the family. In mammals, two EMP genes, *AMBN* and *ENAM* are located adjacent in a same region of the chromosome, a location that suggests tandem duplication. *AMEL*, that was included in the SCPP family on the base of its gene structure and protein function, is located on another chromosome. This strongly suggests that *AMEL* was translocated after it was created from the duplication of a member of the family. The questions were (1) to know whether or not the three EMP genes are phylogenetically linked, and (2) in which order they were created by duplication [9,11]. Protein databases were searched for sequence similarity (psi-blast) using well conserved AMEL sequences deduced from a comparative analysis of tetrapodan sequences. Statistically significant similarities were detected first with AMBN, then ENAM and finally SPARC-L1, suggesting that AMEL (i) had strong relationships with the other EMPs and (ii) was closer to AMBN than to ENAM and SPARC-L1. Then, all available *AMBN, ENAM* and *SPARC-L1* tetrapodan sequences were compiled and the N-terminal regions of the encoded proteins were aligned to the same region of AMEL. The alignment (62 residues) comprised the only region encoded by *AMEL* exons 2, 3, 5 and beginning of exon 6 (the so-called TRAP region) (Figure 2). The phylogenetic analysis revealed that *AMEL* and *AMBN* are sister genes, and that they were probably derived from a duplication of an *ENAM* ancestor, itself being created from *SPARC-L1,* either directly or through an intermediate SCPP gene that remains to be found (Figure 2). A further study revealed that the EMPs could have relationships with two other ameloblast-secreted proteins, ODAM (APIN protein) and amelotin (AMTN), the genes of which are located on the same chromosomal region, as AMBN and ENAM (Figure 3). The *AMEL/AMBN* relationships as well as their link to *ENAM* was strongly supported by this analysis, while those with *ODAM* and *AMTN* were weak, probably because only mammalian sequences were known [11]. *AMEL/AMBN* relationships are also well supported by the gene structure in the 5' region (Figure 2) and the amino acid sequence of the N-ter region. The chromosomal location of *AMBN* and *ENAM* indicates that *AMBN* was created from a tandem duplication of *ENAM.* The three EMP genes are, therefore, paralogs. *AMEL* was created after a duplication of *AMBN*, then translocated on another chromosome. In placental mammals this region is now located in sex chromosomes.

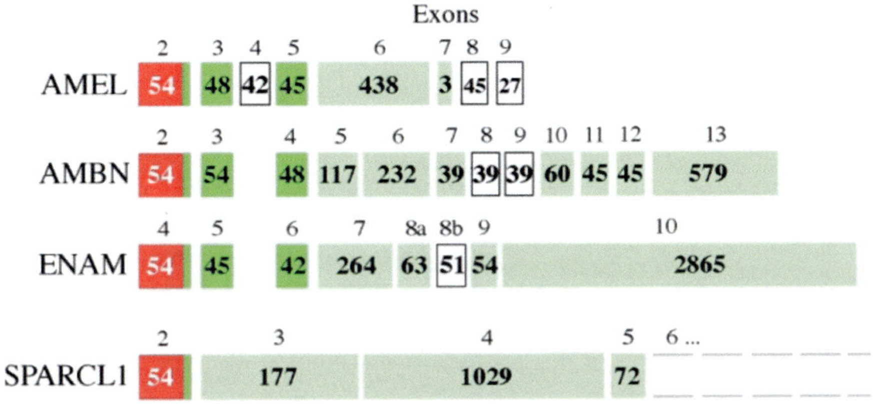

Figure 2: Structure of the coding sequences of the EMP genes (*AMEL*, *AMBN* and *ENAM*) and *SPARC-L1*, the putative ancestor of the secretory calcium-binding phosphoprotein (SCPP) family. Exon name is indicated on top of each box and nucleotide number is indicated within the box. White boxes indicate exons that are not present in the ancestral sequence. *AMEL* exon 4 was acquired in placental mammals while exons 8 and 9 were created in rodents; *AMBN* exons 8 and 9 are repeats of exon 7 in primates; *ENAM* exon 8b was acquired in an amniote ancestor, is still present in reptiles but was lost in mammals except in marsupials (Al-Hashimi et al., submitted). In red: signal peptide; in green: protein sequence. The first coding exon (red) is present in all SCPPs and the dark green exons have been inherited from an ancestral EMP.

AMEL and *AMBN* being paralogous genes, dating the duplication event was possible [11]. Indeed, (i) the two genes are known in mammals (e.g., rodents and humans), sauropsids (crocodile) and amphibians (xenopus), and (ii) the divergence of these lineages is molecularly dated at (around) 90 Ma for primates/rodents, 310 Ma for mammals/sauropsids and 360 Ma for amniotes/amphibians [4]. Taking into account the evolutionary distance of each gene in each lineage, the calculation resulted in a molecular dating of *AMBN* duplication > 600 Ma (Figure 4). This finding confirms the previous, but unrelated, molecular dating by Delgado and colleagues [23] of the origin of *AMEL* by the end of the Precambrian period, during which important rounds of gene duplication occurred [18]. After the duplication, the copy that gave rise to *AMEL* derived through genetic drift until it acquired its new function. Given the high conservation of the N- and C-ter region, this function was already acquired in tetrapod ancestors (see sections 3-2 and 3-4).

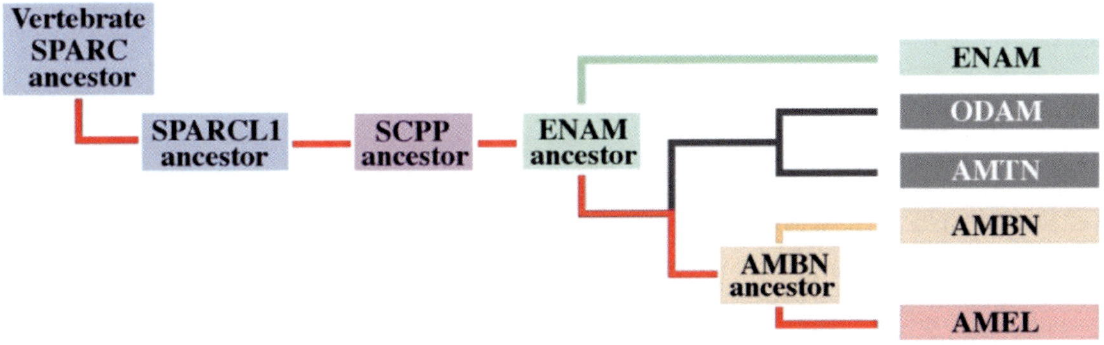

Figure 3: Probable scenario for the origin of *AMEL* (red line). *SPARC-L1*, the putative SCPP gene ancestor was created in early deuterian evolution after the duplication of *SPARC*, that occurred probably during a genome duplication prior vertebrate differentiation. The SCPP ancestor duplicated giving rise to the ancestral *ENAM* from which EMP genes (*AMBN* and *AMEL*), and probably other related ameloblast-expressed genes (*ODAM* and *AMTN*), are derived. In mammals *SPARC-L1, ENAM, AMBN, ODAM* and *AMTN* are located on the same chromosome, with the exception of *AMEL* that was translocated to another chromosome.

Given the relationships between AMEL and AMBN and their structural similarities in the N-ter region we suggest a possible compensation by AMBN when AMEL is mutated. This could explain why enamel is still present (even if hypoplastic or hypomineralized) in AMEL null mice [27,28] and in human mutations [29,30]. Conversely, when AMBN is invalidated, AMEL could also compensate although the enamel width is considerably reduced [31].

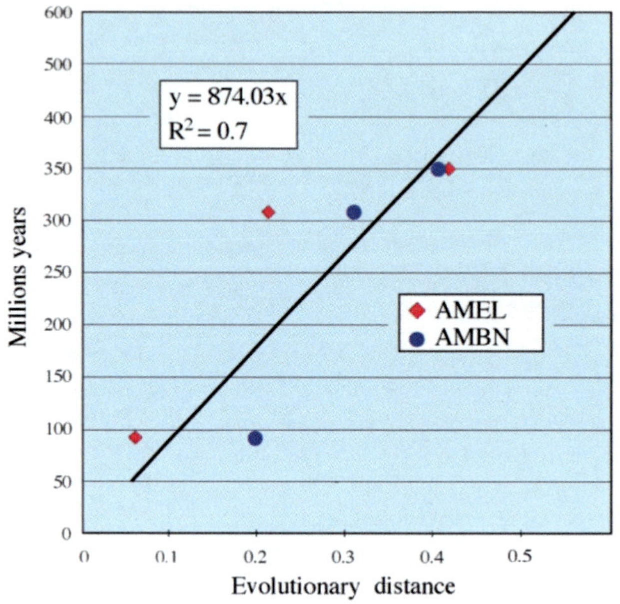

Figure 4: Linear regression of time (millions years) versus evolutionary distance of *AMBN* and *AMEL*. The evolutionary distances were obtained from a phylogenetic analysis of the two gene sequences in human, mouse, crocodile and xenopus. The calibration time was estimated from human/mouse distance = 90 Ma; human/crocodile = 310 Ma; human/xenopus = 350 Ma (Hedges, 2002). This method allowed to estimate the duplication time of *AMBN/AMEL* at a date >600 Ma.

A Gap Still Remains in AMEL Evolution

Although the molecular analyses reported above indicate that EMP genes were present early in vertebrate evolution, our current knowledge of these genes is restricted to the tetrapod level (mammals, sauropsids and lissamphibians), i.e., a period covering around 360 Ma corresponding to the estimated date of the split between amphibians and amniotes. *AMEL* sequences were obtained in two reptiles (a crocodile and a snake) and one amphibian (the African clawed frog) more than 10 years ago [21,22], then *AMBN* was sequenced in a reptile and an amphibian [32,33]. Additional *AMEL* sequences were published in reptiles and amphibians [34-36]. Recently, our research group obtaitned *ENAM* sequences in a crocodile and a lizard, and in the western clawed frog [37]. In contrast, EMP genes are neither known in chondrichthyans (sharks, rays), nor in ray-finned fish (bichirs, teleosts), nor in basal sarcopterygians (lungfish, coelacanths). Thereofore, to date we can only assess that the three EMPs were already present in tetrapod ancestors, i.e., more than 360 Ma but a large gap remains (>100 Ma), separating the supposed date of *AMEL* recruitment in early vertebrates from our limited knowledge in tetrapods (Figure 1). Some structural and immunocytochemical data, however, support that EMPs were present earlier in vertebrate evolution. Indeed, AMEL epitopes have been localized in the enamel layer (ganoin) covering bichir scales and in lungfish tooth enamel [38,39]. These findings indicate that EMPs were present prior the split between the tetrapodan lineage (sarcopterygians) and the ray-finned fish (actinopterygians) that occurred around 420 Ma (Early Devonian). However, these data should be confirmed by sequencing EMP genes in representatives of basal sarcopterygian lineages (e.g., a lungfish and a coelacanth) and in a bichir (polypterid) or a gar pike (lepisosteid), representatives of two basal actinopterygian lineages. Unfortunately, the more the evolutionary distance between living representatives of the vertebrate lineages increases, the more the correlation between the lack of sequenced genomes and the difficulty to obtain EMP gene sequences is strong. Indeed, it is difficult to obtain these genes using PCR because either the conserved regions are encoded by small exons or, when the exons are large the encoded region are highly variable as they belong to the unstructured region of the proteins. It appears that the conservation of gene synteny (as described above), could help but we need genome, or large chromosomal regions to be sequenced to (i) localize well conserved genes that are invariably close to our target gene, and (ii) explore using in silico approach the region of interest. However, one can ask the question whether synteny is conserved in all lineages. Recently, in sauropsids we showed that AMBN and ENAM are located on an other chromosome than that expected when considering the SCPP gene synteny in mammalian genomes [40]. However, this study revealed that the expected synteny is conserved in the clawed toad genome (the only amphibian genome currently available). We have concluded that the DNA region housing EMP genes was translocated onto another chromosome in a sauropsid ancestor. This strategy based on gene synteny was used to localize several SCPP genes in teleost fish genomes [41]. These genes were found to be related to the SIBLING family genes, but no EMP-related genes were found in teleost fish genomes todate. This could mean that either EMP genes are absent in teleosts or they are located on another chromosome.

In summary, more data are needed to complete the AMEL story and to validate the hypothesis that EMPs were present in early vertebrates as the presence of hypermineralized protective tissues (enamel and enameloid) in the fossil record seems to indicate.

AMEL is Enamel Specific: a Demonstration from Various Experiments in Natura

The experimental invalidation of *AMEL* in the mouse results in enamel defaults only [27,28] and several mutations of human *AMEL* leading to amelogenesis imperfecta (see section 4) reveal only hypoplastic or hypomineralized enamel but no collateral effects. Anyway, for years the question of whether or not AMEL, and more generally EMPs, are enamel specific is still debated as there are reports of their expression in loci that are not related to tooth environment [42,43]. However, there was a simple question to ask to close this debate, and its answer is in the natura: what was the fate of AMEL (and EMPs) when teeth and/or enamel were lost in some lineages? If EMPs are enamel specific, their genes has been no longer useful for many millions years and have accumulated mutations leading to pseudogenization. On the contrary, if EMPs are involved in other functions, the genes should be still active.

In the chick, in which the ability to form teeth was lost approximately 100 Ma, our research group demonstrated that chicken *AMEL* is now a pseudogene [44]. Recently, we found in chicken that *ENAM* and *AMBN* were also invalided [40]. In mammals, Déméré et al. [45] have shown hat *ENAM* and *AMBN* genes are pseudogenes in baleen whales, in which the ability to form teeth was lost approximately 40 Ma and, more recently, *ENAM* was found invalidated in various edentate mammalian species (anteaters, pangolins, and aardvark) [46].

In summary, when the ability to develop teeth or enamel was lost in various lineages, EMP genes were always subsequently invalidated. This is a clear demonstration, through unrelated experiments in natura, that these proteins are tooth and/or enamel specific. EMPs play their roles in the only tooth environment, and principally in enamel formation.

THE EVOLUTIONARY ANALYSIS OF AMEL IN TETRAPODS

Although our current knowledge is still restricted to tetrapods, the evolutionary analysis of AMEL allowed to (i) follow its evolution in this lineage during more than 360 Ma in order to know how and when variations and selections have occurred, and (ii) to reveal the residues that were conserved (fixed) and, hence, have a functional importance.

Conservation and Variation of the AMEL Gene Structure During Tetrapod Evolution

We know that *AMEL* was created from a duplication of *AMBN* that occurred probably around 550 Ma but we ignore whether or not the *AMBN* structure was already fixed when the gene was duplicated. One can suppose that the two copies accumulated various, unrelated mutations until they acquired a well defined, but distinct function. They were then subjected to selective pressures (purifying and positive selection) depending on the functional importance of the residues. From what we learnt through the analysis of EMP sequences in tetrapods, the general structure of the three EMPs has not changed during 360 Ma, except minor variations that are interpreted as exon duplications (Figure 2). In passing, the fact that the structure of *ENAM*, *AMBN* and *AMEL* was kept unchanged for 360 Ma witnesses for a long story of these genes prior tetrapod diversification.

AMEL conserved the structure of the 5' coding region, i.e., exons 2, 3 and 5, from the ancestral *AMBN* (currently exons 2, 3, 4), as did the later from *ENAM* (currently exons 4, 5, 6) (Figure 2). Some mutations occurred in these exons but enough similarities were conserved to allow establishing relationships. In contrast, the other exons were subjected to important changes, which strongly suggest that the encoded regions house the specific function of each EMP. *AMEL* exon 6 is probably derived from *AMBN* exon 5 and/or exon 6, the two latter probably being derived probably from *ENAM* exon 7. Indeed, these exons encode a proline rich region.

In tetrapods, the comparison of numerous sequences (> 30 mammals, 5 reptiles, 5 amphibians) reveals that the *AMEL* structure observed in humans (7 exons) and/or rodents (9 exons) is not the structure of the ancestral gene (Figure 2). Six exons (i.e., exons 1,2, 3, 5, 6 and 7) are present in the genome of all species analysed so far and, hence, represent the ancestral tetrapod *AMEL* structure. *AMEL* exon 4 is absent in amphibian, reptilian and basal mammalian (marsupials and monotremes) lineages, but it is present in some placental species (see section 3-2). *AMEL* exons 8 and 9 are only present in rodents. Exon 8 was created in an ancestral rodent through the duplication of a DNA region containing exon 5 and its translocation downstream exon 7, "activating" subsequently the exon 9 (see the review by Li et al., in this book).

In rodents, *AMEL* transcripts are subjected to alternative splicing and 16 different isoforms have been characterized [47]. We don't know whether such an extensive alternative splicing is proper to rodent *AMEL,* but several isoforms were also characterized in various species such as bovine [48], human [49], pig [50], rodents [51-53] and opossum [54]. These findings suggest that such a process is an essential mechanism for AMEL function and that it does occur in other mammalian *AMEL*. In contrast, to our knowledge different isoforms were not reported in reptilian and amphibian *AMEL*. This could suggest either that alternative splicing of *AMEL* was selected during mammalian evolution or that various isoforms do exist in non mammalian *AMEL* but that they were not found because they are expressed in minute amounts.

Therefore, at least two events, that changed a little the gene structure compared to the ancestral condition, have occurred independently during *AMEL* evolution in mammals: (1) exon 4 was created in a mammalian ancestor and (2) in rodents, the DNA region containing exons 4 and 5 was duplicated and inserted downstream in the sequence, after exon 7.

The Origin of AMEL Exon 4 and its Conservation in Mammalian Sequences

The presence of exon 4 was known as soon as the first AMEL sequences were published in rodents, cow, human, etc. [48,49]. It was also established that this exon was (i) present in the two AMEL copies on the sex chromosomes *AMELX* and *AMELY*, but (ii) not included in the major AMEL isoform [55] resulting from its alternative splicing. There is also evidence that the protein containing the region encoded by exon 4 (i.e., the full-length AMEL) could have different function compared to the isoform lacking this region [56]. Exon 4 was not found in marsupial [54], monotreme [22] and all non-mammalian (reptiles and amphibians [21,22]) *AMEL* transcript sequences. This leads to the question on the origin and evolution of *AMEL* exon 4.

A total of 36 gDNA sequences of mammalian *AMEL* were obtained in databases, and the region located upstream exon 5 was explored in order to find exon 4 (Figure 5). Exon 4 was found in all sequences excepted in platypus *AMEL*. However, the analysis reveals that numerous exon 4 are not coding: they either display reading frame shift (indels) or do not possess correct intronic splice sites (Figure 5). Such non coding exon 4 was identified in a primate (marmoset), in several leurasiatherians (dolphin, dog, cat, bats, insectivores), in all afrotherians (elephant, tenrec and hyrax) and in the two marsupials (wallaby and opossum). Given the short evolutionary period (at the geological time) since they were invalidated these exons 4 are still easily recognizable in the DNA sequences as "ghost" exons. A ghost exon 4 was neither found in monotreme nor in non mammalian *AMEL*.

Taken together, these findings indicate that (i) exon 4 has been recruited in an ancestral therian (placentals + marsupials), i.e., after the divergence of the monotreme lineage, around 200 Ma, (ii) it has secondarily been invalidated in the lineages that led to the living species studied. This invalidation indicates that exon 4 function was not important enough for AMEL function in these lineages to be conserved through purifying selection. Mutations have occurred at random and some have probably affected the splice donor site, then the exon 4 sequence accumulated mutations leading sometimes to a reading frame shift. Conversely, it appears that purifying selection has occurred in three lineages, primates, rodents and artiodactyls (cow, pig) as revealed by the conserved sequence of this exon (Figure 5).

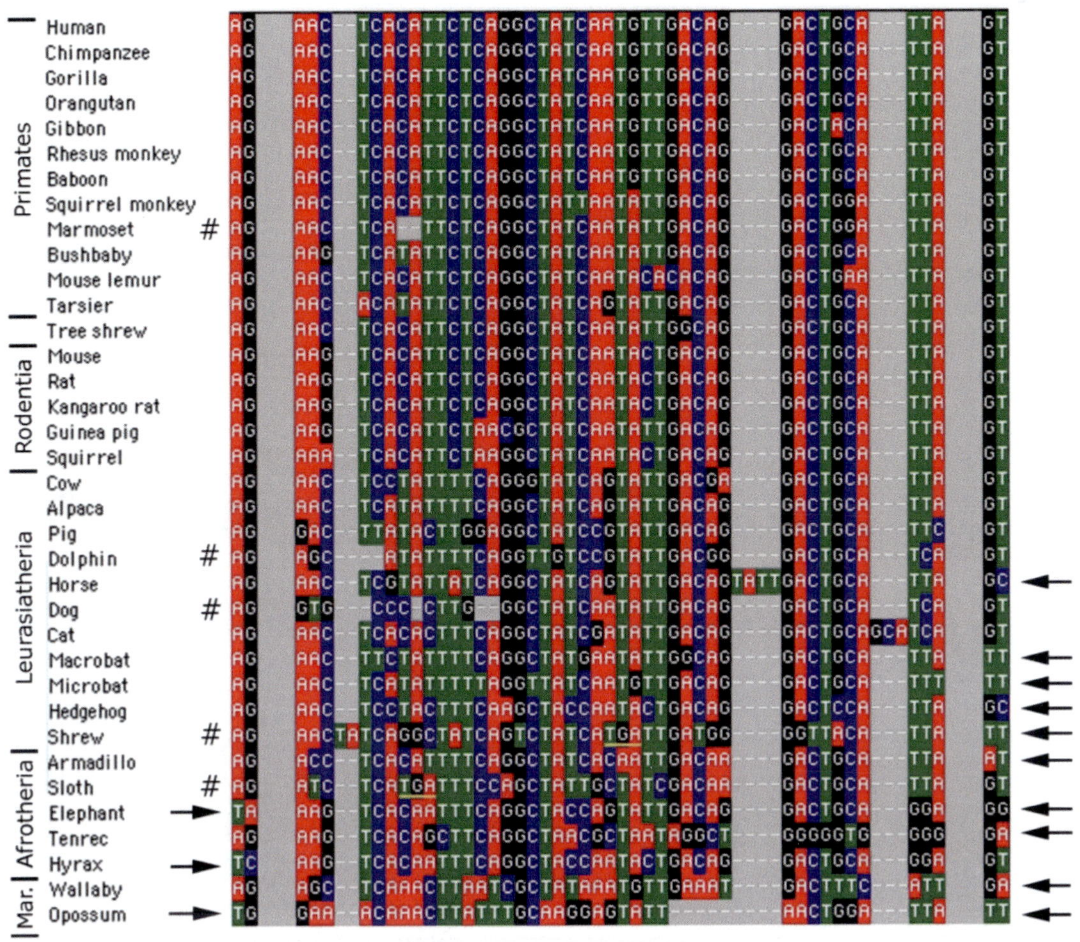

Figure 5: Alignment of the nucleotide sequences of *AMEL* exon 4 in species representative of most mammalian lineages. Exon 4 is not present in monotremes. The two important nucleotides of the donor (left) and acceptor (right) splices are indicated on both sides of the sequence alignment. After its creation in an ancestral therian exon 4 was invalidated in numerous lineages, but it is functional in primates except in marmoset, in all rodents and in a few leurasiatherians, i.e., cow, alpaca, pig and possibly cat. Arrows: splice site mutated; #, reading frame shift or stop codons (underlined). Latin names of species and accession number of sequences used in this study are indicated in the appendix.

Where did exon 4 come from in the ancestral therian *AMEL*? In general, additional exons are recruited through the duplication of a DNA region within a same gene. This region can contain one or several exons, as it involve modules that create new introns of the same phase class at both the 5'- and 3'-ends of the recipient intron. This was the case, for instance, for the creation of exon 8 in rodent *AMEL* (see review by Li et al., this book) and of *AMBN* exons 7 and 8 in primates (Figure 2). It is known that about 10% of all genes contain tandemly duplicated exons and that the vast majority of them are likely to be involved in mutually exclusive alternative splicing events [57,58]. Such an alternative splicing occurs for exon 4. Tandem duplications could play a significant role in gene evolution while alternative splicing also provides a mechanism for the regulation of protein function. Therefore, exon 4 was probably created after tandem duplication of exon 5, as these exons are close one another and have the same size (42 bp). However, sequence comparison of these two exons does not reveal similarities that could support this hypothesis. Immediatly after its creation exon 4 has certainly accumulated a large number of substitutions, which is an expected process occurring after exon duplication, and this could explain why its relationships with another exon are no longer recognizable.

Conserved and Variable AMEL Regions

The evolutionary analysis of AMEL focuses on coding sequences, with the exception of exon 4 (studied above), and exons 8 and 9 that are rodent specific (see review by Li et al., this book). We have seen that the N-terminal region of

AMEL was inherited from AMBN and ENAM, and that its genic structure has not considerably changed during hundreds millions year of evolution. This indicates that this region has probably a similar, crucial function in the three EMPs. As a consequence, the proper role of AMEL (as in other EMPs) has to be found in the region encoded by most of exon 6. These regions and the conserved C-terminal region will be analysed separately, in the three following sub-sections (Figs 6,7,8).

The N-Terminal Region of AMEL Exhibits High Sequence Conservation

The N-ter region of AMEL encoded by exons 2, 3, 5 and beginning of exon 6, i.e. the so-called TRAP (tyrosine rich amelogenin peptide) region, was obtained from 42 *AMEL* sequences available in databases, and aligned using *Se-Al v2.0a11 carbon* software (Figure 6).

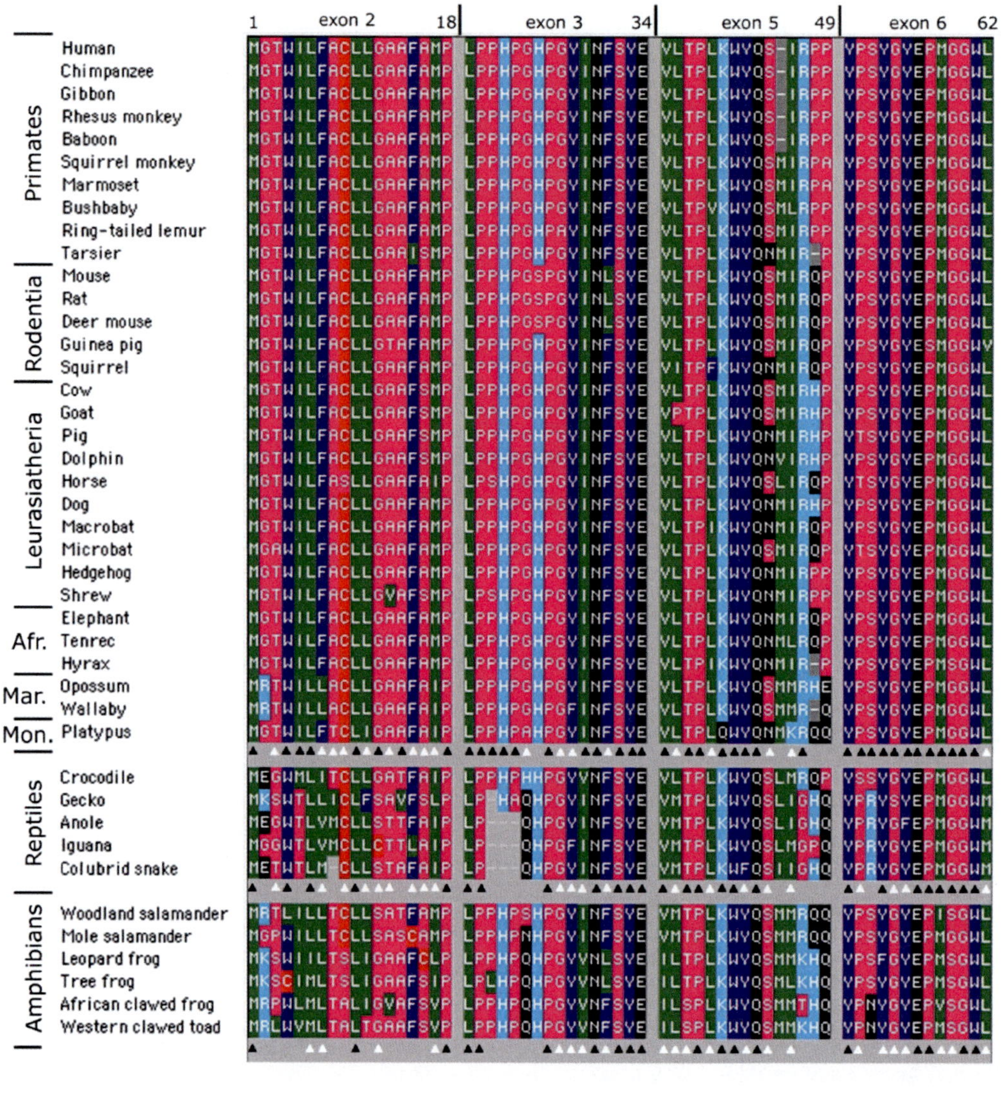

Figure 6: Alignment of the N-terminal sequences of AMEL (62 amino acids encoded by exons 2, 3, 5 and beginning of exon 6) in 42 tetrapods (31 mammals, 5 reptiles, 6 amphibians). The residues composing this region are well conserved, and particularly in mammals, which indicates their important functions. The amino acids were numbered (1-62) from the N-ter methionine in exon 2. Afr. = Afrotheria; Mar. = Marsupiala; Mon. = Monotremata. Black triangles = unchanged positions; white triangles = positions with similar chemical properties. See appendix for latin names of species and sequence accession numbers.

The amino acids (aa) of this region are extremely well-conserved in all mammalian lineages (around 200 Ma of evolution). Out of the 62 aa positions, 57 are conserved: 39 residues are identical (unchanged) and 18 are similar (same chemical properties). Such a high conservation is also found when the analysis is extended to the amniote level (310 Ma), with 26 identical and 22 similar aa, and to the tetrapod level (360 Ma), with 19 identical and 22 similar aa. The analysis reveals that some positions (aa 8, 21-23, 45 and 48) can be deleted without apparent effect on AMEL function in enamel formation. In this region, the constraints onto the residues are apparently stronger in mammalian than in sauropsidan and amphibian AMEL. This can be interpreted either as an increased selective pressure in mammals, or a low rate of substitution in this lineage, or both. The first hypothesis (influence of important selective constraints), would mean that nearly all identical residues must be conserved because they are essential for the correct function of this protein region. This pressure could be related to the loss of tooth replacement in mammals compared to the repeated tooth replacement in most reptiles and amphibians. In other words, a longer time life of enamel could imply the need of a better AMEL structure that was improved by means of natural selection of residues that could have interesting functions (see section 4). This also could indicate a lesser constraint in enamel structure in reptiles and amphibians than in mammals. The second hypothesis (a relatively short evolutionary distance between the lineages) would mean that in theory some positions could be changed without provoking damages of the enamel structure, but that the evolutionary rate was too slow for random substitution operating largely in this region during 200 Ma of mammalian evolution compared to what occurred during 360 Ma of tetrapodan evolution. In this case, the only residues conserved during tetrapod evolution should be considered as really crucial residues for correct enamel formation.

In a previous study devoted to molecular evolution of mammalian *AMEL*, it was demonstrated that the 5' region of exon 5 and the beginning and the end of exon 6 are highly constrained [59].

Most of the Region Encoded by Exon 6 is Variable and Possesses a Hot Spot of Mutation

With the exception of its short N-ter region described above and the C-ter region described in the sub-section below, the region encoded by most of exon 6 is variable as expected for an unstructured region that is theoretically less constrained than a structured region. In each tetrapodan lineages, several residues are substituted and there are deletions and/or insertions of amino acids in virtually all sequences when compared to a putative ancestral sequence [59]. The numerous indels lead to a variable number of residues composing AMEL in various species. Although the presence of this high level of variation, the region encoded by exon 6 can be aligned in mammals. In contrast, alignment of the AMEL region is difficult in reptiles and amphibians due to an high substitution rate. Two important findings result from the evolutionary analysis of this AMEL region in mammals.

First, it was demonstrated that this region was created and extended by means of the insertion of amino acid triplets, i.e. PXQ or/and PXP repeats, through a mechanism called slipped-strand mispairing, which explains tandem repeats of sequence [60]. More than 30 triplets were identified in the putative ancestral mammalian AMEL and these repeats largely contributed to the increase of proline (P) and, to a lesser degree, glutamine (Q) richness of this region [11,59]. Such repeats are also present in reptilian and amphibian AMEL sequences. In crocodile, a preliminary study revealed the presence of at least four repeats of four triplets in the central region (personal results). These findings support the origin of this region from a proline-rich region of *AMBN*, i.e., exons 5 and/or 6. *AMEL* inherited one of these exons. It is worth noting that *AMBN* exons 5 and 6 possess several tyrosines in their N-ter region as does the N-ter of AMEL exon 6. Then, the new exon 6 accumulated PXQ repeats while the rest of the dowstream exons primarily inherited from *AMBN* duplication were lost [11]. This extended PQ-rich region was subsequently conserved during evolution (by means of natural selection) as it brought advantageous properties improving the enamel structure. Because this only region houses the proper function of AMEL in enamel structure, one can deduce that this function resides in its only richness in proline and glutamine, two hydrophylic residues regularly distributed in the sequence. This could explain why the residues in this region are not under a strong functional constraints and can be substituted, provided the PQ-rich sequence is conserved.

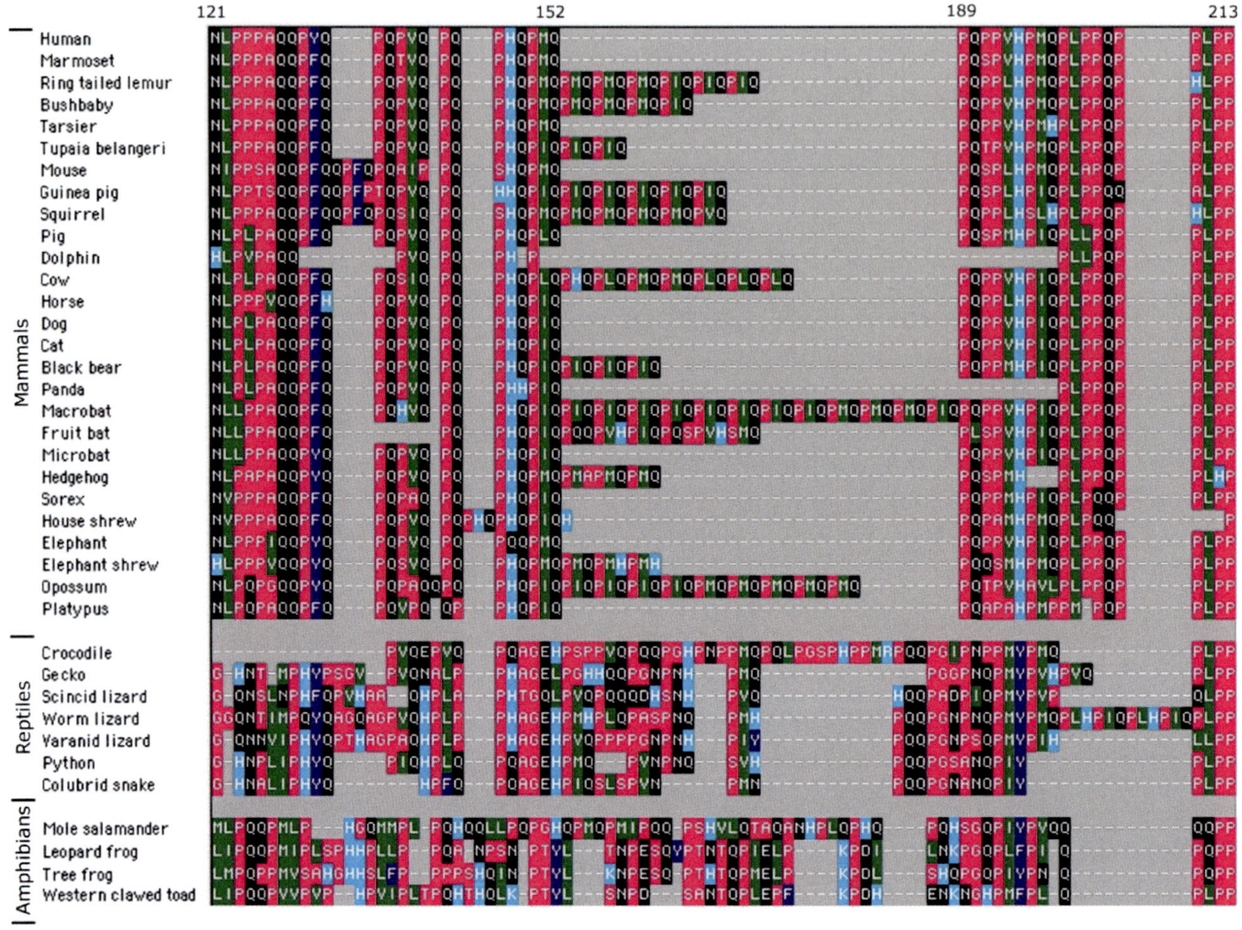

Figure 7: Alignment of 38 tetrapodan amino acid sequences (residues 121-213 in this alignment) in the mid-region of AMEL encoded by exon 6. This region houses a hot spot of mutation as revealed by the numerous deletions and the insertions of triplet repeats. In mammalian AMEL most PXQ repeats are located at the same locus. The reptilian and amphibian sequences are more variable than mammalian AMEL, and they cannot be aligned. See appendix for latin names of species and sequence accession numbers.

The second important result concerning this region encoded by *AMEL* exon 6 consists in the presence of a hot spot of mutation in the mid region of the mammalian sequence. This hot spot of mutation is characterized by the insertion (and less often deletion) of a variable number of PXQ repeats in a same protein locus, but that have occurred independently in virtually all mammalian lineages (Figure 7). In reptilian and amphibian AMELs, this region also houses a large number of deletions and insertions of PXQ repeats but they apparently occurred at more various loci than in mammalian AMEL. In this hot spot of mutation, the selection pressure seems to be relaxed. Could this region be the locus of a biological experiment in natura? At least, it is clearly proved that large insertions of PXQ repeats, such as those occurring in positions 153-188 (e.g., lemur, cow, fruit bat and opossum), are not a problem for enamel formation and structure. These indels are either neutral or could have been selected in some lineages. It is indeed quite interesting to note that most species that possess such large insertions in the mid region of AMEL are "herbivorous", while carnivores does not. We know that an herbivorous diet is highly abrasive. Are these insertions of PXQ repeats advantageous as they reinforce enamel resistance to wear? It would be interesting to compare the enamel microstructure in species in which AMEL houses these insertions and species that do not.

It seems obvious that given (i) AMEL represents around 90% of the forming enamel matrix and (ii) its central region has the proper function in enamel formation, any important change in this region could have an effect on the enamel structure. For instance, we know that mutations affecting this *AMEL* region (stop codons or reading frame shifts) lead to enamel default s(see section 5). In contrast, we don't know whether repeated insertions of PXQ triplets could have a positive effect in, e.g., leading to an improved enamel structure resisting better to enamel abrasion or to microbreaks. However, it is clear that triplet repeats contribute to maintain a high level of prolines (around 30%) and glutamines (around 20%) in this AMEL region, and could improve the interactions with other enamel proteins as it is know that such residues favor protein-protein interactions [61].

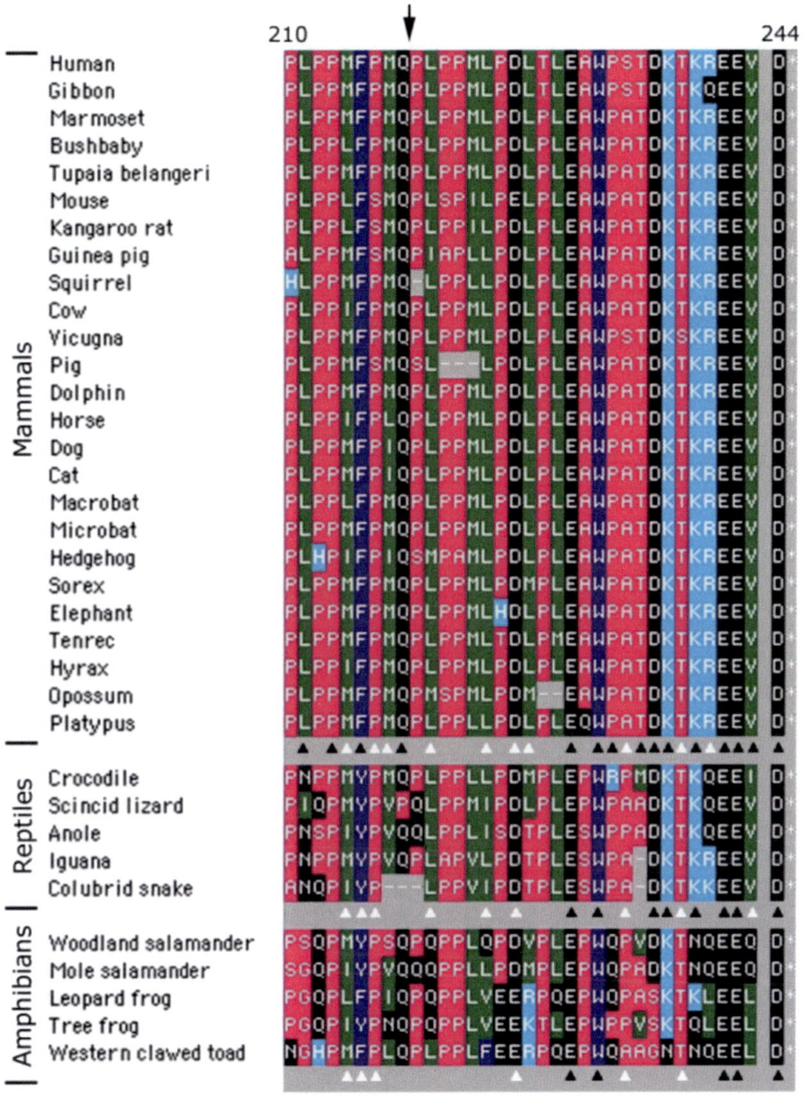

Figure 8: Alignment of 35 tetrapodan C-terminal sequences of AMEL (amino acids 210-244 in this alignment). The 15 last residues of this region are well conserved, and in particular in mammals, which indicates important functions. Triangles as in figure 6. The arrow points to the well-conserved glutamine (Q), which is the intraexonic splice site of LRAP isoform. See appendix for latin names of species and sequence accession numbers.

The C-Terminal Region of AMEL is Well Conserved

The alignment of the C-ter region of tetrapodan AMEL (mostly exon 6 + one residue from exon 7) is easy compared to the mid-region of exon 6. In particular, the 15 last residues are well conserved (Figure 8): in mammals, 11 amino acids are identical and 3 are similar. When extending the analysis to the amniote level, they are 8 and 3, and to the tetrapod level, they are 5 and 2, respectively. Here again, the number of unchanged amino acids is higher when considering mammalian AMEL alone (200 Ma) than when including all tetrapodan sequences. Among the five residues that were unchanged during 360 Ma, four are acidic (one aspartic and three glutamic acids) and one is aromatic (tryptophan). As discussed and commented above for the N-ter region, we don't know whether this high residue conservation in mammalian AMEL is due to an influence of important selective pressures or to a relatively short evolutionary distance between the lineages.

Another interesting feature located in the C-ter region consists in the alternative intraexonic splice site leading to an important isoform called LRAP (leucine rich amelogenin peptide) (Figure 8). The splice site is reported to occur immediately after the glutamine coded by the nucleotides CAG (position 218). This glutamine is unchanged in all mammalian sequences and is also present in some reptilian and amphibian AMEL, which suggests that this isoform could exist in non mammalian species although not reported to date.

SEQUENCE CONSERVATION WITH REGARD TO AMEL FUNCTIONS AND X-LINKED AMELOGENESIS IMPERFECTA

Although all authors agree that AMEL plays a crucial role in enamel structure and mineralization as exemplified by the defaults resulting either from experimental gene invalidation in the mouse [27,28] or from various mutations in human (AIH1) [29,30], the exact function of its various domains is still poorly understood. However, our previous studies have shown clearly that a large number of residues are conserved in the N-terminal region of the protein, encoded by exons 2, 3, 5 and the begining of exon 6, and in the C-ter region encoded by the end of exon 6 [9,59]. From various studies we know that the main functions of the residues in these regions are in cell-matrix and protein-mineral crystal interactions [62-66]. As stated before, these regions have been inherited from AMBN and ENAM, while the rest of AMEL sequence (approximately 110 residues), which is rich in proline and glutamine, possesses its own properties that still remain to be found. We know this variable region is characterized by the presence of PXQ repeats (hot spot of mutation). This feature was selected as it probably represent an advantage for enamel structure. To date at least three mutations in the N-ter region were reported as generating reading frame shifts and premature stop codons resulting in a protein lacking the variable region [29,30,67]. The phenotype was an hypomineralized enamel, indicating that this region is certainly playing a crucial role in enamel mineralization.

Our evolutionary analysis of numerous AMEL sequences (191 residues) reveals that 91 positions were unchanged during 200 Ma of mammalian evolution and 38 were conservative substitutions, i.e., with similar chemical properties (Figure 9). When adding reptilian and amphibian AMEL to our dataset the number of unchanged and conservative residues decreased to 25 and 28, respectively. This means that AMEL is highly constrained in mammals compared to the other tetrapodan lineages, sauropsids and amphibians. These results also point to 25 crucial residues for enamel formation, while the 66 other residues that were unchanged only in mammals could indicate that they play a more important roles for enamel formation in this lineage than in reptiles and amphibians. Three particularly well conserved regions, i.e. playing probably an important role, are identified in tetrapodan AMEL (Figure 9): a 20 aa peptide encoded by the end of exon 3 and most of exon 5 (houses the phosphorylated serine), a 13 aa peptide encoded by the begining of exon 6 (contains the three tyrosines and the TRAP proteolytic site) and a 15 aa peptide at the C-ter extremity characterized by five acidic residues. The intraexonic splice site leading to the LRAP isoform (Q) is conserved in mammals but not in the other lineages.

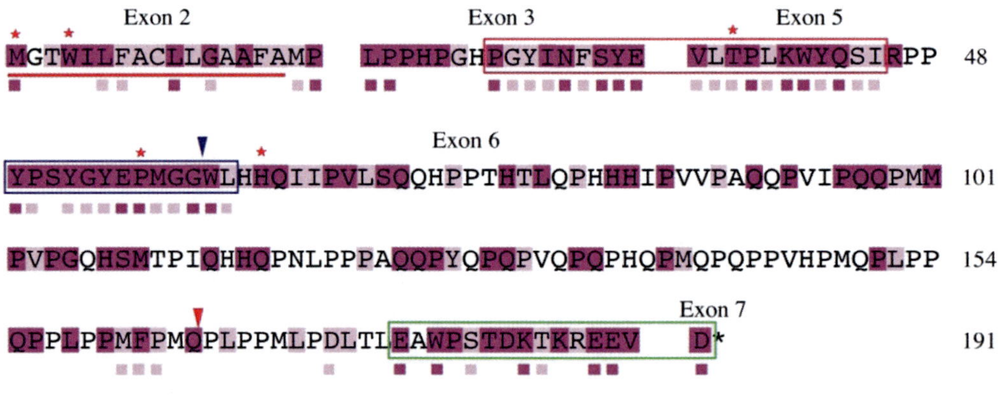

Figure 9: Amino acid sequence of human AMEL encoded by exons 2, 3, 5, 6 and 7, with indication of unchanged (violet background) and chemically conserved (pink background) positions during mammalian evolution (200 Ma). More than 60

mammalian AMEL sequences were used. Violet and pink squares below the positions indicate the conservative status of the sequence at the tetrapod level (360 Ma), i.e., when including reptilian and amphibian AMEL sequences. Three particularly well conserved regions in tetrapods (red, blue, green) are squared. Signal peptide underlined. Blue arrowhead = location of the proteolytic site leading to the TRAP ; red arrowhead = location of the intraexonic splice site leading to the LRAP isoform. Red stars indicate the positions that are known to lead to amelogenesis imperfecta when the residue is changed.

Out of the 15 human mutations leading to AIH1, five concern the only substitution of a single amino acid (Figure 9). They are M1, W4, T37, P56 and H63: p.M1T, p.W4S, p.T51I, p.P70T, p.H77L, respectively in the AIH1 nomenclature. All of them are validated when using the only mammalian dataset, but two of them (p.H77L and p.W4S) are not when using tetrapodan AMEL alignment. However, a similar substitution was not found in tetrapods: histidine (H- basic group) is substituted by glutamine (Q- acid amide) and tryptophane (aromatic) is substituted either by cystein or leucine (hydrophobic).

The results of this evolutionary analysis now allows to validate any human AMEL mutation, which could be suspected for AIH1. The numerous unchanged residues certainly are important for a correct AMEL function, and these positions are predicted to lead to AIH1 when substituted. However, their role still remains to be elucidated.

ACKNOWLEDGEMENTS

I thank Prof. Michel Goldberg for his invitation to participate in this volume. I am indebted to my colleagues, Dr Sidney Delgado and Prof. Marc Girondot, and to MD and PhD students who participated in the studies from which were extracted some information used in this review. This study was financially supported by the CNRS and UPMC.

APPENDIX

Latin names of species and accession number of *AMEL* sequences used in this study.

MAMMALIA

Primates: Human, *Homo sapiens*, NM_182680 - Chimpanzee, *Pan troglodytes*, EF537869 - Gorilla, *Gorilla gorilla*, present study - Orangutan, *Pongo pygmaeus*, EF537870 - Gibbon, *Nomascus leucogenys,* present study - Rhesus monkey, *Macaca mulatta,* EF537871 - Baboon, *Papio hamadryas,* present study - Squirrel monkey, *Saimiri sciureus,* AB091783 - Marmoset, *Callithryx jacchus,* EF537872 - Bushbaby, *Otolemur garnettii,* AB091787 - Ring-tailed lemur, *Lemur catta,* AB091785 - Mouse lemur, *Microcebus murinus,* present study - Tarsier, *Tarsius syrichta,* EF537873.

Scandentia: Tree shrew, *Tupaia belangeri,* EU168855.

Rodentia: Mouse, *Mus musculus*, NM_009666 - Rat, *Rattus norvegicus,* U51195 - Deer mouse, *Peromyscus maniculatus,* present study - Kangaroo rat, *Dipodomys ordii*, present study - Guinea pig, *Cavia porcellus,* AJ012200 - Squirrel, *Spermophilus tridecemlineatus,* EU168861.

Leurasiatheria: Cow, *Bos taurus*, EU168863 - Goat, *Capra hircus,* AF215889 - Alpaca, *Vicugna vicugna,* present study - Pig, *Sus scrofa,* U43405 - Dolphin, *Tursiops truncatus,* AH014446 - Horse, *Equus caballus,* AB032193 - Dog, *Canis lupus familiaris,* EU168873 - Cat, *Felis catus,* EU168880 - Macrobat, *Pteropus vampyrus,* EU168886 - Microbat, *Myotis lucifugus,* EU168887 - Hedgehog, *Erinaceus europaeus,* EU168884 - Shrew, *Sorex araneus,* EU168888.

Afrotheria: Armadillo, *Dasypus novemcinctus*, present study. - Sloth, *Choloepus hoffmanni,* present study - Elephant, *Loxodonta africana,* AY788990 - Tenrec, *Echinops telfairi,* EU168892 - Hyrax, *Procavia capensis,* EU168895 - Opossum, *Monodelphis domestica,* U43407 - Wallaby, *Macropus eugenii,* present study - Platypus, *Ornithorhynchus anatinus,* AF095566.

SAUROPSIDA

Crocodile, *Paleosuchus palpebrosus,* AF095568 - Gecko, *Tarentola americana,* EF202128 - Anole, *Anolis carolinensis,* present study - Scincid lizard, *Chalcides viridanus,* DQ364454 - Worm lizard, *Rhineura floridana,*

EU203600 - Varanid lizard, *Varanus niloticus*, present study - Iguana, *Iguana iguana,* present study - Colubrid snake, *Elaphe quadrivirgata,* AF118568 - Python, *Python reticulatus,* FJ434048.

LISSAMPHIBIA

Woodland salamander, *Plethodon cinereus,* DQ069790 - Mole salamander, *Ambystoma mexicanum,* DQ069791 - Leopard frog, *Rana pipiens,* AY695795 - Tree frog, *Litoria chloris*, DQ069788 - African clawed frog, *Xenopus laevis,* AF095569 - Western clawed toad, *Xenopus tropicalis,* NM_001113681.

REFERENCES

[1] Freeman S, Herron JC. Evolutionary Analysis. Third edition. Prentice Hall, Inc. A Pearson Company. 2003; 816 p.

[2] George RA, Spriggs RV, Bartlett GJ, *et al.* Effective function annotation through catalytic residue conservation. Proc Natl Acad Sci USA 2005; 102(35): 12299-304.

[3] Murphy WJ, Elzirik E, Johnson WE, *et al.* Moleculcar phylogenetics and the origin of placental mammals. Nature 2001; 409: 614-8.

[4] Hedges SD: The origin and evolution of model organisms. Nature Rev Genet 2002; 3: 838-49.

[5] van Rheede T, Bastiaans T., Boone DN, *et al.* The platypus is in its place: nuclear genes and indels confirm the sister group relation of monotremes and Therians. Mol Biol Evol 2006; 23: 587-97.

[6] Ochman H, Wilson AC. Evolution in bacteria: evidence for a universal substitution rate in cellular genomes. J Mol Evol 1987; 26: 74-86.

[7] Welch JJ, Bininda-Emonds ORP, Bromham L. Correlates of substitution rate variation in mammalian protein-coding sequences. BMC Evol Biol 2008; 8: e53.

[8] May RM. How many species are there on earth? Science 1988; 241: 1441-9.

[9] Sire JY, Delgado S, Fromentin D, *et al.* Amelogenin: lessons from evolution. Arch Oral Biol 2005; 50: 205-12.

[10] Sire JY, Delgado S, Girondot M. The amelogenin story: Origin and evolution. Eur J Oral Sci 2006; 114: 64-77.

[11] Sire JY, Davit-Béal T, Delgado S, *et al.* The origin and evolution of enamel mineralization genes. Cells, Tissues Organs 2007; 186: 25-48.

[12] Sire JY, Donoghue PCJ, Vickaryous MK. Origin and evolution of the integumentary skeleton in non-tetrapod vertebrates. J Anat 2009; 214(4): 409-41.

[13] Delgado S, Ishiyama M, Sire JY. Validation of amelogenesis imperfecta inferred from amelogenin evolution. J Dent Res 2007; 86: 326-30.

[14] Subramanian S, Kumar S. Evolutionary anatomies of positions and types of disease-associated and neutral amino acid mutations in the human genome. BMC Genomics 2006; 7: e306.

[15] Davit-Béal T, Allizard F, Sire JY. Enameloid/enamel transition through successive tooth replacements in *Pleurodeles waltl* (Lissamphibia, Caudata). Cell Tissue Res 2007; 328: 167-83.

[16] Davit-Béal T, Chisaka H, Delgado S, *et al.* Amphibian teeth. Current knowledge, unanswered questions, and some directions for future research. Biol Rev 2007; 82: 49-81.

[17] Huysseune A, Sire JY. Evolution of patterns and processes in teeth and tooth-related tissues in non-mammalian vertebrates. Eur J Oral Sci 1998; 106(suppl.1): 437-81.

[18] Gu X, Wang Y., Gu J. Age distribution of human gene families shows significant roles of both large- and small-scale duplications in vertebrate evolution. Nature Genet 2002; 31: 205-9.

[19] Huysseune A, Sire JY, Witten PE. Evolutionary and developmental origins of the vertebrate dentition. J Anat 2009; 214: 465-76.

[20] Girondot M, Sire JY. Evolution of the amelogenin gene in toothed and tooth-less vertebrates. Eur J Oral Sci 1998; 106(suppl. 1): 501-8.

[21] Ishiyama M, Mikami M, Shimokawa H, *et al.* Amelogenin protein in tooth germs of the snake *Elaphe quadrivirgata*: immunohistochemistry, cloning and cDNA sequence. Arch Histol Cytol 1998; 61: 467-74.

[22] Toyosawa S, O'Huigin C, Figueroa F, *et al.* Identification and characterization of amelogenin genes in monotremes, reptiles, and amphibians. Proc Natl Acad Sci USA 1998; 95: 13056-61.

[23] Delgado S, Casane D, Bonnaud L, *et al.* Molecular evidence for Precambrian origin of amelogenin, the major protein of vertebrate enamel. Mol Biol Evol 2001; 18: 2146-53.

[24] Shu DG, Conway Morris S., Han J, *et al.* Head and backbone of the Early Cambrian vertebrate *Haikouichthys*. Nature 2003; 421: 526-9.
[25] Kawasaki K, Weiss KM. Mineralized tissue and vertebrate evolution: The secretory calcium-binding phosphoprotein gene cluster. Proc Natl Acad Sci USA 2003; 100: 4060-5.
[26] Kawasaki K, Suzuki T, Weiss KM. Genetic basis for the evolution of vertebrate mineralized tissue. Proc Natl Acad Sci USA 2004; 101: 11356-61.
[27] Gibson CW, Yuan ZA, Hall B, *et al.* Amelogenin-deficient mice display an amelogenesis imperfecta phenotype. J Biol Chem 2001; 276: 31871-5.
[28] Prakash SK, Gibson CW, Wright JT, *et al.* Tooth enamel defects in mice with a deletion at the Arhgap 6/Amel X locus. Calc Tissue Int 2005; 77(1): 23-9.
[29] Hart PS, Hart TC, Simmer JP, *et al.* A nomenclature for X-linked amelogenesis imperfecta. Arch Oral Biol 2002; 47: 255-60.
[30] Hart PS, Aldred M, Crawford P, *et al.* Amelogenesis imperfecta phenotype-genotype correlations with two amelogenin gene mutations. Arch Oral Biol 2002; 47: 261-5.
[31] Hatakeyama J, Fukumoto S, Nakamura T, *et al.* Synergistic roles of amelogenin and ameloblastin. J Dent Res 2009; 88(4): 318-22.
[32] Shintani S, Kobata M, Toyosawa S, *et al.* Identification and characterization of ameloblastin gene in a reptile. Gene 2002; 283: 245-54.
[33] Shintani S, Kobata M, Toyosawa S, *et al.* Identification and characterization of ameloblastin gene in an amphibian, *Xenopus laevis*. Gene 2003; 318: 125-36.
[34] Delgado S, Couble ML, Magloire M, *et al.* Cloning, sequencing and expression of the amelogenin gene in two scincid lizards. J Dent Res 2006; 85: 138-43.
[35] Wang X, Fan JL, Ito Y., *et al.* Identification and characterization of a squamate reptilian amelogenin gene: *Iguana iguana*. J Exp Zool (Mol Dev Evol) 2006; 306B: 393-406.
[36] Diekwisch TG, Jin T, Wang X, *et al.* Amelogenin Evolution and Tetrapod Enamel Structure. In: Koppe T, Meyer G, Alt KW, Eds. Comparative Dental Morphology. Front Oral Biol 2009; 13: 74-9.
[37] Al-Hashimi N, Sire JY, Delgado S. Evolutionary analysis of mammalian enamelin, the largest enamel protein, supports a crucial role for the 32 kda peptide and reveals selective adaptation in rodents and primates. J Mol Evol 2009; 69: 635-56.
[38] Zylberberg L, Sire JY, Nanci A. Immunodetection of amelogenin-like proteins in the ganoine of experimentally regenerating scales of *Calamoichthys calabaricus*, a primitive actinopterygian fish. Anat Rec 1997; 249: 86-95.
[39] Satchell PG, Shuler CF, Diekwisch TGH. True enamel covering in teeth of the Australian lungfish *Neoceratodus forsteri*. Cell Tissue Res 2000; 299: 27-37.
[40] Al-Hashimi N, Lafont AG, Delgado S, *et al.* The enamelin gene in lizard, crocodile and clawed toad, and the pseudogene in the chick. Submitted
[41] Kawasaki K, Suzuki T, Weiss KM. Phenogenetic drift in evolution: the changing genetic basis of vertebrate teeth. Proc Natl Acad Sci USA 2005; 102: 18063-8.
[42] Spahr A, Lyngstadaas SP, Slaby I, *et al.* Ameloblastin expression during craniofacial bone formation in rats. Eur J Oral Sci 2006; 114: 504-11.
[43] Haze A, Taylor AL, Blumenfeld A, *et al.* Amelogenin expression in long bone and cartilage cells and in bone marrow progenitor cells. Anat Rec 2007; 290: 455-60.
[44] Sire JY, Delgado S, Girondot M. Hen's teeth with enamel cap: from dream to impossibility. BMC Evol Biol 2008; 8: e246.
[45] Deméré TA, McGowen MR, Berta A, *et al.* Morphological and molecular evidence for a stepwise evolutionary transition from teeth to baleen in mysticete whales. Syst Biol 2008; 57: 15-37.
[46] Meredith RW, Gatesy J, Murphy WJ, *et al.* Molecular decay of the tooth gene Enamelin (ENAM) mirrors the loss of enamel in the fossil record of placental mammals. PLoS Genet 2009; 5(9): e1000634.
[47] Bartlett JD, Ball RL, Kawai T, *et al.* Origin, splicing, and expression of rodent amelogenin exon 8. J Dent Res 2006; 85: 894-9.
[48] Gibson C, Golub E, Herold R, *et al.* Structure and expression of the bovine amelogenin gene. Biochemistry 1991; 30: 1075-9.
[49] Salido EC, Yen PH, Koprivnikar K, *et al.* The human enamel protein gene amelogenin is expressed from both the X and the Y chromosomes [see comments]. Am J Hum Genet 1992; 50: 303-16.

[50] Yamakoshi Y, Tanabe T, Fukae M, *et al*. Porcine amelogenins. Calc Tissue Int 1994; 54: 69-75.

[51] Simmer JP, Hu CC, Lau EC, *et al*. Alternative splicing of the mouse amelogenin primary RNA transcript. Calcif Tissue Int 1994; 55: 302-10.

[52] Bonass WA, Kirkham J, Brookes SJ, *et al*. Isolation and characterisation of an alternatively-spliced rat amelogenin cDNA: LRAP- a highly conserved, functional alternatively-spliced amelogenin? Biochim Biophys Acta 1994; 1219: 690-2.

[53] Li R, Li W, DenBesten PK. Alternative splicing of amelogenin mRNA from rat incisor ameloblasts. J Dent Res 1995; 74: 1880-5.

[54] Hu CC, Zhang C, Qian Q, *et al*. Cloning, DNA sequence, and alternative splicing of opossum amelogenin mRNAs. J Dent Res 1996; 75: 1728-34.

[55] Veis A. Amelogenin gene splice products: potential signaling molecules. Cell Mol Life Sci 2003; 60: 38-55.

[56] Jegat N, Septier D, Veis *et al*. Short-term effects of amelogenin gene splice products A+4 and A-4 implanted in the exposed rat molar pulp. Head Face Med 2007; 3: 40.

[57] Kondrashov FA, Koonin EV. Origin of alternative splicing by tandem exon duplication. Human Mol Genet 2001; 10(23): 2661-9.

[58] Letunic I, Copley RR, Bork P. Common exon duplication in animals and its role in alternative splicing. Hum Mol Genet 2002; 11(13):1561-7.

[59] Delgado S, Girondot M, Sire JY. Molecular evolution of amelogenin in mammals. J Mol Evol 2005; 60: 12-30.

[60] Levinson G, Gutman GA. Slipped-strandmispairing: a major mechanism for DNA sequence evolution. Mol Biol Evol 1987; 4: 203-21.

[61] Williamson MP. The structure and function of proline-rich regions in proteins. Biochem J 1994; 297: 249-60.

[62] Paine ML, Luo W, Zhu D-H, *et al*. Functional domains for amelogenin revealed by compound genetic defects. J Bone Min Res 2003; 18: 466-72.

[63] Paine ML, Wang H-J, Snead ML. Amelogenin self-assembly and the role of the proline located within the carboxyl-telopeptide. Connect Tissue Res 2003; 44(suppl 1): 52-57.

[64] Ravindranath RMH, Basilrose RM, Ravindranath NH, *et al*. Amelogenin interacts with cytokeratin-5 in ameloblasts during enamel growth. J Biol Chem 2003; 278: 20293-302.

[65] Ravindranath RM, Moradian-Oldak J, Fincham AG. Tyrosyl motif in amelogenins binds N-acetyl-D-glucosamine. J Biol Chem 1999; 274: 2464-71.

[66] Snead M. Amelogenin protein exhibits a modlar design: Implications for form and function. Connect Tissue Res 2003; 44(suppl): 47-51.

[67] Kim JW, Simmer JP, Hu YY, *et al*. Amelogenin p.M1T and p.W4S mutations underlying hypoplastic X-linked amelogenesis imperfecta. J Dent Res 2004; 83: 378-83.

CHAPTER 2

Amelogenin Gene Regulation

Megan K. Pugach and Carolyn W. Gibson

Department of Anatomy and Cell Biology; University of Pennsylvania School of Dental Medicine; 240 S. 40th Street, Philadelphia, PA, 19104 USA; Email: Megan Pugach: mpugach@biochem.dental.upenn.edu or Carolyn Gibson: gibson@biochem.dental.upenn.edu

Abstract: The amelogenin genes encode the conserved amelogenin proteins, which are expressed at a high level during the secretory stage of amelogenesis by ameloblast cells in the developing tooth. Most of the amelogenin genes studied to date have 7 exons, however exons 8 and 9 have been identified in some rodents. Amelogenin genes are localized to X and Y chromosomes in human, bovine, and several other species, while in rodents, the single gene is X-chromosomal, and is autosomal in monotremes. Promoter and intron analyses of murine and bovine genes have revealed regulatory regions, and alternative splicing of the primary RNA transcript is a prominent feature in all species analyzed. The X-chromosomal amelogenin (*Amelx*) gene is nested within an intron of the *Arhgap6* gene in human, mouse, bovine, dog and horse, generally in the opposite orientation. Amelogenin mRNA and protein have also been detected at low levels in dental pulp cells and in several non-dental tissues, including brain, bone and stem cells. Future research is expected to address down-regulation at the end of the secretory stage of amelogenesis, mechanisms related to regulation of alternative RNA splicing and stability during development, and expression patterns and consequences of amelogenin expression in non-dental cell types.

Key Words: Amelogenin, Gene Structure, Gene Expression, RNA Alternative Splicing

INTRODUCTION

Amelogenin genes have been identified in more than 52 mammalian species, and sequence analysis revealed a conserved gene structure and amino acid sequence [1,2]. The N- and C-termini of the secreted amelogenin proteins are the most highly conserved domains in the vertebrates studied [2], and homology between the coding regions of mouse and human X-chromosomal amelogenin genes is 92%, excluding exon 4 [3,4]. Because a high level of homology can reveal a conserved function, it became important to examine the pattern of gene expression, which is the topic of this chapter. We will consider regulatory regions within the gene, effects of intron size, nested gene structure, mechanisms to determine stability of the message and species differences. Since several reviews have recently covered some aspects of these topics, the reader will be referred to them where appropriate.

GENE STRUCTURE AND IMPLICATIONS FOR EXPRESSION

In general amelogenin genes have 7 exons, with the exception of some rodents which have, in addition, exons 8 and 9 [5], (Table 1). Translation initiation invariably occurs in exon 2, exon 4 is frequently skipped or does not exist, exon 6 is the largest exon with internal sites for RNA alternative splicing, and exon 7 encodes the final amino acid and the translation termination codon [6]. In mouse and rat, when exon 7 is skipped, termination of translation occurs in exon 9 with the addition of 24 amino acids at the amelogenin C-terminus [5].

Table 1: Amelogenin Genes with Exons 8 and 9.

Species	GenBank Accession Number
Mouse	NM_001081978; AY842498
Rat	U51195

Although highly conserved, several differences in gene structure have been reported, as amelogenin genes are localized to both the X and Y chromosomes in human and some primates, bovine, horse and pig, but only to the X chromosome in mouse, rat and several other species (Table 2). Human X and Y chromosomal genes are expressed at different levels and have approximately 87% homology to each other within the coding regions [7,3]. The amelogenin gene is autosomal in several species including platypus, opossum and crocodile (Table 2).

Table 2: Amelogenin Gene Localization.

Species	GenBank Accession Number
Both X and Y chromosome	
Human	NC_000023.1; NC_000024.1
Chimpanzee	NC_006491.2; NC_006492.2
Macaque	NC_007878.1; FJ527010
Bovine	NC_007331.3; AB091790.1
Horse	NC_009175.2; AB032194
Porcine	AB091791; AB091792
Only X chromosome	
Mouse	NC_000086.6
Rat	NC_005120.2
Dog	NC_006621.2
Western clawed frog (*Xenopus tropicalis)*	NM_001113681
Autosome	
African clawed frog (*Xenopus laevis)*	AF095569 (amel-a); AF095570 (amel-b)
Platypus (*Ornithorynchus anatinus)*	NW_001794395.1; NW001747921.1; AF095566
Opossum (*Monodelphis domestica)*	U43407
Leopard frog (*Rana pipiens)*	AY695795
Spiny anteater (*Tachyglossus aculeatus)*	AF095567
Crocodile (*Paleosuchus palpebrosus)*	AF118568
Rat snake (*Elaphe quadrivirgata)*	AF095568
Lizard (*Chalcides viridanus)*	DQ364454

The amelogenin gene was shown to be "nested", that is, physically located within another gene [8]. In mouse, *Amelx* is within intron 1 of the *Arhgap6* gene in the opposite orientation, and a similar relationship exists in several other species [8], (Table 3). Since *Arhgap6* is expressed in most tissues, but *Amelx* expression is cell specific, it has been difficult to determine whether this nested position has implications for regulation of gene expression [9].

Table 3: Amelogenin Genes Nested in Arhgap6.

Species	GenBank Accession Number
Human	NC_000023.1
Mouse	NC_000086.6
Chimpanzee	NC_006491.2
Bovine	NC_007331.3
Macaque	NC_007878.1
Canine	NC_006621.2
Horse	NC_009175.2

It is frequently an advantage to have access to an annotated gene sequence so that gene structure may be studied and compared between species. Table 4 lists the current sequences for genes in species from human and mouse to horse, cow and pig.

Table 4: Annotated Amelogenin Genes.

Species	GenBank Accession Number
Human AMELX	NC_000023.1; NG_012040.1; AY040206**
Human AMELY	NG_008011.1
Mouse Amelx	NC_000086.6
Rat Amelx	NC_005120.2
Bovine AMELX	NC_007331.3
Bovine AMELY	AB091790
Chimp AMELX	NC_006491.2
Chimp AMELY	NC_006492.2
Macaque AMELX	NC_007878.1
Horse AMELX	NC_009175.2
Porcine AMELX	AB091791

Annotated sequences include exons and introns only.

** Includes promoter and downstream sequence

AMELOGENIN EXPRESSION IN TEETH

Regulation of gene expression has been evaluated *in vivo* in teeth and in ameloblast-like cells in culture, with studies of the relative importance of the promoter, the first and fourth introns, and message stability, as described below.

Amelogenin expression by ameloblasts has been extensively evaluated at the level of messenger RNA by *in situ* hybridization and by RT-PCR. Using *in situ* hybridization, RNA transcripts were detected at birth in a bilaterally symmetric pattern in murine left and right molars, and with a complementary pattern when comparing maxillary to mandibular teeth [10]. By the more sensitive RT-PCR approach, amelogenin mRNA was detected in mouse mandibles at embryonic day 15 during the cap stage [11]. Using anti-amelogenin antibodies, amelogenin proteins were not detectable at the cap stage, but appeared later in ameloblasts at the time of birth [12,13] . Expression levels are elevated during the secretory stage, and then diminish during transition and maturation stages.

In order to identify the regulatory regions of the amelogenin gene able to provide signals for the normal pattern of ameloblast expression, transgenic mice were generated with a 3.5 kb bovine X-chromosomal amelogenin gene upstream region linked to the beta-galactosidase reporter gene [14]. These mice expressed the reporter gene in ameloblasts beginning at birth, but not in tissues other than teeth, as was predicted. Another transgenic mouse demonstrated proper developmental regulation using only 2.2 kb of the upstream murine amelogenin gene region [15]. Evaluation of these mouse lines revealed that additional regions of the amelogenin gene are necessary in the transgene for endogenous levels of expression to be observed.

More recently transgenic vectors have included 5.5 kb of the upstream amelogenin gene region, intron 1 and 500 bp of 3' genomic sequence, and these mice expressed the transgene at times and levels more closely resembling that seen in wild-type molars [16,17]. These experiments led to the conclusion that the genomic sequences included the necessary components for proper expression of *Amelx* in molars *in vivo*. In some cases, results were unexpected, as some transgenes with bovine regulatory regions led to much higher levels of transgenic expression in molars compared to incisors [18]. It is possible that this is related to the pattern of the bovine dentition, which lacks maxillary incisors. An advantage of the bovine system is that it allows determination of phenotype with different transgene expression levels within a single animal.

In vitro approaches are used to identify regulatory transcription factors in transfected cells. Cultured LS8 ameloblast-like cells have been used in transfection studies with promoter constructs to further define regulatory regions [19]. The regulation of *Amelx* transcription in murine ameloblasts has been evaluated by examination of upstream genomic sequence for predicted domains bound by regulatory transcription factors, by gel shift and using domain deletion approaches. This work has been recently summarized, and transcription factors CCAAT/enhancer binding protein alpha, NF-Y and Msx2 are thought to play important regulatory roles in ameloblasts [20-23].

AMELOGENIN RNA ALTERNATIVE SPLICING IN TEETH

The amelogenin primary RNA transcript is subject to extensive alternative splicing, and the most abundant amelogenin message includes exons 1, 2, 3, 5, 6 and 7. Internal splicing is seen within the largest exon 6 at several locations, but the reading frame is always kept intact. Although at least fifteen mRNAs are produced by alternative selection of exons or regions of exons [24-26] and the abundance of the different mRNAs varies considerably, relatively little is currently understood about the regulation of splice site choice.

Because exon 4 is frequently not included in bovine, murine and human species, its skipping has been studied mechanistically. A segment of bovine *Amelx* genomic DNA that included part of exon 3, intron 3, exon 4, intron 4 and part of exon 5 was generated by PCR and inserted in-frame into the Green Fluorescent Protein coding region of plasmid pGreenLantern [27]. When this plasmid was transfected into cultured cells, exon 4 was skipped in the mRNA as expected. We observed that bovine intron 4 is very small at 63 base pairs, and predicted to be too small to participate in normal splicing of adjacent exons. When intron 4 was increased in size by the insertion of 250 base pairs or 1000 base pairs of heterologous DNA, the inclusion of exon 4 was enhanced, indicating that small intron 4 size is an inhibitory factor for inclusion of exon 4 in bovine amelogenin mRNA [28]. Murine intron 4 includes 96 base pairs and human intron 4 is 91 base pairs in length; both of these small intron sizes may act to inhibit exon 4 inclusion but not as severely as in bovine, where we have yet to detect its normal presence by RT-PCR.

The inclusion of certain exons varies during the course of development. For example, in mRNA from bovine teeth, the inclusion of exon 3 changes during development while mRNA encoding a small but abundant amelogenin, leucine rich amelogenin peptide (LRAP), is constant from fetal day 140 through day 200 [29]. In murine molars, additional RT-PCR products were detected in late bell stage [30], and various splice products have been localized both temporally and spatially [31].

AMELOGENIN EXPRESSION IN OTHER TISSUES

Although amelogenin has traditionally been considered an enamel protein, expression has been reported in dental pulp cells by several groups [32-35]. Furthermore, expression was observed at a low level in non-dental cell types, including stem cells, bone cells, brain and other soft tissues [36-39], (see review in [23]. Extra-ameloblast expression at low levels may be linked to the proposed signaling functions of several of the amelogenin proteins [40] as described in another chapter of this book.

REGULATION OF MESSAGE STABILITY

Investigators have reported that dental epithelial cells take up amelogenin proteins and propose that these intracellular amelogenins can bind differentially to amelogenin mRNAs, altering message stability [41,42]. Uptake is through the LAMP family of amelogenin receptor proteins [43].

CONCLUSION

Initially amelogenins were thought to be tissue-specific enamel proteins, but currently there is agreement that expression also occurs in other tissues. Expression in non-mineralizing tissues may indicate additional functions such as a role in signal transduction. Regulatory mechanisms have been reported for transcription and alternative splicing in murine ameloblasts, but little information is available for regulation of expression in other cell types and for inclusion of exons other than exon 4. The implications of gene nesting have not been described, and the mechanism for reducing the expression level at the end of the secretory stage is drawing interest. There is still much to learn about expression of these interesting proteins that are critical for the formation of normal dental enamel [43].

ACKNOWLEDGMENTS

This work was supported by the National Institute of Dental and Craniofacial Research of the NIH by grant DE011089 and grant DE019968. We acknowledge present and past members of the Gibson lab and collaborators who contributed to the work described in this chapter.

REFERENCES

[1] Fincham AG, Belcourt AB, Termine JD, *et al.* Amelogenins; sequence homologies in enamel-matrix proteins from three mammalian species. Biochem J 1983; 211:149-54.
[2] Delgado S, Ishiyama M, Sire JY. Validation of amelogenesis imperfecta inferred from amelogenin evolution. J. Dent Res 2007; 86:326-30.
[3] Salido EC, Yen PH, Koprivnikar K, *et al.* The human enamel protein gene amelogenin is expressed from both the X and Y chromosomes. Am J Hum Genet 1992; 50: 303-16.
[4] Oida S, Miyazaki H, Iimura T, *et al.* Molecular structure of the mouse amelogenin genomic DNA. DNA Sequence-The Journal of Sequencing and Mapping 1996; 6:307-10.
[5] Li W, Mathews C, Gao C, *et al.* Identification of two additional exons at the 3' end of the amelogenin gene. Archs Oral Biol 1998; 43:497-504.
[6] Gibson CW. Regulation of amelogenin gene expression. Crit Rev Euk Gene Expr 1999; 9:45-57.
[7] Nakahori Y, Takenaka O, Nakagome Y. A human X-Y homologous region encodes "amelogenin". Genomics 1991; 9:264-69.
[8] Prakash SK, Paylor R, Jenna S, *et al.* Functinal analysis of ARHGAP6, a novel GTPase-activating protein for RhoA. Human Molec Genet 2000; 9:477-88.
[9] Gibson CW, Thomson NH, Abrams WR, *et al.* Nested genes: biological implications and use of AFM for analysis. Gene 2005; 350:15-23.
[10] Snead ML, Luo W, Lau EC, *et al.* Spatial- and temporal-restricted pattern for amelogenin gene expression during mouse molar tooth organogenesis. Development 1988; 104:77-85.
[11] Zeichner-David M, Vo H, Tan H, *et al.* Timing of the expression of enamel gene products during mouse tooth development. Int J Dev Biol 1997; 41:27-38.
[12] Slavkin HC, Zeichner-David M, MacDougall *et al.* Antibodies to murine amelogenins: localization of enamel proteins during tooth organ development in vitro. Differentiation 1982; 23:73-82.
[13] Snead ML, Lau EC, Zeichner-David M, *et al.* Relationship of the ameloblast biochemical phenotype to morpho- and cyto-differentiation. Molecular Approaches to Developmental Biology 1987; 641-52.
[14] Chen E, Piddington R, Decker S, *et al.* Regulation of amelogenin gene expression during tooth development. Dev Dyn 1994; 199:189-98.
[15] Snead ML, Paine ML, Chen LS, *et al.* The murine amelogenin promoter: developmentally regulated expression in transgenic animals. Connect Tissue Res 1996; 35:41-7.
[16] Chen E, Yuan ZA, Wright JT, *et al.* The small bovine amelogenin LRAP fails to rescue the amelogenin null phenotype. Calc Tiss Int 2003; 73:487-95.
[17] Gibson CW, Yuan ZA, Li Y, *et al.* Transgenic mice that express normal and mutated amelogenins. J Dent Res 2007; 86:331-5.
[18] Li Y, Suggs C, Wright JT, *et al.* Partial rescue of the amelogenin null dental enamel phenotype. J Biol Chem 2008; 283:15056-62.
[19] Chen LS, Couwenhoven RI, Hsu D, *et al.* Maintenance of amelogenin gene expression by transformed epithelial cells of mouse enamel organ. Arch Oral Biol 1992; 37:710-8.
[20] Zhou YL, Snead ML. Identification of CCAAT/enhancer binding protein alpha as a transactivator of the mouse amelogenin gene. J Biol Chem 2000; 275:12273-80.

[21] Zhou YL, Lei Y, Snead ML. Functional antagonism between Msx2 and CCAAT/enhancer binding protein alpha in regulating the mouse amelogenin gene expression is mediated by protein-protein interaction. J Biol Chem 2000; 275:29066-75.
[22] Xu Y, Zhou YL, Luo W, *et al.* NF-Y and CCAAT/enhancer-binding protein alpha synergistically activate the mouse amelogenin gene. J Biol Chem 2006; 281:16090-8.
[23] Gibson CW. The amelogenin "enamel proteins" and cells in the periodontium. Crit Rev Euk Gene Expres 2008; 18:345-60.
[24] Gibson CW, Collier PM, Yuan ZA, *et al.* Regulation of amelogenin gene expression. Dental Enamel, Wiley, Chichester, Ciba Foundation Symposium 205; 1997; pp. 187-99.
[25] Simmer JP, Hu CC, Lau EC, *et al.* Alternative splicing of the mouse amelogenin primary RNA transcript. Calcif Tissue Int 1994; 55:302-10.
[26] Hu CC, Ryu OH, Qian Q, *et al.* Cloning, characterization and heterologous expression of exon 4-containing amelogenin mRNAs. J Dent Res 1997; 76:641-7.
[27] Gibson CW, Yuan ZA, Chen E. Ameloblast-specific splicing factors are not required for correct splicing of exons 3 through 5 in amelogenin RNA. Proceedings of the Sixth International Conference of Chemistry and Biology of Mineralized Tissues, M. Goldberg, A Boskey, C Robinson, eds., American Academy of Orthopaedic Surgeons, Rosemont IL, 2000; pp 199-203.
[28] Yuan ZA, Chen E, Gibson CW. Model system for evaluation of alternative splicing: exon skipping. DNA and Cell Biology 2001; 20:807-13.
[29] Yuan ZA, Collier PM, Rosenbloom J, *et al.* Analysis of amelogenin mRNA during bovine tooth development. Archs Oral Biol 1996; 41:205-13.
[30] Couwenhoven RI, Snead ML. Early determination and permissive expression of amelogenin transcription during mouse mandibular first molar development. Dev Biol 1994; 164:290-9.
[31] Iacob S, Veis A. Identification of temporal and spatial expression patterns of amelogenin isoforms during mouse molar development. Eur J Oral Sci 2006; 114 Suppl 1:194-200.
[32] Oida S, Nagano T, Yamakoshi Y, *et al.* Amelogenin gene expression in porcine odontoblasts. J Dent Res 2002; 81:103-8.
[33] Nagano T, Oida S, Ando H, *et al.* Relative levels of mRNA encoding enamel proteins in enamel organ epithelia and odontoblasts. J Dent Res 2003; 82:982-6.
[34] Papagerakis P, MacDougall M, Hotton D, *et al.* Expression of amelogenin in odontoblasts. Bone 2003; 32:228-40.
[35] Ye L, Le TQ, Zhu L, *et al.* Amelogenins in human developing and mature dental pulp. J Dent Res 2006; 85:814-8.
[36] Warotayanont R, Zhu D, Snead ML, *et al.* Leucine-rich amelogenin peptide induces osteogenesis in mouse embryonic stem cells. Biochem Biophys Res Comm 2008; 367:1-6.
[37] Haze A, Taylor AL, Blumenfeld A, *et al.* Amelogenin expression in long bone and cartilage cells and in bone marrow progenitor cells. Anat Rec 2007; 290:455-60.
[38] Deutsch D, Haze-Filderman A, Blumenfeld A, *et al.* Amelogenin, a major structural protein in mineralizing enamel, is also expressed in soft tissues: brain and cells of the hematopoietic system. Eur J Oral Sci 2006; 114 Suppl 1:183-9.
[39] Li Y, Yuan ZA, Aragon MA, *et al.* Comparison of body weight and gene expression in amelogenin null and wild-type mice. Eur J Oral Sci 2006; 114 (Suppl 1): 190-3.
[40] Veis A. Amelogenin gene splice products: potential signaling molecules. Cell Mol Life Sci 2003: 60:38-55.
[41] Xu L, Harada H, Tamaki TY, *et al.* Reuptake of extracellular amelogenin by dental epithelial cells results in increased levels of amelogenin mRNA through enhanced mRNA stabilization. J Biol Chem 2006a; 281:2257-62.
[42] Xu L, Harada H, Taniguchi A. The exon 6ABC region of amelogenin mRNA contributes to increased levels of amelogenin mRNA through amelogenin protein-enhanced mRNA stabilization. J Biol Chem 2006b; 281:32439-44.
[43] Xu L, Harada H, Taniguchi A. The effects of LAMP1 and LAMP3 on M180 amelogenin uptake, localization and amelogenin RNA induction by amelogenin protein. J Biochem 2008; 144:531-7.
[44] Gibson CW, Yuan ZA, Hall B, *et al.* Amelogenin-deficient mice display an amelogenesis imperfecta phenotype. J Biol Chem 2001; 276:31871-5.

CHAPTER 3

Lessons from the Amelogenin Knockout Mice

Naoto Haruyama[1,2,4,*], Junko Hatakeyama[3,4], Yuji Hatakeyama[3], Carolyn W. Gibson[5] and Ashok B. Kulkarni[4,*]

[1]Global Center of Excellence Program, International Research Center for Molecular Science in Tooth and Bone Diseases, [2]Maxillofacial Orthodontics, Department of Maxillofacial Reconstruction and Function, Division of Maxillofacial/Neck Reconstruction, Graduate School, Tokyo Medical and Dental University, Tokyo, Japan; [3]Functional Structures Section, Department of Morphological Biology, Division of Biomedical Sciences, Fukuoka Dental College, Fukuoka, Japan; Functional Genomics Section, Laboratory of Cell and Developmental Biology, National Institute of Dental and Craniofacial Research, National Institutes of Health, Department of Health and Human Services, Bethesda, MD, USA and [5]Department of Anatomy and Cell Biology, School of Dental Medicine, University of Pennsylvania, Philadelphia, PA, USA; [*]Email: Naoto Haruyama (haruyama.gcoe@tmd.ac.jp) or Ashok Kulkarni (ak40m@nih.gov)

Abstract: Although others and we have earlier reported that the amelogenins play critical roles in proper enamel formation, the *in vivo* functions of each of the amelogenin isoforms have not been clearly defined because of their heterogeneity and complexity. This chapter will review the current information on the functions of amelogenin splice isoforms, full length amelogenin and leucine rich amelogenin peptide (LRAP), in enamel formation. We will also discuss the emerging evidence for the additional role of LRAP as a signaling molecule in mesenchymal cells of the periodontal tissues. We believe that further insights into the signaling pathway modulated by the multifunctional amelogenin proteins will lead to development of new therapeutic approaches to treat dental diseases and disorders.

Key Words: Amelogenin, Mouse Model, M180, Leucine rich Amelogenin Peptide (LRAP), Signaling Molecules.

COMPLEXITY OF AMELOGENIN PROTEINS AND SPLICE ISOFORMS

Ameloblasts synthesize and secrete amelogenins as the most abundant extracellular matrix proteins into the developing enamel [1]. Amelogenins are transcribed from the Amelx gene located on the X chromosome. At least 15 mutations in AMELX were found in the amelogenin coding sequences in patients with the most common genetic disorder affecting enamel, amelogenesis imperfecta (AI). The spectrum of AI phenotype varies, ranging from deficiencies in the thickness of enamel (hypoplastic AI) to defects in the enamel maturation (hypomaturation AI) [2]. Six mutations in the coding region at the N-terminus showed enamel hypomaturation/hypomineralization with some degree of hypoplasia [3-8]. Some of these mutations are adjacent to a region that harbors a specific site for a proteinase-mediated cleavage of amelogenin protein. All mutations in the C-terminus of the amelogenin protein are associated with smooth hypoplastic enamel (hypoplastic AI) [5, 7, 9-11]. AMELX mutations in the signal peptide for protein secretion, which may lead to a total loss of amelogenin, resulted in severe reduction in enamel thickness (hypoplastic AI) with normal mineralization [6, 10, 12].

The amelogenin gene is highly conserved in at least 26 mammalian species, particularly in the hydrophilic N-terminal and C-terminal regions including the leucine rich amelogenin peptide (LRAP) splicing site [13]. The N-terminal region includes amino acids that may be involved in various functions- a phosphorylation site at serine 16 [14], and a tyrosyl motif which binds N-acetyl glucosamine and keratins [15-17].

The 'A-domain' at the N-terminus and the 'B-domain' at the C-terminus of the amelogenins have important but different roles in organization and growth of enamel apatite crystals through the process of self-assembly of amelogenin nanospheres [18, 19].

Amelogenin genes in some species, including bovine and human, are located on both X (*Amelx*) and Y (*Amely*) chromosomes. The two genes have similar, but differing specific amino acid sequences resulting in two distinct protein isoforms in the enamel of the males. The amount of transcripts from *AMELY* is about 10% of those of *AMELX* [20]. Moreover, by alternate splicing at least 15 mRNAs are generated in the ameloblasts from a mouse *Amelx* gene [21-23], which consists of 9 exons. M180, the most abundant amelogenin isoform, is the product of exons 2,3,5,6 and 7 [24]. Exon 6 is the largest one and it contains three internal splice acceptor sites. The major cryptic splice deletion removes most of the 5-prime end of exon 6, resulting in one of the two most abundant isoforms- leucine rich amelogenin peptide (LRAP) [25], also known as M59 [21] or A-4 [24]. Moreover, the spliced isoforms undergo orderly proteolysis by matrix metalloproteinase 20 (MMP20) and kallikrein 4 (KLK4) during enamel secretion and maturation [26-28].

Although many reports suggest that the amelogenins have critical roles in proper enamel formation, the functions of each amelogenin isoform has not been clearly delineated because of their heterogeneity and complexity. Mice have only a single *Amelx* gene and no corresponding gene on the Y chromosome [29], and serve as a good animal model to study the functions of *Amelx* under the condition that excludes effects of amelogenins encoded from the Y chromosome.

In order to begin to understand amelogenin function, we generated a targeted deletion within the murine X-chromosomal amelogenin gene. The teeth from these null mice have a chalky-white discoloration indicating a disturbance in the enamel mineral. The incisors and molars display attrition and scanning electron microscopic (SEM) examination indicated a hypoplastic enamel phenotype, which was disorganized and lacked a prismatic structure [30]. In these amelogenin null (KO) mice, none of the amelogenin proteins were expressed and the phenotype was similar to X-linked human hypoplastic AI, confirming an important role of amelogenins in enamel formation [30]. Interestingly, the amelogenin KO mice did secrete a thin layer of mineralized enamel (10-20% thickness of normal enamel), suggesting that the amelogenins are not required for the initiation of enamel mineralization, but are essential for proper formation and elongation of enamel crystals, as well as for proper enamel thickness and volume. Interestingly, a recent report suggests that enamelin, another enamel protein, is critical for initiation of enamel mineralization [31].

THE ROLE OF M180 AND LRAP IN ENAMEL FORMATION

In order to understand the role of individual amelogenin proteins, transgenic mice were generated that expressed a single amelogenin, e.g. the M180 amelogenin which is the most abundant isoform in vivo, or LRAP, the second most abundant amelogenin, under the control of the bovine amelogenin promoter [32, 33].

Molars from the M180 transgenic mouse lines with wild-type background (TgM180) were grossly similar to wild-type teeth [33]. TgLRAP mice harbor the bovine LRAP cDNA transgene. TgLRAP mice with wild-type background showed little change in the enamel structure except pitting on the enamel surface. Although the TgLRAP mice express abundant LRAP protein, their enamel thickness and structure are normal [32]. These results indicate the robust nature of amelogenesis.

The TgM180 or TgLRAP mice could then be mated with the *Amelx* KO mice to determine whether a single amelogenin was able to rescue the KO enamel phenotype. When KO females were mated with TgM180 males, male offspring that were TgM180 with amelogenin null background (TgM180KO) have none of the endogenous amelogenin proteins, but only the transgenic M180 protein, showed evidence of 60% rescue of the thickness, density and volume of enamel produced [34]. Because complete rescue was not observed, it was assumed that some of the other amelogenin isoforms are also required for a normal enamel layer. By mating the amelogenin KO female with a TgLRAP male, introduction of bovine LRAP into the amelogenin KO enamel was achieved in male offspring. The TgLRAP with amelogenin KO background (TgLRAPKO) showed a subtle changes in enamel. SEM images of etched TgLRAPKO incisors showed that some prismatic structure was evident in etched enamel [35]. However, the enamel thickness in TgLRAPKO was basically unchanged compared to amelogenin KO mice, suggesting that LRAP may function cooperatively with other amelogenins such as M180. Another possibility is that the 6 amino acid difference of bovine LRAP from murine LRAP may have affected the susceptibility of amelogenin to the murine MMP20 or KLK4 proteases.

Under physiological conditions, amelogenin self-assembles into nanospheres of 15-20 nm in diameter, consisting of multiple monomers [36]. The amelogenin nanospheres align in beaded rows along the c-axis of the developing hydroxyapatite in enamel [37]. The formation and c-axial orientation of hydroxyapatite on the self-assembled full-length amelogenin was observed in vitro, suggesting the mechanism of full-length amelogenin function as a scaffold during enamel biomineralization [38]. The C-terminus of LRAP is also suggested to orient itself next to the hydroxyapatite [39], implying the involvement of LRAP in crystal growth. However, a recent in vitro study showed that only M180 (full-length) amelogenin enhanced mineral formation although both M180 and LRAP formed nanospheres [40]. Supporting this in vitro experiment and as mentioned above, TgM180KO mice showed partial rescue of the AI phenotype [34]. However, the component parts of nanospheres in vivo have not been determined although they do include amelogenin proteins.

INCREASED ROOT RESORPTION FOUND IN AMELOGENIN-DEFICIENT MICE

Although enamel proteins have been considered as an important part of enamel development for a long time, it has been recently shown that LRAP can also play a role as an intercellular signaling molecule [24, 41]. We will discuss the roles of amelogenin in non-enamel tissues, particularly the periodontal tissues, in the following sections.

Amelogenins are predominantly expressed in ameloblasts. However, amelogenin expression outside of enamel tissues such as in periodontal tissues- cementoblasts, periodontal ligament cells (PDLs) or Hertwig's epithelial root sheath (HERS) [42-45] has been reported by utilizing immunohistochemisrty or in situ hybridization. Other groups reported that the amelogenin signal was not detected either in periodontal tissues or HERS [46]. Using RT-PCR, two amelogenin alternative splice isoforms, M180 and LRAP, were identified in molar cementoblast/PDL cells from wild-type mice [47]. This discrepancy in detection of amelogenin expression in periodontal tissues may be caused by a combination of the difference in detection methods, species, and developmental stages of the animals analyzed. However, these reports support the idea that enamel-related proteins may be involved in cementum formation and/or homeostasis of periodontal tissue through an intercellular signaling role.

Therefore, we performed detailed phenotypic analysis of the periodontal tissues in *Amelx* null mice. The null mice showed increased formation of cementicles, irregular calcified globules on the root surface, compared to wild type. Moreover, the area of root resorption and number of osteoclasts (odontoclasts) on the root surface were significantly increased by six months to one year of age in the *Amelx* null tooth root. The osteoclastogenesis was concomitant with the increased expression of receptor activator of nuclear factor-kappa B ligand (RANKL) in PDL, suggesting that the loss of amelogenin in periodontal tissues (cementoblast and HERS) lead the cementum defects and increased number of osteoclasts by changing the signal mediated by RANK-RANKL pathway in *Amelx* null mice [47].

THE ROLE OF AMELOGENIN IN PERIODONTAL TISSUES

The co-cultures of wild-type osteoclast-progenitors with *Amelx* null cementoblast/PDL cells displayed an increased number of tartrate-resistant acid phosphatase (TRAP) positive cell formation [48]. Consistent with the increased RANKL expression near the cementum of the *Amelx* null mice, the *Amelx* null cementoblast/PDL cells also showed increased RANKL expression compared to wild-type cementoblast/PDL cells. However, the expression of RANKL in *Amelx* null cementoblast/PDL cell culture was reduced in the medium exogenously supplemented with porcine LRAP, but not in the medium supplemented with P172 (porcine full length amelogenin). In addition, decrease in migration of cementoblast/PDL cells was found in the cells derived from *Amelx* null mice compared to the cementoblast/PDL cells derived from the wild-type mice. The mouse embryo fibroblasts (MEF) did not show any change in the cell migration in the presence of LRAP, suggesting specificity to periodontal cells [48]. These findings suggest that LRAP may confer protection to the cementum from abnormal osteoclastogenesis, and that the LRAP is important for the development and maintenance of the periodontal tissues.

Emdogain® (EMD; Straumann, Switzerland) is now commonly used to regenerate the periodontal tissues in patients with periodontitis [49-52]. The majority of EMD is considered as amelogenin proteins collected from porcine tooth germ, although growth factors are also detected in EMD [53]. EMD treatment has been reported to suppress the expression of RANK and RANKL in rat experimental periodontitis [54]. The mouse and porcine full-length amelogenin significantly decreased the cultured osteoclast numbers, although the amelogenin dose in the reports is much higher than that we used in our co-culture system [55, 56]. All these reports suggest that amelogenin application suppresses root resorption by inhibiting osteoclastogenesis (odontoclastogenesis). On the other hand, reduced expression of bone sialoprotein (BSP) in *Amelx* mice was observed in the root surfaces and alveolar bone [57]. The lowest dose of full-length amelogenin enhanced BSP expression in OCCM-30 (immortalized murine cementoblast) cells, but the high dose of amelogenin did not. The full-length amelogenin stimulated BSP expression through the fibroblast growth factor 2 (FGF2) response element and transforming growth factor-β1 (TGF-β1) activation element in the promoter of the BSP gene using a rat osteosarcoma cell line [58]. Experiments in which tyrosine rich amelogenin peptide (N-terminal cleavage fragment of amelogenin) and LRAP were added to OCCM-30 cells demonstrated the increased expression of osteopontin (OPN) and the decreased expression of osteocalcin (OCN) [59, 60]. Application of recombinant human full-length amelogenin after periodontitis showed recruitment of mesenchymal progenitor cells, resulting in the regeneration of alveolar bone and PDL cells [61].

The functional differences between full-length amelogenin and other isoforms such as LRAP to the anabolic effect on alveolar bone and PDL cells remain to be elucidated.

SUMMARY

Recently, LRAP treatment of wild-type and amelogenin null embryonic stem (ES) cells showed elevated mineral matrix formation accompanied with significant increase in BSP and osterix gene expression [62]. It was also reported that mouse LRAP or full-length amelogenin induced the activation of the Wnt pathway in either ES cells or osteoblast/PDLs, respectively [63, 64]. Interestingly, two splice products of amelogenin (M73; LRAP + exon 4 and M59; LRAP) have been shown to bind to a 95 kDa transmembrane protein identified as lysosomal membrane protein-1 (LAMP-1) [65]. Furthermore, amelogenin was also shown to bind to CD63, a member of the tetraspanin family, LAMP-1, and LAMP-2 by using yeast two-hybrid system [66, 67]. LAMPs are highly glycosylated proteins, associated with vesicular structures of the endocytic pathway. These proteins are especially implicated as binding proteins functioning in a scavenger or protein uptake process after the degradation of amelogenin protein in tooth development [68]. The downstream signaling mediated by LAMPs or the relationship between LAMP and Wnt signaling still remains to be elucidated. However, it is conceivable that the LAMP receptors or other binding partners may have specific roles in cell signaling through the uptake of amelogenins.

Table 1: The potential roles of amelogenin isoforms

	M180	LRAP
Amelogenin isoform	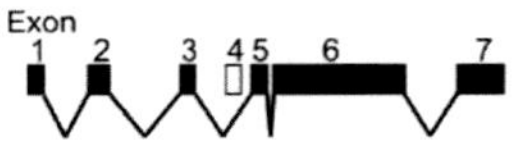	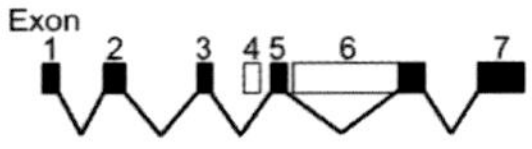
Impact on enamel thickness	High	Low or none
Impact on enamel structure	High	Low
Osteoclastogenesis	Inhibition	Inhibition
Mesenchymal cell proliferation & migration	Induction	Induction
Mesenchymal cell differentiation into mineralizing tissues	Induction ?	Induction ?

In conclusion, the earlier studies linked M180 and LRAP function mainly to enamel formation. The isoforms play distinct roles on enamel development and thickness in vivo. On the other hand, the emerging evidence suggests that LRAP has an additional role as a signaling molecule not only in epithelial but also in mesenchymal cells including periodontal tissues (Table 1). The multifunctional nature of amelogenin proteins may explain the effectiveness of EMD. Further insights into the signaling pathway modulated by amelogenin will lead to new therapeutic approaches to treat dental diseases and disorders.

ACKNOWLEDGEMENTS

We would like to thank Dr. Yoshihiko Yamada for critical reading of this chapter and Shelagh Powers for editorial assistance. This work was supported by the Division of Intramural Research, the national Institute of Dental and Craniofacial Research, the National Institutes of Health.

REFERENCES

[1] Termine JD, Belcourt AB, Christner PJ, *et al.* Properties of dissociatively extracted fetal tooth matrix proteins. I. Principal molecular species in developing bovine enamel. J Biol Chem 1980; 255:9760-8.

[2] Wright JT. The molecular etiologies and associated phenotypes of amelogenesis imperfecta. Am J Med Genet A 2006; 140:2547-55.

[3] Aldred MJ, Crawford PJ, Roberts E, *et al.* Identification of a nonsense mutation in the amelogenin gene (AMELX) in a family with X-linked amelogenesis imperfecta (AIH1). Hum Genet 1992; 90: 413-6.

[4] Lench NJ, Brook AH, Winter GB. SSCP detection of a nonsense mutation in exon 5 of the amelogenin gene (AMGX) causing X-linked amelogenesis imperfecta (AIH1). Hum Mol Genet 1994;3:827-8.

[5] Lench NJ, Winter GB. Characterisation of molecular defects in X-linked amelogenesis imperfecta (AIH1). Hum Mutat 1995;5:251-9.

[6] Lagerstrom-Fermer M, Landegren U. Understanding enamel formation from mutations causing X-linked amelogenesis imperfecta. Connect Tissue Res 1995;32:241-6.

[7] Hart PS, Aldred MJ, Crawford PJ, *et al.* Amelogenesis imperfecta phenotype-genotype correlations with two amelogenin gene mutations. Arch Oral Biol 2002; 47:261-5.

[8] Kida M, Sakiyama Y, Matsuda A, *et al.* A novel missense mutation (p.P52R) in amelogenin gene causing X-linked amelogenesis imperfecta. J Dent Res 2007 ;86:69-72.

[9] Kindelan SA, Brook AH, Gangemi L, *et al.* Detection of a novel mutation in X-linked amelogenesis imperfecta. J Dent Res 2000;79:1978-82.

[10] Sekiguchi H, Alaluusua S, Minaguchi K, *et al.* A new mutation in the amelogenin gene causes X-linked amelogenesis imperfecta. J Dent Res 2001;80 (617): (Abstract 0722).

[11] Greene SR, Yuan ZA, Wright JT, *et al.* A new frameshift mutation encoding a truncated amelogenin leads to X-linked amelogenesis imperfecta. Arch Oral Biol 2002;47:211-7.

[12] Kim JW, Simmer JP, Hu YY, *et al.* Amelogenin p.M1T and p.W4S mutations underlying hypoplastic X-linked amelogenesis imperfecta. J Dent Res 2004;83:378-83.

[13] Delgado S, Girondot M, Sire JY. Molecular evolution of amelogenin in mammals. J Mol Evol 2005;60:12-30.

[14] Fincham AG, Hu Y, Lau EC, *et al.* Amelogenin post-secretory processing during biomineralization in the postnatal mouse molar tooth. Arch Oral Biol 1991;36:305-17.

[15] Ravindranath RM, Moradian-Oldak J, Fincham AG. Tyrosyl motif in amelogenins binds N-acetyl-D-glucosamine. J Biol Chem 1999 22;274:2464-71.

[16] Ravindranath RM, Tam WY, Bringas P, Jr., *et al.* Amelogenin-cytokeratin 14 interaction in ameloblasts during enamel formation. J Biol Chem 2001;276:36586-97.

[17] Ravindranath RM, Tam WY, Nguyen P, *et al.* The enamel protein amelogenin binds to the N-acetyl-D-glucosamine-mimicking peptide motif of cytokeratins. J Biol Chem 2000 ;275:39654-61.

[18] Paine ML, Zhu DH, Luo W, *et al.* Enamel biomineralization defects result from alterations to amelogenin self-assembly. J Struct Biol 2000;132:191-200.

[19] Moradian-Oldak J, Goldberg M. Amelogenin supra-molecular assembly in vitro compared with the architecture of the forming enamel matrix. Cells Tissues Organs 2005;181:202-18.

[20] Salido EC, Yen PH, Koprivnikar K, *et al.* The human enamel protein gene amelogenin is expressed from both the X and the Y chromosomes. Am J Hum Genet 1992; 50:303-16.

[21] Hu CC, Ryu OH, Qian Q, *et al.* Cloning, characterization, and heterologous expression of exon-4-containing amelogenin mRNAs. J Dent Res 1997;76:641-7.

[22] Bartlett JD, Ball RL, Kawai T, *et al.* Origin, splicing, and expression of rodent amelogenin exon 8. J Dent Res 2006; 85:894-9.

[23] Li Y, Yuan ZA, Aragon MA, *et al.* Comparison of body weight and gene expression in amelogenin null and wild-type mice. Eur J Oral Sci 2006;114 Suppl 1:190-3; discussion 201-2, 381.

[24] Veis A. Amelogenin gene splice products: potential signaling molecules. Cell Mol Life Sci 2003;60:38-55.

[25] Fincham AG, Belcourt AB, Termine JD, *et al.* Amelogenins. Sequence homologies in enamel-matrix proteins from three mammalian species. Biochem J 1983;211:149-54.

[26] Bartlett JD, Simmer JP. Proteinases in developing dental enamel. Crit Rev Oral Biol Med 1999;10:425-41.

[27] Simmer JP, Hu JC. Expression, structure, and function of enamel proteinases. Connect Tissue Res 2002;43:441-9.

[28] Lu Y, Papagerakis P, Yamakoshi Y, *et al.* Functions of KLK4 and MMP-20 in dental enamel formation. Biol Chem 2008;389:695-700.

[29] Lau EC, Mohandas TK, Shapiro LJ, *et al.* Human and mouse amelogenin gene loci are on the sex chromosomes. Genomics 1989;4:162-8.

[30] Gibson CW, Yuan ZA, Hall B, *et al.* Amelogenin-deficient mice display an amelogenesis imperfecta phenotype. J Biol Chem 2001;276:31871-5.

[31] Hu JC, Hu Y, Smith CE, *et al.* Enamel defects and ameloblast-specific expression in Enam knock-out/lacz knock-in mice. J Biol Chem 2008;283:10858-71.

[32] Chen E, Yuan ZA, Wright JT, *et al.* The small bovine amelogenin LRAP fails to rescue the amelogenin null phenotype. Calcif Tissue Int 2003 73:487-95.

[33] Gibson CW, Yuan ZA, Li Y, *et al.* Transgenic mice that express normal and mutated amelogenins. J Dent Res 2007;86:331-5.

[34] Li Y, Suggs C, Wright JT, *et al.* Partial rescue of the amelogenin null dental enamel phenotype. J Biol Chem 2008;283:15056-62.

[35] Gibson CW, Li Y, Daly B, *et al.* The leucine-rich amelogenin peptide alters the amelogenin null enamel phenotype. Cells Tissues Organs 2009;189:169-74.

[36] Moradian-Oldak J, Paine ML, Lei YP, *et al.* Self-assembly properties of recombinant engineered amelogenin proteins analyzed by dynamic light scattering and atomic force microscopy. J Struct Biol 2000;131:27-37.

[37] Fincham AG, Moradian-Oldak J, Diekwisch TG, *et al.* Evidence for amelogenin "nanospheres" as functional components of secretory-stage enamel matrix. J Struct Biol 1995;115:50-9.

[38] Du C, Falini G, Fermani S, *et al.* Supramolecular assembly of amelogenin nanospheres into birefringent microribbons. Science 2005 Mar 4;307(5714):1450-4.

[39] Shaw WJ, Campbell AA, Paine ML, *et al.* The COOH terminus of the amelogenin, LRAP, is oriented next to the hydroxyapatite surface. J Biol Chem 2004;279:40263-6.

[40] Habelitz S, DenBesten PK, Marshall SJ, *et al.* Self-assembly and effect on crystal growth of the leucine-rich amelogenin peptide. Eur J Oral Sci 2006;114 Suppl 1:315-9; discussion 27-9, 82.

[41] Veis A, Tompkins K, Alvares K, *et al.* Specific amelogenin gene splice products have signaling effects on cells in culture and in implants in vivo. J Biol Chem 2000;275:41263-72.

[42] Slavkin HC, Bessem C, Fincham AG, *et al.* Human and mouse cementum proteins immunologically related to enamel proteins. Biochim Biophys Acta 1989;991:12-8.

[43] Hammarstrom L. The role of enamel matrix proteins in the development of cementum and periodontal tissues. Ciba Found Symp 1997;205:246-55; discussion 55-60.

[44] Fong CD, Hammarstrom L. Expression of amelin and amelogenin in epithelial root sheath remnants of fully formed rat molars. Oral Surg Oral Med Oral Pathol Oral Radiol Endod 2000;90:218-23.

[45] Sonoyama W, Seo BM, Yamaza T, *et al.* Human Hertwig's epithelial root sheath cells play crucial roles in cementum formation. J Dent Res 2007;86:594-9.

[46] Diekwisch TG. The developmental biology of cementum. Int J Dev Biol 2001;45:695-706.

[47] Hatakeyama J, Sreenath T, Hatakeyama Y, *et al.* The receptor activator of nuclear factor-kappa B ligand-mediated osteoclastogenic pathway is elevated in amelogenin-null mice. J Biol Chem 2003;278:35743-8.

[48] Hatakeyama J, Philp D, Hatakeyama Y, *et al.* Amelogenin-mediated regulation of osteoclastogenesis, and periodontal cell proliferation and migration. J Dent Res 2006;85:144-9.

[49] Hammarstrom L, Heijl L, Gestrelius S. Periodontal regeneration in a buccal dehiscence model in monkeys after application of enamel matrix proteins. J Clin Periodontol 1997;24(9 Pt 2):669-77.

[50] Gestrelius S, Andersson C, Lidstrom D, *et al.* In vitro studies on periodontal ligament cells and enamel matrix derivative. J Clin Periodontol 1997;24(9 Pt 2):685-92.

[51] Cardaropoli G, Leonhardt AS. Enamel matrix proteins in the treatment of deep intrabony defects. J Periodontol 2002;73:501-4.

[52] Velasquez-Plata D, Scheyer ET, Mellonig JT. Clinical comparison of an enamel matrix derivative used alone or in combination with a bovine-derived xenograft for the treatment of periodontal osseous defects in humans. J Periodontol 2002;73:433-40.

[53] Suzuki S, Nagano T, Yamakoshi Y, *et al.* Enamel matrix derivative gel stimulates signal transduction of BMP and TGF-{beta}. J Dent Res 2005;84:510-4.

[54] Fujishiro N, Anan H, Hamachi T, *et al.* The role of macrophages in the periodontal regeneration using Emdogain gel. J Periodontal Res 2008;43:143-55.

[55] Nishiguchi M, Yuasa K, Saito K, *et al.* Amelogenin is a negative regulator of osteoclastogenesis via downregulation of RANKL, M-CSF and fibronectin expression in osteoblasts. Arch Oral Biol 2007;52:237-43.

[56] Yagi Y, Suda N, Yamakoshi Y, *et al.* In vivo application of amelogenin suppresses root resorption. J Dent Res 2009 ; 88:176-81.

[57] Viswanathan HL, Berry JE, Foster BL, *et al.* Amelogenin: a potential regulator of cementum-associated genes. J Periodontol 2003;74:1423-31.

[58] Shimizu E, Saito R, Nakayama Y, *et al.* Amelogenin stimulates bone sialoprotein (BSP) expression through fibroblast growth factor 2 response element and transforming growth factor-beta1 activation element in the promoter of the BSP gene. J Periodontol 2005;76:1482-9.

[59] Boabaid F, Gibson CW, Kuehl MA, *et al.* Leucine-rich amelogenin peptide: a candidate signaling molecule during cementogenesis. J Periodontol 2004;75:1126-36.

[60] Swanson EC, Fong HK, Foster BL, *et al.* Amelogenins regulate expression of genes associated with cementoblasts in vitro. Eur J Oral Sci 2006;114 Suppl 1:239-43; discussion 54-6, 381-2.

[61] Haze A, Taylor AL, Haegewald S, *et al.* Regeneration of bone and periodontal ligament induced by Recombinant amelogenin after periodontitis. J Cell Mol Med 2009 Feb 17.

[62] Warotayanont R, Zhu D, Snead ML, *et al.* Leucine-rich amelogenin peptide induces osteogenesis in mouse embryonic stem cells. Biochem Biophys Res Commun 2008;367:1-6.

[63] Warotayanont R, Frenkel B, Snead ML, *et al.* Leucine-rich amelogenin peptide induces osteogenesis by activation of the Wnt pathway. Biochem Biophys Res Commun 2009; 387:558-63.

[64] Matsuzawa M, Sheu TJ, Lee YJ, *et al.* Putative signaling action of amelogenin utilizes the Wnt/beta-catenin pathway. J Periodontal Res 2009;44:289-96.

[65] Tompkins K, George A, Veis A. Characterization of a mouse amelogenin [A-4]/M59 cell surface receptor. Bone. 2006;38:172-80.

[66] Wang H, Tannukit S, Zhu D, *et al.* Enamel matrix protein interactions. J Bone Miner Res 2005; 20:1032-40.

[67] Zou Y, Wang H, Shapiro JL, *et al.* Determination of protein regions responsible for interactions of amelogenin with CD63 and LAMP1. Biochem J 2007; 408:347-54.

[68] Shapiro JL, Wen X, Okamoto CT, *et al.* Cellular uptake of amelogenin, and its localization to CD63, and Lamp1-positive vesicles. Cell Mol Life Sci 2007; 64:244-56.

CHAPTER 4

Amelogenins: A Review of Formative and Degradative Aspects, and Transgene Expression in Bone Cells

Rima Wazen, Sylvia Francis Zalzal and Antonio Nanci

Laboratory for the Study of Calcified Tissues and Biomaterials, Faculty of Dentistry, Université de Montréal, Montreal, Quebec, Canada

Abstract: The cells that form calcified tissues produce various matrix proteins that foster a favourable environment for the regulated and structured deposition of calcium and phosphate ions into a carbonated form of apatite mineral. Differing from collagen-based calcified tissues, the organic matrix of enamel is produced by epithelially-derived cells – the ameloblasts, and consists of two major classes of proteins, amelogenins (AMEL) and nonamelogenins [1]. The AMEL class comprises full-length proteins, truncated isoforms resulting from alternative mRNA splicing, and fragments generated by extracellular proteolytic processing [1]. Enamel is distinctive from other calcified tissues because its organic matrix must ultimately be almost totally removed for it to achieve its full mineralization status. Thus, amelogenesis involves both formative and degradative processes. Studies over the past few years have revealed unexpected potentials for AMEL beyond structuring and organizing mineral at the surface of teeth, in particular their apparent capacity to influence osteogenic events. The objective of this mini-review is to highlight some key features of AMEL as related to both processes, and briefly go over our efforts to introduce enamel protein transgenes in bone forming cells.

Key Words: Amelogenins, Ameloblasts, Secretion, Degradation, Dental Mineralization, Bone Formation.

OVERVIEW OF AMELOGENESIS

Enamel development can be subdivided into three major functional stages, pre-secretion, secretion and maturation [2]. Throughout these stages, ameloblasts undergo a number of distinct morphological changes related to their function. During presecretion, differentiating ameloblasts acquire their phenotype, change polarity, and develop their protein synthetic apparatus. In the secretory stage, ameloblasts actively produce an organic matrix, and elaborate and organize the full thickness of an enamel layer that is partially mineralized. The extremely long enamel crystals attain their maximum length but must still grow in width and thickness. A cytoplasmic extension, the Tomes' process, part of which extends into the forming enamel layer, develops at the apical extremity of ameloblasts (Figure 1A). The cells synthesise, modify posttranslationally the various enamel proteins (nonamelogenins more so than AMEL), and package them in secretory granules that are targeted for constitutive release at two distinct secretory sites along Tomes' process. Differential matrix release at these two sites gives rise to interrod and rod enamel patterns [3]. Finally, during the maturation stage, ameloblasts no longer have a Tomes' process and undergo cyclic changes in the morphology of their apical surface from a smooth to a ruffled border (Figure 1B). This so-called modulation affects the "leakiness" of the cells allowing them to periodically flush the enamel fluid space of protein fragments generated by bulk enzymatic degradation [4-8]. The removal of the organic matrix creates space that allows the apatite crystals to grow in width and thickness. This growth results in production of excess acid (H^+ ions) that must be neutralized to prevent reverse demineralisation of crystals and maintain an optimal pH for the functioning of matrix degrading enzymes [9]. To achieve this, ruffle-ended ameloblasts release bicarbonate ions [9;10]. The change in leakiness during the ruffled-smooth-ruffled transition may also contribute to the overall buffering process. Finally, for reasons that are not yet clear, about half of the ameloblast population undergoes apoptosis, at least in rodents [11-13].

Michel Goldberg (ED)

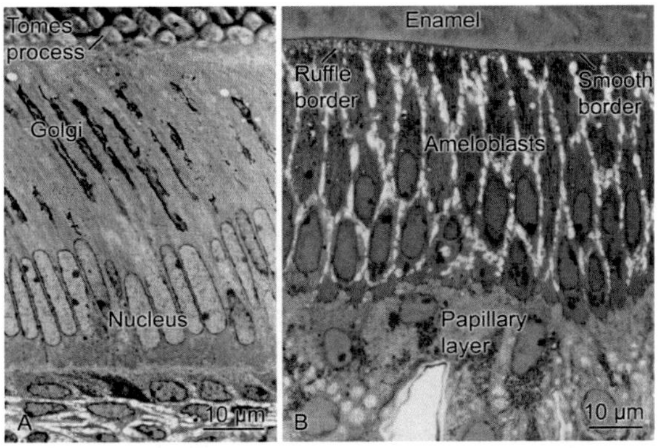

Figure 1: **(A)** As illustrated in this cytochemical preparation for an acid phosphatase, the Golgi apparatus in secretory stage ameloblasts is an extensive organelle that occupies much of the supranuclear compartment. At this stage, ameloblasts have an apical extension, called Tomes' process, that extends into the forming enamel layer. **(B)** During the maturation stage, ameloblasts undergo cyclic changes in the morphology to exhibit either a smooth or ruffled border.

AMELOGENINS ARE SECRETED BEFORE ACCRETION OF THE ENAMEL LAYER

It was originally believed that presecretory stage ameloblasts were cells preparing for active secretion, hence that do not yet produce enamel matrix proteins. However, several studies have now shown that synthesis and secretion of enamel proteins is not restricted to the secretory stage and begins earlier than suspected. Indeed, AMEL are immunodetected very early on during tooth development in the forming mantle predentin (Figure 2) and this before other enamel proteins such as ameloblastin are [14]. If fact, ameloblastin seems to appear extracellularly slightly later, at about the time formation and mineralization of the enamel layer initiate [14]. Amelogenin is also transiently expressed by differentiating odontoblasts [15-17]. The precocious expression of AMEL raises the possibility that members of this protein class may have additional functions to building enamel, including perhaps epithelio-mesenchymal signalling. Amelogenins are first immunodetected in association with the *lamina fibroreticularis* of the basement membrane separating differentiating ameloblasts (Figure 2) where they could be in a position to influence the spatial redistribution of fibronectin that is believed to participate in final odontoblast differentiation and polarization [18]. However, to date publications on AMEL knockout mice [19;20] have not reported abject defects in tooth crowns or roots that would be consistent with defective signalling, suggesting no implication of AMEL in the process or the existence of redundant and/or compensatory mechanisms. So, whether AMEL are multifunctional or not still remains to be demonstrated.

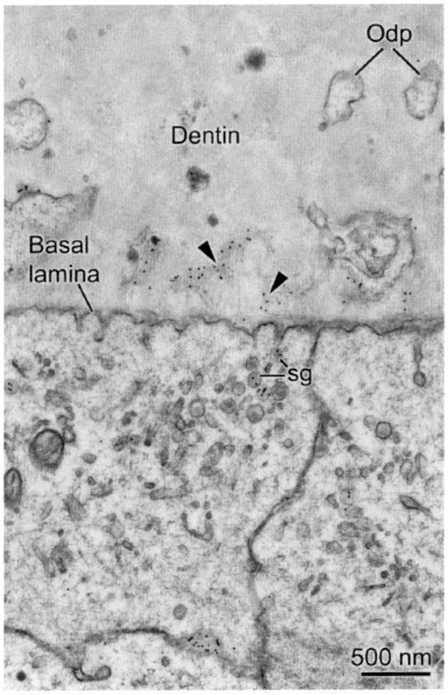

Figure 2: Immunocytochemical preparation illustrating the production of amelogenins by differentiating ameloblasts during the presecretory stage and their early extracellular release (arrowheads) prior to mantle dentin mineralization. sg, secretory granule; Odp, odontoblast process.

THE SECRETORY PATHWAY OF AMELOGENINS

Ameloblasts have an ultrastructural organization that is consistent with an intense synthetic and secretory activity. In particular, the Golgi complex is extensive and organized as a cylindrical organelle that is surrounded by abundant cisternae of rough endoplasmic reticulum and that occupies a large portion of the supranuclear compartment (Figures 1A, 3). Proteins are translocated from rough endoplasmic reticulum to the Golgi apparatus and then progress through the stack of Golgi saccules where they condense and undergo further posttranslational modification (Figures 4A, 5A). They are packaged into secretory granules that bud off from the mature face of the Golgi (Figure 5A), and subsequently targeted to secretory surfaces along Tomes' process where they fuse with the cell membrane and release their content into the forming enamel layer (Figure 5B). Secretion is constitutive in the sense that secretory granules are not stored for prolonged periods and their release is continuous. A question that was still until recently unanswered is whether the various enamel proteins are sorted and secreted differentially or whether they co-localized within the same granule. The double-immunogold labelling approach has been advantageously applied to quantitatively address this question (Figure 5B) [21]. The results showed that in the majority of cases (~70%) both AMEL and ameloblastin, a nonamelogenin, are packaged within the same secretory granule but there is also a smaller percentage (~13%) of granules that contain only ameloblastin [21]. This suggests the existence of a regulatory mechanism at the level of the Golgi apparatus for sorting and packaging AMEL and nonamelogenins. The apparent start of enamel build-up as ameloblastin (and perhaps other nonamelogenins) joins pre-existent AMEL, thereafter co-secretion of both protein classes [21], and the significant reduction in AMEL expression in a mutant mouse model expressing a truncated form of ameloblastin [22] is consistent with a functional association between these two proteins related to sustaining enamel formation.

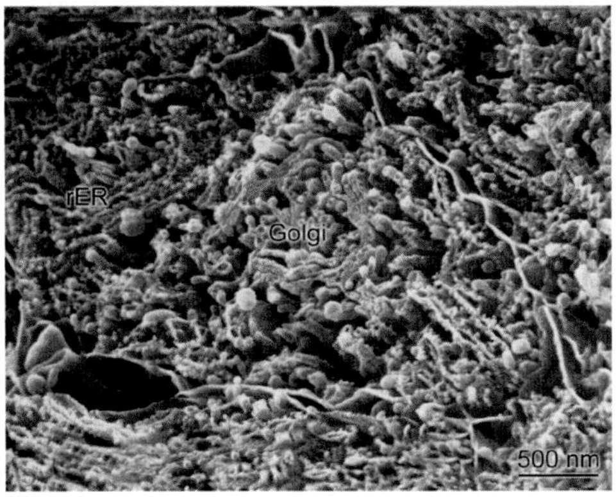

Figure 3: Scanning electron microscope view of cross-fractured secretory stage ameloblast showing the Golgi apparatus surrounded by rough endoplasmic reticulum (rER).

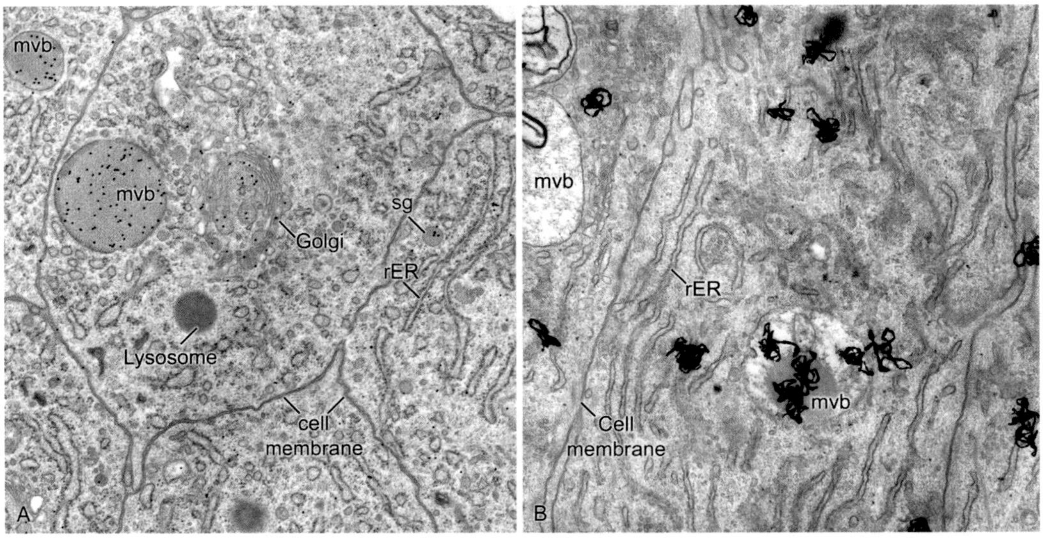

Figure 4: (A) Immunogold preparation of secretory stage ameloblasts showing the presence of amelogenins in multivesicular bodies (mvb) that are elements of the degradative endosomal/lysosomal system. **(B)** As judged by radioautography at 20 minutes following injection of ^{3}H-methionine, these proteins are newly-synthesized. rER, rough endoplasmic reticulum; sg, secretory granules.

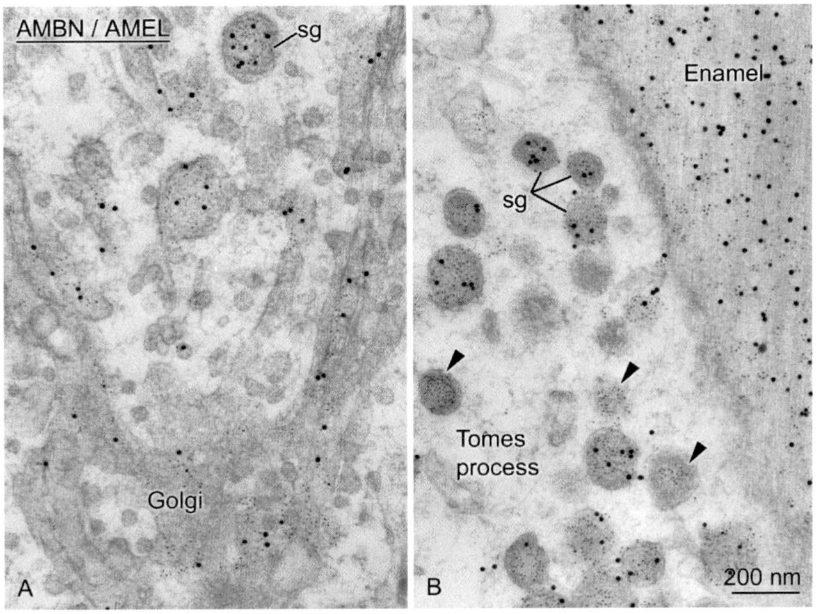

Figure 5: Dual immunogold labelling for amelogenin (AMEL, large gold particles) and ameloblastin (AMBN, small gold particles). **(A)** Labelling for both AMBN and AMEL can be found within the saccules of the Golgi apparatus and in some of the secretory granules (sg) that bud off from the mature face of the Golgi. **(B)** Most of the secretory granules that accumulate in Tomes' process are immunoreactive for both proteins but some of them (arrowheads) contain only AMBN.

EXTRACELLULAR DISTRIBUTION OF AMELOGENINS IN FORMING ENAMEL

Radiolabeling studies have shown that enamel proteins slowly diffuse away from secretory surfaces, intermix, and randomize across the forming enamel layer over time [23]. However, the situation is more complex; following release from the cell, AMEL and nonamelogenins assume differential distributions that appear to correlate with their proposed functions [14]. Mapping of their extracellular distribution using immunogold cytochemistry revealed the presence of intact AMEL and/or their fragments throughout the forming enamel layer but the density of labeling is lowest at enamel growth sites [14;24]. In contrast, nonamelogenins generally show an inverse distribution pattern. That is, newly secreted molecules temporarily accumulate at enamel growth sites where crystals actively elongate and are then found in lower concentration deeper within the enamel layer, mainly as fragmented forms [14;25;26]. The presence of AMEL among the enamel crystals throughout the layer is consistent with a role in regulating the growth in width and thickness of crystals [14;27]. It should be recalled here that AMEL must be removed in order for such growth to take place. Possible mechanisms for achieving the observed protein distributions include "boosted" secretion from secretory granules enriched in ameloblastin [21], and differences in molecular behaviors along the plasma membrane at secretory surfaces [28] and at the growing extremity of enamel crystals. Indeed, it may not be desirable to have high concentration of growth-limiting AMEL at enamel growth sites where crystals are actively forming on all axes. A more simplistic yet plausible explanation would be that there is not enough space for both proteins to co-exist at high concentration at the enamel growth sites and AMEL must wait for nascent nonamelogenins to breakdown to "normalize" their concentration around the lengthening extremity of the enamel crystals.

THERE IS NO BULK UPTAKE OF WHOLE-LENGTH OR RELATIVELY INTACT AMELOGENINS BY AMELOBLASTS

For a certain time, maturation stage ameloblasts were viewed as cells that resorb intact or partially degraded enamel proteins directly from maturing enamel and dispose of them within their lysosomes, and were as such compared to osteoclasts. This was before it was discovered that ameloblasts secrete enzymes for the degradation of extracellular matrix [28]. Amelogenins undergo both short- and long-term extracellular processing into lower molecular weight proteolytic products [29;30]. The C-terminal end of AMEL is cleaved after its secretion by matrix metalloproteinase-20, and the remaining protein is degraded into smaller fragments by a serine proteinase during the maturation stage. In contrast, nonamelogenins undergo very rapid extracellular processing and do not accumulate over time in the forming enamel layer. In some species, fragments from enamel matrix proteins leave the enamel layer quickly while in other N- and C-terminal portions of nonamelogenins persist along with processed AMEL [14;23;25;31]. The comparison to osteoclasts was likewise abandoned as it became evident that osteoclasts do not phagocytose bulk organic matrix but rather secrete enzymes that degrade bone matrix proteins extracellularly, uptake the fragmented proteins and transcytose them into the extracellular space [32]. Also, rather than producing protons to dissolve mineral like osteoclasts, ameloblasts must neutralize the acid pH generated during crystal growth [9;27;33]. This said, ameloblasts at all stages do possess an extensive endosomal/lysosomal system and various enamel proteins have been immunodetected in them (Figures 4, 6) [14;34]. So where do these proteins come from? A key to answering this question resides in the age of the proteins – are they recently-produced or older proteins that have been in the enamel layer for some time?

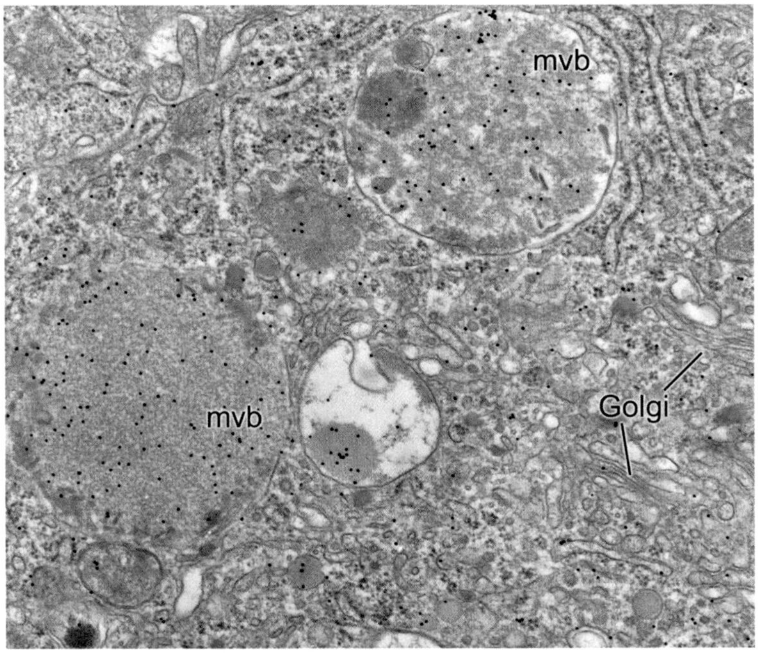

Figure 6: At the start of the maturation stage, ameloblasts still exhibit some immunogold labelling for amelogenin over the Golgi apparatus. These cells characteristically also show prominent multivesicular bodies (mvb) whose content is also immunoreactive.

There are different possible origins for the enamel proteins found in lysosomal elements of ameloblasts and likely more than one is operative. First of all, it must be emphasized that radioautographic studies indicate that much of the material accumulating within lysosomal elements of ameloblasts corresponds to newly formed proteins (Figure 4B) [35;36]. During the secretory stage, patches of enamel proteins that are immunoreactive for AMEL are found along the basolateral surfaces of ameloblasts. These derive either from ectopic secretion and/or diffusion away from the enamel layer of protein fragments created by short term processing [14;37]. Hence they comprise relatively young proteins/fragments that may subsequently be reincorporated by the cell through fluid phase endocytosis [38]. It is also known that certain cell types, such as fibroblasts, degrade a portion of their newly-synthesized secretory products intracellularly prior to their release [39]. This maybe a mechanism for fine-regulation of the secretory output and may be particularly relevant for cells with constitutive secretion such as ameloblasts. Indeed, ameloblasts appear to synthesize more proteins than are secreted at the "start" and "end" of the secretory stage, and the excess proteins are rapidly degraded [35]. While enamel protein production is maximal during the secretory stage, ameloblasts in the maturation stage continue to produce AMEL, albeit at a much reduced rate and for a short time (Figure 6) [14]. These proteins are not needed, and may be shunted to the lysosomal system prior to their secretion, or secreted, immediately reinternalized and targeted to lysosomes (Figures 4B, 6).

There is no major increase in cellular radiolabeling in maturation stage ameloblasts at times when aged, radiolabeled enamel proteins are lost from maturing enamel [35;40;41]. Thus proteins originating from the enamel layer do not seem to be major contributors to the radiolabeling seen in cells. Smooth-ended ameloblasts possess leaky distal junctions and as ruffle-ended cells transform into smooth-ended ones, fragmented forms of enamel proteins can leave the enamel layer. These fragments may diffuse laterally among ameloblasts to be endocytosed along basolateral surfaces for degradation in lysosomes. Some fragments may also leach out beyond the ameloblast layer through the leaky basal junctions that characterize ruffle-ended cells and diffuse throughout the papillary layer and perhaps beyond. Indeed, enamel proteins are occasionally immunodetected deep within the papillary layer or the connective tissue surrounding the tooth [42]. Some uptake through the apical surface of ameloblasts also cannot be excluded. In any case, endocytosed enamel proteins appear to be rapidly degraded into by-products that are returned to the general circulation.

CAN EXPRESSION OF AMELOGENINS BE ACHIEVED IN OSTEOGENIC CELLS?

Systematic comparison of cellular and matrix events during development and the fact that enamel organ cells can produce noncollagenous proteins found in bone, cementum and dentin [43;44] raise interesting questions about the relationship among these calcified tissues. Interestingly, it was also reported that exon 2 of the AMEL gene was recruited from the duplication of exon 2 of a osteonectin/SPARC gene, most likely during the Precambrian period, about 100 million years before the appearance of mineralization in the fossil record [45]. Since noncollagenous matrix proteins in calcified tissues, in general, may share functional features [42], conceptually one could take advantage of the properties of proteins found in enamel, for instance, to influence cell behavior, matrix organization and potentially be able to alter activity in other mineralized tissues such as bone.

Based on the premise that AMEL may have a signalling role during tooth root formation and cementogenesis [46-48], a concept which still remains to be demonstrated, enamel matrix derivatives, consisting essentially of fragmented AMEL, have been developed and used as an alternative approach for periodontal regeneration for over a decade [49-51]. Ultimately, treatment with enamel matrix derivatives, by yet unclear mechanisms, appears to favor bone formation around teeth [49;52]. Studies attempting to elucidate how this is achieved have shown that AMEL influence the activity of osteogenic cells [53-58], participate in pulp healing and dentin repair/regeneration [59-64] and induce changes in the gene expression profile of osteoblasts [65;66]. Some studies have reported the transient presence of enamel proteins in embryonic bone [67], long bone cells, cartilage cells, cells of the epiphyseal growth plate and in bone marrow stromal cells [68]. We have also reported cross-reactivity of an antibody to bovine AMEL [69] with noncollagenous compartments in rat bone [70]. Furthermore, Veis et al. [71] have shown that low molecular weight AMEL splice products, extracted from the collagen-based dentin, induced Cbfa1 mRNA expression by cultured embryonic rat muscle fibroblasts, and bone sialoprotein and mineral deposition at the site of implantation of recombinant peptides. Animal studies have further demonstrated the ability of enamel matrix derivatives to affect bone regeneration in osseous defects [72].

Based on these findings, we have undertaken lentiviral gene transfer experiments to introduce enamel protein transgenes in bone forming cells, both in vitro and by local administration in animals. In vitro, we have been able to introduce the genes for both AMEL and ameloblastin in osteogenic cells (Figure 7), and demonstrated that expression of the ameloblastin transgene does not significantly affect production of other major proteins by the cells [73]. Most importantly, our studies have shown that in vivo the tooth organ and the cells that form and maintain bone – osteoblasts and osteocytes – can be stably and efficiently transfected for both secreted and cytoplasmic proteins. These results open the door to studies aimed at determining whether the introduction of AMEL and nonamelogenins in the bone matrix can advantageously influence bone formation and remodelling, as well as the biomechanical properties of bone. Such a capacity would be of clinical relevance for both bone repair and reduction/prevention of excessive bone loss in diseases such as osteoporosis where targeting of major anatomical sites could be achieved by local gene transfer.

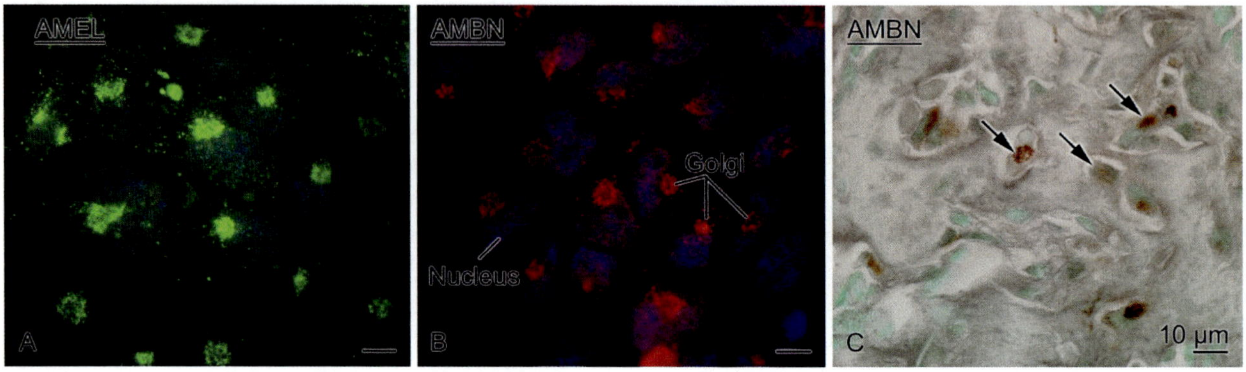

Figure 7: Lentiviruses encoding for either **(A)** amelogenin (AMEL) or **(B)** ameloblastin (AMBN) can be used to successfully infect human osteogenic sarcoma cells (SaOS-2). Immunofluorescence reveals the presence of both proteins in the perinuclear region of the cells where the Golgi is found. **(C)** Using infusion of lentivirus encoding for AMBN through a 'bony window' in the rat hemimandible, osteoblasts and osteocytes (arrows) in bone near the drill site can be made to express the transgene, here revealed by immunoperoxidase labelling. Nuclei in A and B are stained blue using Hoechst.

ACKNOWLEGEMENTS

Funded by the Canadian Institutes of Health Research

REFERENCES

[1] Hu JC, Yamakoshi Y, Yamakoshi F, *et al.* Proteomics and genetics of dental enamel. Cells Tissues Organs 2005;181(3-4):219-31.
[2] Nanci A. Enamel: Composition, formation, and structure. In: Nanci A, editor. Ten Cate's Oral Histology: Development, Structure, and Function. 7 ed. St-Louis: Mosby Elsevier; 2007. p. 141-90.
[3] Nanci A, Warshawsky H. Characterization of putative secretory sites on ameloblasts of the rat incisor. Am J Anat 1984;171:163-89.
[4] Leblond CP, Warshawsky H. Dynamics of enamel formation in the rat incisor tooth. J Dent Res 1979;58B:950-75.
[5] Smith CE. Ameloblasts: Secretory and resorptive functions. J Dent Res 1979;58(B):695-706.
[6] Sasaki T. Tracer, cytochemical, and freeze-fracture study on the mechanisms whereby secretory ameloblasts absorb exogeneous proteins. Acta Anat 1984;118:23-33.
[7] Sasaki T. Endocytotic pathways at the ruffled borders of rat maturation ameloblasts. Histochemistry 1984;80:263-8.
[8] Robinson C, Kirkham J. Dynamics of amelogenesis as revealed by protein compositional studies. In: Butler WT, editor. The chemistry and biology of mineralized tissues. 1 ed. Birmingham: EBSCO Media, Inc.; 1985. p. 248-63.
[9] Smith CE. Cellular and chemical events during enamel maturation. Crit Rev Oral Biol Med 1998;9(2):128-61.
[10] Lacruz RS, Nanci A, Kurtz I, *et al.* Regulation of pH during amelogenesis. Calcif Tissue Int 2009;DOI 10.1007/s00223-009-9326-7.
[11] Smith CE, Warshawsky H. Quantitative analysis of cell turnover in the enamel organ of the rat incisor. Evidence for ameloblast death immediately after enamel matrix secretion. Anat Rec 1977;187:63-98.
[12] Kaneko H, Ogiuchi H, Shimono M. Cell death during tooth eruption in the rat: surrounding tissues of the crown. Anat Embryol (Berl) 1997 May;195(5):427-34.
[13] Moe H. Physiological cell death of secretory ameloblasts in the rat incisor. Cell Tissue Res 1979 Apr 12;197(3):443-51.
[14] Nanci A, Zalzal S, Lavoie P, *et al.* Comparative immunochemical analyses of the developmental expression and distribution of ameloblastin and amelogenin in rat incisors. J Histochem Cytochem 1998;46(8):911-34.
[15] Oida S, Nagano T, Yamakoshi Y, *et al.* Amelogenin gene expression in porcine odontoblasts. J Dent Res 2002 Feb;81(2):103-8.

[16] Papagerakis P, MacDougall M, Hotton D, *et al.* Expression of amelogenin in odontoblasts. Bone 2003;32:228-40.
[17] Nagano T, Oida S, Ando H, *et al.* Relative levels of mRNA encoding enamel proteins in enamel organ epithelia and odontoblasts. J dent Res 2003 Dec;82(12):982-6.
[18] Meyer J-M, Lesot H, Staubli A, *et al.* Immunoperoxidase localizaton of fibronectin during odontoblast differentiation. An ultrastructural study. BSM 1989;2:19-24.
[19] Gibson CW, Yuan ZA, Hall B, *et al.* Amelogenin-deficient mice display an amelogenesis imperfecta phenotype. J Biol Chem 2001 Aug 24;276(34):31871-5.
[20] Hatakeyama J, Philp D, Hatakeyama Y, *et al.* Amelogenin-mediated regulation of osteoclastogenesis, and periodontal cell proliferation and migration. J Dent Res 2006 Feb;85(2):144-9.
[21] Zalzal SF, Smith CE, Nanci A. Ameloblastin and amelogenin share a common secretory pathway and are co-secreted during enamel formation. Matrix Biol 2008 May;27(4):352-9.
[22] Fukumoto S, Kiba T, Hall B, *et al.* Ameloblastin is a cell adhesion molecule required for maintaining the differentiation state of ameloblasts. J Cell Biol 2004 Dec 6;167(5):973-83.
[23] Smith CE, Nanci A. The protein dynamics of amelogenesis. Anat Rec 1996;245:186-207.
[24] Nanci A, Hashimoto J, Zalzal S, *et al.* Transient accumulation of proteins at interrod and rod enamel growth sites. Adv Dent Res 1996;10(2):135-49.
[25] Uchida T, Murakami C, Dohi N, *et al.* Synthesis, secretion, degradation and fate of ameloblastin during the matrix formation stage of the rat incisor as shown by immunocytochemistry and immunochemistry using region-specific antibodies. J Histochem Cytochem 1997;45(10):1329-40.
[26] Dohi N, Murakami C, Tanabe T, *et al.* Immunocytochemical and immunochemical study of enamelins, using antibodies against porcine 89-kDa enamelin and its N-terminal synthetic peptide, in porcine tooth germs. Cell Tissue Res 1998;293(2):313-25.
[27] Simmer JP, Fincham AG. Molecular mechanisms of dental enamel formation. Crit Rev Oral Biol Med 1995;6(2):84-108.
[28] Bartlett JD, Ganss B, Goldberg M, *et al.* 3. Protein-protein interactions of the developing enamel matrix. Curr Top Dev Biol 2006;74:57-115.
[29] Bartlett JD, Simmer JP. Proteinases in developing dental enamel. Crit Rev Oral Biol Med 1999;10(4):425-41.
[30] Fincham AG, Hu Y, Lau EC, *et al.* Amelogenin post-secretory processing during biomineralization in the postnatal mouse molar tooth. Arch Oral Biol 1991;36:305-17.
[31] Yamakoshi Y, Tanabe T, Oida S, *et al.* Calcium binding of enamel proteins and their derivatives with emphasis on the calcium-binding domain of porcine sheathlin. Arch Oral Biol 2001 Nov;46(11):1005-14.
[32] Nanci A. Bone. In: Nanci A, Ed. Ten Cate's Oral Histology: Development, Structure, and Function. 7 ed. St-Louis: Mosby Elsevier; 2007. p. 108-40.
[33] Simmer JP, Snead ML. Molecular biology of the amelogenin gene. In: Robinson C, Kirkham J, Shore R, editors. Dental enamel, formation to destruction.Boca Raton: CRC Press, Inc.; 1995. pp. 59-83.
[34] Nanci A, Slavkin HC, Smith CE. Application of high-resolution immunocytochemistry to the study of the secretory, resorptive, and degradative functions of ameloblasts. Adv Dent Res 1987;1:148-61.
[35] Smith CE, Nanci A. Secretory activity as a function of the development and maturation of ameloblasts. Connect Tissue Res 1989;22:147-56.
[36] Nanci A, Bitton GM, Ahluwalia JP, *et al.* Degradation of newly formed enamel proteins in relation to the secretory activity of ameloblasts. In: Fearnhead RW, editor. Tooth enamel V.Yokohama: Florence Publishers; 1989. p. 69-73.
[37] Nanci A, Smith CE. Development and calcification of enamel. In: Bonucci E, editor. Calcification in Biological Systems.Boca Raton: CRC Press, Inc.; 1992. p. 313-43.
[38] Nanci A, Fortin M, Ghitescu DL. Endocytotic functions of ameloblasts and odontoblasts: Immunocytochemical and tracer studies on the uptake of plasma proteins. Anat Rec 1996;245:219-34.
[39] Bienkowski RS. Intracellular degradation of newly synthesized secretory proteins. Biochem Pharmacol 1983;214:1-10.
[40] Smith CE, Borenstein S, Fazel A, *et al.* In vitro studies of the proteinases which degrade amelogenins in developing rat incisor enamel. In: Fearnhead RW, Ed. Tooth enamel V.Yokohama: Florence Publishers; 1989. p. 286-90.
[41] Smith CE, Pompura JR, Borenstein S, *et al.* Degradation and loss of matrix proteins from developing enamel. Anat Rec 1989;224:292-316.

[42] Nanci A, Smith CE. Matrix-mediated mineralization in enamel and the collagen-based hard tissues. In: Goldberg M, Boskey A, Robinson C, Eds. Chemistry and Biology of Mineralized Tissues.Rosemont: J.Am.Acad.Orthop.Surg.; 1999. p. 217-24.

[43] Bosshardt DD, Nanci A. Immunodetection of enamel- and cementum-related (bone) proteins at the enamel-free area and cervical portion of the tooth in rat molars. J Bone Miner Res 1997;12(3):367-79.

[44] Bosshardt DD, Nanci A. Immunolocalization of epithelial and mesenchymal matrix constituents in association with inner enamel epithelial cells. J Histochem Cytochem 1998;46(2):135-42.

[45] Delgado S, Casane D, Bonnaud L, *et al.* Molecular evidence for precambrian origin of amelogenin, the major protein of vertebrate enamel. Mol Biol Evol 2001 Dec;18(12):2146-53.

[46] Hammarstrom L. Enamel matrix, cementum development and regeneration. J Clin Periodontol 1997 Sep;24(9):658-68.

[47] Slavkin HC, Bessem C, Fincham AG, *et al.* Human and mouse cementum proteins immunologically related to enamel proteins. Biochim Biophys Acta 1989;991:12-8.

[48] Sonoyama W, Seo BM, Yamaza T, *et al.* Human Hertwig's epithelial root sheath cells play crucial roles in cementum formation. J Dent Res 2007 Jul;86(7):594-9.

[49] Bosshardt DD. Biological mediators and periodontal regeneration: a review of enamel matrix proteins at the cellular and molecular levels. J Clin Periodontol 2008 Sep;35(8 Suppl):87-105.

[50] Hammarstrom L, Heijl L, Gestrelius S. Periodontal regeneration in a buccal dehiscence model in monkeys after application of enamel matrix proteins. J Clin Periodontol 1997 Sep;24(9 Pt 2):669-77.

[51] Lyngstadaas SP, Wohlfahrt JC, Brookes SJ, *et al.* Enamel matrix proteins; old molecules for new applications. Orthod Craniofac Res 2009 Aug;12(3):243-53.

[52] Venezia E, Goldstein M, Boyan BD, *et al.* The use of enamel matrix derivative in the treatment of periodontal defects: a literature review and meta-analysis. Crit Rev Oral Biol Med 2004;15(6):382-402.

[53] Warotayanont R, Frenkel B, Snead ML, *et al.* Leucine-rich amelogenin peptide induces osteogenesis by activation of the Wnt pathway. Biochem Biophys Res Commun 2009 Sep 25;387(3):558-63.

[54] Warotayanont R, Zhu D, Snead ML, *et al.* Leucine-rich amelogenin peptide induces osteogenesis in mouse embryonic stem cells. Biochem Biophys Res Commun 2008 Feb 29;367(1):1-6.

[55] Jegat N, Septier D, Veis A, *et al.* Short-term effects of amelogenin gene splice products A+4 and A-4 implanted in the exposed rat molar pulp. Head Face Med 2007;3:40.

[56] Haze A, Taylor AL, Haegewald S, *et al.* Regeneration of bone and periodontal ligament induced by Recombinant amelogenin after periodontitis. J Cell Mol Med 2009 Feb 17.

[57] Shimizu E, Saito R, Nakayama Y, *et al.* Amelogenin Stimulates Bone Sialoprotein (BSP) Expression Through Fibroblast Growth Factor 2 Response Element and Transforming Growth Factor-beta1 Activation Element in the Promoter of the BSP Gene. J Periodontol 2005 Sep;76(9):1482-9.

[58] Nishiguchi M, Yuasa K, Saito K, *et al.* Amelogenin is a negative regulator of osteoclastogenesis via downregulation of RANKL, M-CSF and fibronectin expression in osteoblasts. Arch Oral Biol 2007 Mar;52(3):237-43.

[59] Nakamura Y, Hammarstrom L, Matsumoto K, *et al.* The induction of reparative dentine by enamel proteins. Int Endod J 2002 May;35(5):407-17.

[60] Lacerda-Pinheiro S, Marchadier A, Donas P, *et al.* An In vivo Model for Short-Term Evaluation of the Implantation Effects of Biomolecules or Stem Cells in the Dental Pulp. Open Dent J 2008;2:67-72.

[61] Lacerda-Pinheiro S, Jegat N, Septier D, *et al.* Early in vivo and in vitro effects of amelogenin gene splice products on pulp cells. Eur J Oral Sci 2006 May;114 Suppl 1:232-8.

[62] Goldberg M, Lacerda-Pinheiro S, Jegat N, *et al.* The impact of bioactive molecules to stimulate tooth repair and regeneration as part of restorative dentistry. Dent Clin North Am 2006 Apr;50(2):277-98, x.

[63] Nakamura Y, Gestrelius S, Hammarström L, *et al.* Enamel matrix derivative induces reparative dentine formation. J dent Res 2001;80:652.

[64] Nakamura Y, Hammarstrom L, Lundberg E, *et al.* Enamel matrix derivative promotes reparative processes in the dental pulp. Adv Dent Res 2001 Aug;15:105-7.

[65] Reseland JE, Reppe S, Larsen AM, *et al.* The effect of enamel matrix derivative on gene expression in osteoblasts. Eur J Oral Sci 2006 May;114 Suppl 1:205-11.

[66] Carinci F, Piattelli A, Guida L, *et al.* Effects of Emdogain on osteoblast gene expression. Oral Dis 2006 May;12(3):329-42.

[67] Spahr A, Lyngstadaas SP, Slaby I, *et al.* Ameloblastin expression during craniofacial bone formation in rats. Eur J Oral Sci 2006 Dec;114(6):504-11.
[68] Haze A, Taylor AL, Blumenfeld A, *et al.* Amelogenin expression in long bone and cartilage cells and in bone marrow progenitor cells. Anat Rec (Hoboken) 2007 May;290(5):455-60.
[69] Seyer JM, Glimcher MJ. Isolation, characterization and partial amino acid sequence of a phosphorylated polypeptide (E4) from bovine embryonic dental enamel. Biochim Biophys Acta 1977 Aug 23;493(2):441-51.
[70] Nanci A, Wazen R, Nishio C, *et al.* Immunocytochemistry of matrix proteins in calcified tissues: functional biochemistry on section. Eur J Histochem 2008 Oct;52(4):201-14.
[71] Veis A, Tompkins K, Alvares K, *et al.* Specific amelogenin gene splice products have signaling effects on cells in culture and implants *in vivo*. J Biol Chem 2000;275(52):41263-72.
[72] Kawana F, Sawae Y, Sahara S, *et al.* Porcine enamel matrix derivative enhances trabecular bone regeneration during wound healing of injured rat femur. Anat Rec 2001 Dec 1;264(4):438-46.
[73] Wazen RM, Moffatt P, Zalzal SF, *et al.* Local gene transfer to calcified tissue cells using prolonged infusion of a lentiviral vector. Gene Ther 2006 Nov;13(22):1595-602.

CHAPTER 5

The Non-Amelogenins: Ameloblastin and Enamelin

Yong-Hee P. Chun[1,2], Jan C-C Hu[2] and James P. Simmer[2]

[1]Department of Periodontics, University of Texas Health Science Center at San Antonio, 7703 Floyd Curl Drive San Antonio, Texas 78229, [2]Department of Biologic and Materials Science University of Michigan, School of Dentistry, 1011 North University, Ann Arbor, MI 48109-1078

Abstract Ameloblastin *(AMBN)* and enamelin (*ENAM)* are two of the 23 secretory calcium-binding phosphoprotein (SCPP) genes on human chromosome 4q. They are members of the proline and glutamine rich group. Both ameloblastin and enamelin function specifically during tooth formation, and probably both are only critical for dental enamel formation. Both genes have been shown to degenerate in mammals that have lost the ability to make dental enamel during evolution. In mice that cannot express functional ameloblastin or enamelin during tooth formation the mineralization front along the secretory portion of the ameloblast plasma membrane fails to generate enamel mineral ribbons. A non-functional mineral crust forms over dentin that readily abrades away when the teeth erupt into function. Ameloblasts undergo pathological changes, such as mineralization of the cell layer, disorganization, and apoptosis. In this chapter we review what is known about ameloblastin structure and function and conclude that enamelin and ameloblastin are both critical for the formation of enamel mineral ribbons during the secretory stage of amelogenesis and that their primary function is at the mineralization front.

Key Words: Enamel, Enamelin, Amelogenin, Ameloblastin, Amelogenesis Imperfecta, Biomineralization, Tooth Formation

INTRODUCTION

Dental enamel is the most highly mineralized tissue in the body. Mature enamel contains less than 1% organic material. It is acellular, contains no collagen, and has no biological means to repair itself. Enamel forms in an extracellular space lined by ameloblasts, tightly connected epithelial cells that control the ionic and the organic contents of the enamel extracellular space [1]. Dental enamel is the product of ameloblasts [2-5]. Enamel mineral is mainly calcium hydroxyapatite, but the dimensions and organization of its crystallites are unlike any observed outside of amelogenesis. The crystals grow in bundles called rods, with about 10,000 crystallites/rod [6]. Individual enamel crystals are ~25 nm thick and ~65 nm wide, and those in rods appear to extend from the dentino-enamel junction (DEJ) to the surface of the tooth, a distance of ~2 mm [7].

Dental enamel forms in two main stages: secretory and maturation. At the onset of the secretory stage, the basal lamina beneath the ameloblasts is degraded and replaced by a dynamic (rapidly turning over) layer of secreted enamel proteins that together function to initiate and lengthen thin enamel mineral "ribbons". An important component in the degrading basal lamina is laminin-5, which is comprised of three polypeptides: alpha-3 (*LAMA3*), beta-3 (*LAMB3*) and gamma-2 (*LAMC2*). *LAMB3* defects cause junctional epidermolysis bullosa, an inherited syndrome that includes enamel malformations as a feature [8]. The initiation of enamel protein secretion coincides with the degradation of laminin 5 [9]. Enamel crystals form at a mineralization front just outside of the ameloblast plasma membrane where the basal lamina used to be.

The genes encoding enamel proteins belong to the secretory calcium-binding phosphoprotein (SCPP) gene family, which arose from a single common ancestral gene (*SPARCL1*) by iterative gene duplications [10-12]. *SPARCL1* in turn arose from *SPARC* (secreted protein, acidic, cysteine-rich; osteonectin or BM-40), which encodes a basal lamina protein[13]. The defining features of SCPP genes are a conserved signal peptide, one or more serines phosphorylated by Golgi casein kinase, and type 0 splice junctions (where introns do not split codons). Golgi casein kinase phosphorylates serine residues in the context Ser-X-Glu/Ser(P) [14]. In humans there are 23 SCPP genes. All localize to chromosome 4q, except the two amelogenin genes (*AMELX* and *AMELY*) on the sex chromosomes. There are two SCPP subfamilies. The older is the "dentin/bone" or "acidic" gene cluster, which includes five genes: dentin sialophosphoprotein (*DSPP*), dentin matrix acidic phosphoprotein 1 (*DMP1*), integrin-binding sialoprotein (*IBSP*), matrix extracellular phosphoglycoprotein (*MEPE*), and secreted phosphoprotein 1 (*SPP1*). This group is also known

Michel Goldberg (ED)

as the SIBLINGs (Small Integrin-Binding LIgand, N-linked Glycoprotein) [15]. The second is the "enamel/milk/saliva" or "proline-glutamine-rich" subfamily, which contains the enamel group, including amelogenin (*AMELX/AMELY*), ameloblastin (*AMBN*), enamelin (*ENAM*), amelotin (*AMTN*), and odontogenic, ameloblast associated (*ODAM*). The amino acid compositions of human enamelin, ameloblastin, and amelogenin are shown in Table 1.

Table 1: Amino acid compositions, calculated isoelectric points (pI), and calculated molecular weights (MW) of human enamelin, ameloblastin, and amelogenin. Note that enamelin alone has cysteine (Cys), and that all three proteins are proline (Pro) and glutamine (Gln) rich.

Human	Enamelin		Ameloblastin		Amelogenin	
AA	Res./ 1103	Res./ 1000	Res./ 396	Res./ 1000	Res./ 175	Res./ 1000
Ala	35	32	34	86	3	17
Cys	6	5	0	0	0	0
Asp	42	38	11	28	3	17
Glu	80	73	23	58	5	29
Phe	41	37	16	40	2	11
Gly	86	78	39	99	6	34
His	31	28	11	28	14	80
Ile	31	28	9	23	7	40
Lys	49	44	9	23	3	17
Leu	50	45	36	91	13	74
Met	19	17	15	38	10	57
Asn	89	81	14	35	2	11
Pro	154	140	61	154	49	280
Gln	86	78	31	78	24	137
Arg	60	54	15	38	2	11
Ser	91	83	25	63	6	34
Thr	58	53	19	48	7	40
Val	32	29	16	40	9	51
Trp	15	14	3	8	3	17
Tyr	48	44	9	23	7	40
MW	124.5 kDa		42.5 kDa		19.9 kDa	
pI	6.8		5.4		6.5	

Amelotin and odam are components of the basal lamina beneath maturation stage ameloblasts [16,17]. Amelogenin, ameloblastin, and enamelin are not considered to be components of a basal lamina, for it is generally held that there is no basal lamina along the distal membrane of secretory stage ameloblasts. Secretory stage enamel proteins, however, may associate following their secretion with the ameloblast membrane where they form a mineralization front. The mineralization front is a place of continual protein turnover where the enamel ribbons, comprised initially of amorphous calcium phosphate [18], grow in length. Given the association between the mineralization front and the secretory surface of the ameloblast cell membrane, secretory stage enamel proteins may be thought of as having some features of a basal lamina. While the mechanism of dental enamel formation and the functions of amelogenin, ameloblastin, and enamelin are at present, unknown, it seems likely that their central role is to generate and elongate an array of parallel mineral ribbons at the mineralization front, along the secretory surface of the ameloblast plasma membrane.

In this chapter we review the "non-amelogenin" proteins: ameloblastin and enamelin. When either of these two sister proteins are absent, there is a failure of the mineralization front and a progressive deterioration of ameloblasts [19-21].

AMELOBLASTIN

Ameloblastin was discovered by scientists in Japan as they isolated proteins from the immature enamel of porcine developing teeth and determined their amino acid compositions [22-25]. Polyclonal antibodies raised against a group 13 to 17 kDa proteins specifically immunostained the sheath space at the perimeter of enamel rods [26]. A partial protein sequence of the 15 kDa peptide was determined [27], which proved that this protein was not amelogenin and therefore was a novel enamel protein. The cDNAs of rat, pig, mouse and human ameloblastin were characterized [28-31] , and revealed that two Ambn isoforms are expressed from alternatively spliced mRNA transcripts [30]. The cDNA variants differ by the deletion or inclusion of 45 nucleotides from the 5' end of exon 6, so one isoform is 15 amino acids larger than the other. Numerous amelogenin isoforms are generated by alternative splicing, while enamel transcripts are not alternatively spliced [32].

Enamel proteins can accept relatively large insertions with no apparent loss of function. The insertions typically take the form of tandem repeats. Human ameloblastin has an insertion of 26 amino acids relative to mammalian homogues due to the tandem duplication of an exon (exons 7, 8, 9) (Figure. 1) [33,34]. The ameloblastin gene is also expressed in reptiles and amphibians [35-37].

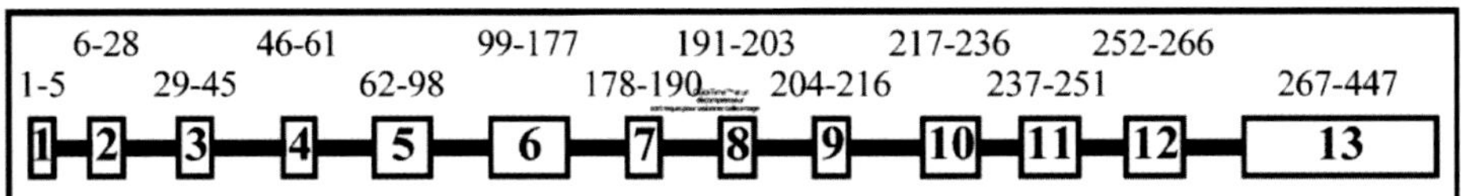

Ex/Int	Nucleotides	Amino Acids	Ex/Int	Nucleotides	Amino Acids
Exon 1	**90: 2-91**	**5: Met^{1}-Lys^{5}**	**Exon 7**	**39: 10342-10380**	**13: Leu^{178}-Ser^{190}**
Intron 1	953: 92-1044		Intron 7	135: 10381-10515	
Exon 2	**69: 1045-1113**	**23: Ile^{6}-Pro^{28}**	**Exon 8**	**39: 10516-10554**	**13: Leu^{191}-Ser^{203}**
Intron 2	3603: 1114-4716		Intron 8	135: 10555-10689	
Exon 3	**51: 4717-4767**	**17: Phe^{29}-Glu^{45}**	**Exon 9**	**39: 10690-10728**	**13: Leu^{204}-Thr^{216}**
Intron 3	3603: 1114-4716		Intron 9	249: 10729-10977	
Exon 4	**48: 6074-6121**	**16: Thr^{46}-Gln^{61}**	**Exon 10**	**60: 10978-11037**	**20: Ile^{217}-Pro^{236}**
Intron 4	3014: 6122-9135		Intron 10	96: 11038-11133	
Exon 5	**111: 7254-7364**	**37: Tyr^{62}-Gln^{98}**	**Exon 11**	**45: 11134-11178**	**15: Leu^{237}-Leu^{251}**
Intron 5S	1771: 7365-9135		Intron 11	416: 11179-11594	
Intron 5L	1816: 7365-9180		**Exon 12**	**45: 11595-11639**	**15: Asn^{252}-Ala^{266}**
Exon 6L	**237: 9136-9372**	**79: Phe^{99}-Glu^{177}**	Intron 12	2263: 11640-13902	
Exon 6S	**192: 9181-9372**	**64: Pro^{114}-Glu^{177}**	**Exon 13**	**1103: 13903-15005**	**182: Gly^{267}-Pro^{447}**
Intron 6	1169: 9173-10341				

Figure 1: *AMBN* Gene Structure (ref seqs: cDNA, NM_016519.4; and gene, NC_000004.11). The human ameloblastin gene on chromosome 4q21 is 15,005 bp in length. Exons are indicated by numbered boxes. The number of amino acids encoded by each exon is shown below the box. The range of amino acids is shown above. The *AMBN* gene is divided into 13 exons, and according to the official assignment of the translation initation codon, all are coding. For referencing polymorphisms and disease associated mutations, amino acids are numbered starting with the translation initation site. For Ambn, the signal peptide is cleaved after Ala^{26}, so the secreted protein is 26 amino acids shorter than the amino acid sequence deduced from the reference sequence. Alternative splicing can delete a shorter (intron 5S) or longer (intron 5L) segment for intron 5 resulting longer (exon 6L) or shorter (exon 6S) segments for exon 6, respectively. The numbers to the left of colons are the total numbers of nucleotides or amino acids in an exon or intron, the ranges of numbers to the right of the colons correspond to the numbers of the nucleotides or amino acids in the AMBN genomic reference sequence.

Ameloblastin Post-Translational Modifications

The deduced amino acid sequences show that ameloblastin does not have any N-linked glycosylations; however, Ambn is O-glycosylated. Virtually all of what we know about the ameloblastin protein and its post-translational modifications has been learned from investigations on pig enamel. The two porcine ameloblastin isoforms are secreted as 395 and 380 amino acid proteins. The amino acid numbers used through the text correspond to those of the secreted proteins and do not include the signal peptide sequences. The extra 15 amino acids in the Ambn^{395} isoform extend from Tyr^{73} to Gln^{87} (YEYSLPVHPPPLPSQ). Ser^{86} in this segment is glycosylated so, in a sense, alternative splicing determines the glycosylation state of ameloblastin [38]. This Ambn segment is highly conserved throughout phylogeny (Figure 2). Porcine ameloblastin is also O-glycosylated in its C-terminal domain, which is cleaved into products having apparent molecular weights of 13, 15, 27 and 29 kDa [39]. Thr^{348} has a sulphated O-linked glycosylation containing galactose and N-acetylgalactosamine. Other post-translational modifications found in porcine ameloblastin are the hydroxylations of Pro^{11} [30] and Pro^{324} [39] and the phosphorylation of Ser^{17} [38].

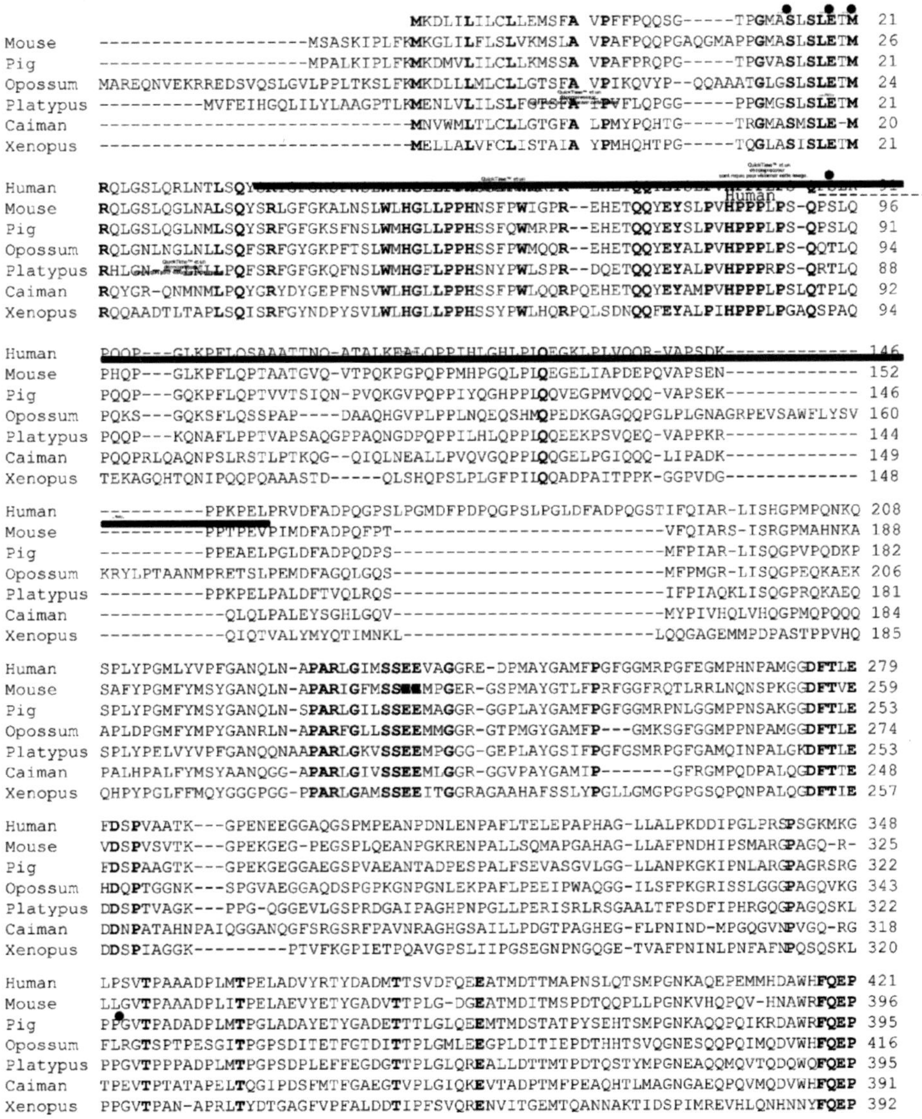

Figure 2: Alignment of ameloblastin protein sequences from Human (*Homo sapiens*; NM_016519.4), Mouse (*Mus musculus*; BC087927.1), Pig (*Sus scrofa*; NM_214037.1), Opossum (*Monodelphis domestica*; XM_001368805.1), Platypus (*Ornithorhynchus anatinus*; XM_001512271.1), Caiman (*Caiman crocodilus*; AY043290.1), and Frog (*Xenopus laevis*; NM_001090021.1). Amino acids conserved in all seven sequences are in bold. Dots mark putative hydroxyprolines and Golgi casein kinase phosphorylation sites. A dark line marks the sequence deleted in the Ambn knock-out. Gray shaded area marks the 15 amino acid segment that is deleted by alternative mRNA splicing to make the shorter Ambn isoform.

Ameloblastin (~62 kDa) is hydrolyzed by Mmp-20 into smaller products that accumulate in the secretory stage enamel matrix [40]. It is not known if ameloblastin cleavage products perform a necessary function, but Mmp-20 [41] , which catalyzes the processing of enamel proteins during the secretory stage [42], is critical for proper dental enamel formation [43,44].

Ameloblastin Cleavage Products.

The N-terminal Ambn cleavage products (13, 15, 17 kDa) are relatively resistant to further degradation [45]. These products concentrate in the sheath space [27, 30, 46]. N-terminal cleavage products from the larger, glycosylated isoform ($Ambn^{395}$) are likely responsible for the observed lectin-staining properties of the porcine sheath space [47]. The 27 kDa and 29 kDa porcine Ambn C-terminal cleavage products bind calcium [25, 46] and are degraded into smaller O-glycosylated, sulfated peptides having apparent molecular weights of 13 kDa and 15 kDa [39, 48] . These O-glycosylated C-terminal fragments of ameloblastin have a higher calcium binding affinity than amelogenin and the 32 kDa enamelin [39]. The N-terminal 129 amino acids of porcine Ambn have a calculated pI of 10.6, while the C-terminal 66 amino acids have a calculated pI of 4.5, suggesting the protein is "bipolar" [30]. Immunohistochemistry of the Ambn N-terminal cleavage products in developing pig enamel shows a honeycomb pattern (highlighting the sheath space) all the way down to the dentino-enamel junction, while the Ambn C-terminal fragments show a reverse honeycomb immunolocalization pattern (highlighting the rods) and are only present at the enamel surface [46]. An *ab initio* 3D model of the human ameloblastin is consistent with ameloblastin being a bipolar protein, with the N- and C-terminal domains being connected by an unstructured interfacing link that is susceptible to proteolytic cleavage [49].

Conservation of Ameloblastin Sequences

An alignment of Ambn deduced amino acid sequences from diverse species is shown in Figure 2. For discussion, we will break the Ambn sequence into four regions. The first region is the signal peptide. There is some disagreement as to proper assignment of the Ambn translation initiation site, so the actual length of the signal peptide is ambiguous. A proper Kozak consensus sequence requires a purine in the -3 position before the ATG [50]. This condition is not met by start codon used in the *AMBN* reference sequence (NM_016519.4). We suspect that the proper translation initation site for Ambn is the fixed (conserved in all species) Methionine that is sixteen amino acids upstream of the signal peptide cleavage site. The sixteen amino acid signal peptide is well conserved, both in length and sequence homology. A quarter of the amino acids in the signal peptide (4/16) are fixed. Region 2 is the Ambn N-terminal domain (human Val^1 to Gln^{86}), which is the most conserved part of ameloblastin. More than a third of its amino acids (31/86) are identical in the alignment going back to amphibians. Two of the fixed residues are in the appropriate context for phosphorylation by Golgi casein kinase (human Ser^{15} and Ser^{17}). Region 3 of Ambn (from human Pro^{87} to Leu^{226}) is encoded by human exon 6S (6 short) through exon 11. This poorly conserved segment has only a single fixed amino acid (human Gln^{130}) and appears to be susceptible to proteolytic processing. This segment contains obvious insertions in the human and opossum Ambn sequences, suggesting that this part of the protein can vary significantly without affecting Ambn function. The final segment (human Asn^{227}-Pro^{421}) is encoded by exons 12 and 13. It contains two fixed potential Golgi casein kinase phosphorylation sites (human Ser^{236} and Ser^{237}) in a highly conserved amino acid context. The last four amino acids (Phe-Gln-Glu-Pro) at the Ambn C-terminus are fixed.

Ameloblastin is expressed predominantly or exclusively in developing teeth [28, 29, 48, 51-57]. Not only is Ambn expression closely associated with tooth formation, but in baleen whales, mammals that have lost the ability to make dental enamel during evolution, the *Ambn* gene has degenerated into a nonfunctional pseudogene [58]. The restriction of Ambn expression in developing teeth, the lack of selection for maintenance of the *Ambn* gene in mammals that no longer make enamel, and localization of the *AMBN* gene in the critical region for *amelogenesis imperfecta* (AI) [59] all make *AMBN* a strong candidate gene for AI (which by the strict definition only affects teeth). However, extensive characterization of dozens of families with AI has failed to identify a single *AMBN* disease-associated mutation [60].

Ambn null mice make no true enamel, while *Ambn* heterozygous mice have a nearly normal enamel layer [19]. No defects outside of the enamel layer were observed. A surprising feature of the *Ambn* null mice was obvious pathology in the ameloblast layer, which is also seen in the *Enam* null mouse [20]. It has recently been demonstrated that the *Ambn* knock-out mouse only deletes exons 5 and 6 of the *Ambn* gene [19] and secretes a shortened *Ambn* protein lacking this region [21, 61]. The deleted region extends from mouse Tyr^{41} through Glu^{157}, which is a highly conserved part of the protein. The truncated *Ambn* protein secreted by the *Ambn* null mouse is 279 amino acids in length and has clearly lost function, but it is not known if expression of the nonfunctional protein affects the null phenotype in these mice.

Ameloblastin Function

It is apparent from the lack of true enamel in mice lacking a functional *Ambn* gene that ameloblastin is critical for proper formation of the mineralization front and that an understanding of Abmn function will require investigating events at the mineralization front. Ameloblastin has been proposed to function in the maintenance of rod integrity [30], but the specific localization of Ambn cleavage products to the sheath space in pig and cattle has was not observed in rat [54]. Ameloblastin is thought to function as a cell attachment protein [19, 29], but the cell attachment motifs are not well conserved in the growing number of Ambn sequences available. Recently the cell attachment property of recombinant Ambn was reported to relate to heparin binding possibly involving a Val-Thr-Ly-sGly heparin binding motif [62], but such a motif is not conserved in other Ambn sequences. The observation that ameloblasts seem to detach in the Ambn defective mice does not implicate ameloblastin directly in cell attachment because the enamel layer, which the cells attach to, is absent. The same thing seems to happen in *Enam* null mice which do not make an enamel layer. At present, the specific function of ameloblastin is unclear, but it seems certain to be a critical component of the mineralization front.

ENAMELIN

Like ameloblastin, enamelin was initially discovered by scientists in Japan during analyses of porcine enamel extracts. The first published protein sequences were from the N-termini of the 89 kDa (MPMNMPRMPGFSPKREPM) [63] and 32 kDa (LXHVPGRIPPGYGRPPTP) enamelin cleavage products [64]. Affinity purified anti-peptide antibodies were raised against the 32 kDa enamelin were highly specific for developing enamel [65]. Western blots revealed that the 32 kDa enamelin must be the cleavage product of a larger protein as slower-migrating protein bands on SDS-PAGE from porcine enamel extracts reacted against the 32 kDa antibody [66]. Knowledge of porcine enamelin protein sequences led directly to the cloning and characterization of the first full-length enamelin cDNAs from pig [66,67] mouse [68], and human [69]. Enamelin deduced amino acid sequences are now available from 36 mammalian species [70] and include representatives from placental mammals, marsupials, and monotremes and frog [71].

Enamelin Post-Translational Modifications

The C-terminal region of enamelin is notable because it is only observed at the mineralization front and contains six highly conserved cysteines (human: Cys^{835}, Cys^{836}, Cys^{919}, Cys^{946}, Cys^{1018}, and Cys^{1098}). In contrast, amelogenin and ameloblastin have no cysteines at all. It seems likely that the cysteines in enamelin participate in disufide bridges. These bridges could be intramolecular (within a single enamelin protein) or intermolecular (binding two or more enamelin proteins together, or binding enamelin to an unknown protein, perhaps associated with the ameloblast cell membrane). Asparagine (Asn, N) residues in the context Asn-X-Ser/Thr (where X is any amino acid but Pro) are often glycosylated in the endoplasmic reticulum. Human enamelin has eleven Asn residues in this context: N^{75}KT, N^{87}QT, N^{206}ST, N^{213}ST, N^{226}DT, N^{233}ST, N^{257}AS, N^{428}KS, N^{495}QS, N^{895}SS, and N^{1001}ES. Six of the asparagines are strongly conserved among mammals. The three conserved Asn residues in the 32 kDa enamelin cleavage product are known to be glycosylated in pig (Asn^{207}, Asn^{214}, Asn^{227}) [66] A defining feature of SCPP proteins is phosphorylation by Golgi casein kinase, which phosphorylates serine residues in the context Ser-X-Glu/Ser(P) [14]. Four serines in human enamelin (Ser^{13}, Ser^{15}, Ser^{152}, Ser^{177}) are in the appropriate context for phosphorylation by Golgi casein kinase. The two serines in the porcine 32 kDa enamelin cleavage product are phosphorylated (Ser^{153}, Ser^{178}) [66] The last known post-translational modification is the hydroxylation of porcine Pro^{509} (human Pro^{514}), which was identified while sequencing the 25 kDa enamelin cleavage product [66] Although the enamelin sequence is not highly conserved among tetrapods, sites of putative post-translational modifications are often well conserved (Figure 3). As expected, both enamelin and ameloblastin share greater sequence similarity with organisms that are more closely related evolutionarily, but time might not be the only factor influencing the sequence conservation. There are regions of these proteins that might have gained or changed functions during evolution, with conservation of the altered sequences only being observed in their decendents. Thus, even though *Ambn* and *Enam* genes are expressed in species that make enameloid, this finding does not exclude key roles for these proteins in the production of true enamel. Tandem duplications at the gene level have lengthened the enamelin protein in some species, such as mouse [68].

```
Human MLVLRCRLGTSFPKLDNLVPKGK MKILLVF LGLLGN SVA M P--MHMPRMPGFSSKSEEMMRYNQFNFM NGPHMAHLGPFFGNG--------LPQQFPQY QMPM  54
Pig   -MLLSCRHGASSPKLDNLVPSGK MKILLVF LGLLCY SAA M P--MQMPRMPGFSSKSEEMMRYGHFNFM NAPHMAHLGTLYGNGM------QLPQFFPQY QMPM  56
Mouse MLLLQCRNPTSPPKPCGLVPNVK MS-LLVF LGLLGV SAA M PFQMPMPRMPGFSSKSEEMMRYNQFNFM NAPPMMPMGP-YGNGMPMP--PHMPPQYPPY QMPM  61
Platy                 (115) MKSFLLF LGLFGA STA M P--MHMPRMPGFGSKSEEMMPYGQYNFM NSPHMAQLGPLYGYG------LQLPQFFQPP QMPP  56
Frog                      M MVPIILL LCFLIS SNS V P--MHFSHM---SSNSEEGMPYGPYGYQ N-PQMPGIGSMYGLGFPHYSQMIQLQQAFGR QPSS  58

Human WPQPPPNTWHPRKSSAP----KRHNKTDQTQETQKPNQTQSKKP----PQKRP------LKQ PSHNQPQPEEEAQP PQAFPPFGNGLFPYQQPPWQIPQRLPPP 144
Pig   WPQPPPNKKHPQKPSAS----KQQSKTDPAPESQKPNQPQPKTP----TPKQP------LNE PSPTPTQPEEETQT PQAFPPFGNGLFPYQQPLWHVPHRIPP- 145
Mouse WPPPVPNGWQQPPMP------NFPSKTDQTQETAKPNQTNPQEPQ---PQKQP------LKE PPNEAARAKDDAQP PQPFPPFGNGLYPYPQPPWPIPQRGPPT 150
Platy WPQPPPNGWPAQNPGPPQGG-KPQAKPGQSQNTKQPNPSQPKKPPQQQPPKQA------AKQ PAPGPSKPTEETRQ PQMYPPFGNGFFPFQLQPWQIPPQMPP- 152
Frog  WLPQNIARTQQIHKETIPLNLPRFHLQPVQSQLSQLPAPPVQQPQLNPPQSKSNYVTKQPHQ PLQLPPAPDQQAQA PMMFPPFSNIMNPYQ-PYWQQPFMH--- 158

Human GY GRPPTSNEEGGNPYFGYFGYHGFGGRPPYYSEEMFEQDFEKPKEEDPPKAESPG-----TEPTA NSTVTETNSTQ---PNPKGSQ GGNDTSP---TGNSTPG 237
Pig   GY GRPPTSNEEGGNPYFGFFGYHGFGGRPPYYSEEMFEQDFEKPKEKDPPKTETPA-----TEPSV NTTVPETNSTQ---PNAPNPR G-NDTSP---TGTSGQG 237
Mouse AF GRPKFSNEEG-NPYYAFFGYHGFGGRP-YYSEEMFE-DYEKPKEKDPPKPEDPPPDDPPPEAST NSTVPDANATQ------SIPE GGNDTSP---IGNTGPG 242
Platy GY GRPPGSNEEGGNPYFGYFGHQGFGGRPPYYSEEMKEE------EKESPKEDSPS-----PEPTA NSTVAETNSTQPSGPSQAGSQ GGNATDPGQSAGNGSPA 245
Frog  GF GRPPNSNE-GNGNYFGFFG---MGGRAPYNSEEINEDEEPAKAEKESPKTESP------VAETS NTTIADNNSTT-----ISQSQ G-NATTNNESMAGDITQ 246

Human LNTGNNPPAQ NGIGPL PAVNASGQGGPGSQIPWRPS--QPNIRENHPYPNIR-NF PSGRQWY------------FTGTVM GHRQNRPFYRNQQVQRGPR-W NFF 325
Pig   PNPRSNPTGQ NG---- PAVNVSGQGVPRSQSPWGPR--QTIIHENYPNPNIR-GF PARRQWR------------PPGPAM GHRRNGPFYRNQQIQRGPR-W NSF 321
Mouse PNAGNNPTVQ NGVFPP PKVNVSGQGVPKSQIPWRPS--QPNIYENYPYPN----Y PSERQWQ------------TTGT-Q GPRQNGPGYRNPQVERGPQ-W NSF 326
Platy QTPGHGTVPD NGEPPG PLLNASDHGGARGPKPTGPGPGQPPFRGRPANPNAAPGF PAGRQRRPFVHPFGRPFDRPVGRPV GRRDHGPTYGNTPKARGPLRW NAV 349
Frog  SSTIALN-AQ NGHIEG PPVIAVVHNKHKNTLHGASRQAHYVVRAPNPDTILSNHQ PHQKYHIVD---------KILVGRG GFPSQNTIYHQEQITGKVPLT NIH 340

Human AWERKQVARPGNPVYHKAY-PPTSRGNYPNYAGNPANLRRKPQGPNK---------------------------------------------------------  371
Pig   TLEGKQAVRPGYPTYRRVY-GSTARSNPPNYAGNSANLRRKPEGPNK---------------------------------------------------------  367
Mouse AWEGKQATRPGNPTYGKPP-SPTSG---VNYAGNPVHFGRNLPGPNKPFVGANPASNKPFVGANPASNKPFVGANPASNKPFVGANPASNKPFVGANPASNKPY  426
Platy TSEGKRVARPGYPMYRRPFPVAAPGRGFPNRAGNPLNLRKNPQAPAK---------------------------------------------------------  396
Frog  TEKSSYIRHVPQTNSDKIPLRTVATKDGDSFVREARGMHFDPTMNNTIG--------------------------------------------------------  388

Human --------------------------------------------------------------------------------------HPVGTTVAPLGPKPGPVV  389
Pig   --------------------------------------------------------------------------------------NPMVTNVAPPGPKHGTVD  385
Mouse VGANPASNKPFIGANPAANKPSIGTNPAANKPSIGTNPAANKPFVRNNVGANKPFVGTNPSSNQPFLRSNQASNKPFMRSNQASNKPFVGTNVASVGPKQVTVS  530
Platy -------------------------------------------------------------------------------------HPGEANSGPVYSQRGGLMA  414
Frog  -------------------------------------------------------------------------------------------NDAIQQIYRNNVP  401

Human RNEKIQNPK EKPLGPKEQIIV PTKNPTSPWRNSQQYEVNKSNYKLPHS EGYMPVPNFNSVDQHENS YYPRGDS--RKVPNSDGQTQSQNLPKGIVLGSRRMPYE  491
Pig   QNENIQNPR EKQVSQKERTVV PTRDPSGPWRNSQDYGINKSNYKLPQP EDNMLVPNFNSIDQRENS YYPRGES--KRAPNSDGQTQTQIIPKGIVLEPRRIPYE  487
Mouse HNMKTQNPK EKSLGQKERTVT PTKDASNPWRSAKQYGINNPNYNLPRS EGSMVGPNFNSFDQQENS YFSKGAS--KRVPSPNIQIQSQNLPKGIALEPRRTPFQ  632
Platy PREPVASPQ ENPPSPREKPSF PTRGPAVPWRKPQNYGPGKPVYRPPLS EGRPADPGPSPFDPRENP YYPRGDATDRRFLSSGGSAPGRHFPEGIVLKP------  513
Frog  DNASPKVDN EHLSFLVNKNKT PNRKIILVQHQGREHFPGHIMESVIES EYAPRGIFSS--HRNTPS YTQINKEDQKLSVPNNGDNSGNINTAHIKSEDLFRGGE  503

Human SETNQSELKHSSYQPAVYPEEIPSPAKEHFPAGRNTWDHQEISPPFKEDPGRQEEH LPHPSHGSRGSVFYPEYNPYDPRENSPYLRG NTWDERDDSPNTMGQKE  595
Pig   SETNQPELKHSAYQP-VYTEGIPSPAKEHFPAGRNTWNQQEISPPFKEDPGRQEEH LPHLSHGSRVHVYYPDYNPYDPRENSPYLRS NTWYERDDSPNTMGQPE  590
Mouse SETKKPELKHGTHQP-AYPKKIPSPTRKHFPAERNTWNRQKILPPLKEDYGRQDEN LRHPSYGSRGNIFYHEYTNPYHNEKSQYIKS NPWDK--SSPSTMMRPE  733
Platy -EDDQPPSKQKPFHP-VTSERTPREPSPTKP-QR---TSPEPPPPLEEGPGRQDKS LTYPPISPRSGIPYPDHHPYDP--KGTWDEG NEPTP--SSGPAEQPGR  607
Frog  FFQHNGENAALYQKE-GTASDIGTASDIG--------TAYDIGTAYDIGTATTGQQ LESIYLVKHFPTNHFQVYGDNNPKNPSHLLS NTWQKKPDQLESPRNN-  597

Human SPLYPINTPDQKEIVP YNEEDPVDPTGD EVFPGQNRWG-EELSFKGGPTVRHYEGEQYTSNQPKEYLPYSLDN--PSKPREDFYYSEFYPWSPDENFPSYNTAS  696
Pig   NPHYPMNTPDPKETIP YNEEDPIDPTGD EHFPGQSRWDMEELSFKEDPTVRHYEGEQYTSNQPKEYLPYSLDN--PSKPREDFLYGEFYPWNPEENFPSYNTAP  692
Mouse NPQYTMTSLDQKETEQ YNEEDPIDPNED ESFPGQSRWGDEEMNFKGNPTVRQYEGEHYASTLAKEYLPYSLSN--PPKPSEDFPYSEFYPWNPQETFPIYNPGP  835
Platy QPSPCSPRMGQRGEVP YNEEDPVDPTGD EPNLGPGPWEETANG-KEDPSRYHKSP-QYPQSRATEPQDYPPYPEGGLEKHRDFPYGDFYPRGPEDNLQPYNGAD  709
Frog  -------LLGQKEIYL YPDTELYHQTNN ELPLGKQHWDNEIDFSAVQFENPGSSTYYMKDSQRQKQWPTASNNRVELDRQPTDQPKYLLISKLDPAKNTDVSTF  694

Human TMPP PIESRG YYVNNAAGPEESTLFP SRNSWDHRIQAQGQRERR PYFNRNIWDQATHLQ KAPARPPDQKGNQPYYSNTPAGLQKNPIWHEGENLNYGMQITRMN  800
Pig   TVSS PVESRG YYANNAVGQEESTMFP SWSSWDPRIQAQGQKEGR PYLNRNFWDQSTNLY KTPTSSPHQKENQPYSNNSPAGLQKNPTWHEGENLNYGMQITRLN  796
Mouse TIAP PVDPRS YYVNNAIGQEESTLFP SWTSWDHRNQAERQKESE PYFNRNVWDQSINLH KSNIP------NHPYSTTSPARFPKDPTWFEGENLNYDLQITSLS  933
Platy QL-- PVEGRG YYTHDAVGQGGPLQFP SRDSWDWGLRSAAQERRA PYDERDSWDHAINSP KSTAG---ATETLSPSHSVPAGIRGKPHEESVDWSYRGGQVSDLG  808
Frog  TTNE PMAQNG YITNQEA-YLQSPNNK SPFIFNK--PSTDGILYI PIDELHDSQNNPVHL KLTPY------SKAHSENHSPGVFRSLQEVNPNIYPSSLRRQSLN  789

Human SPEREHSSFPNFIPPSY PSGQKEAHLFHLSQR-GS CCAGSSTGPKDNPL ALQDYTPSYGLAPGENQDTSPLYTDGSHTKQTRDII SPTSILPGQR NSSEK---R  900
Pig   SPERDHLAFPDLIPPDY PGGQKESHVFHLSQR-GP CCAGGSMWPKNNPL ALQDYTQSFGLAPGENPDTSIGYAEDSHIKYARQTV SPTSIVPGQR NSSEKILPG  899
Mouse PPEREQLAFPDFLPQSY PTGQNEAHLFHQSQR-GS CCIGGSTGHKDNVL ALQDYTSSYGLPPRKNQETSPVHTESSYIKYARPNV SPASILPSQR NISENKLTA 1036
Platy VPEAEGPALMEPVARSD PADPREASSYPVAVARSS CCAGGSPGPRDPPL APQDYSSPLGLSLWELQVGGPRSPGGSRSRHVQQAA SPVGYPAIRR NGTEEAPPT  912
Frog  PRKTGHYSCTIPLTGVD PTLEHSNALIL------V CCKLNDMG-QSHPS ANEDNVHHLKVVLNEYKESVPHQDQTHRQHTRDVIE SP---KFSIQ NNVMTVRPN  883

Human ESQNP--FRDDVSTLRRNT PCSIKNQLGQKEIMPFP EASSLQS KNTP CLKNDLG GDGNNILEQVFEDNQLNERTVDLTPEQLVIGT PDEGSNPEGIQSQVQENE 1002
Pig   ESQNPSPFKDDVSTLRRST PCSVKSQLSQRGIMPLP EANSLQS KNTP CLTSDLG GDGNNVLEQIFEGNQLNERTVDLTPEQLVFGT PDKEPRPEGIPNEMQGNE 1003
Mouse ESPNPSPFGDGVPTVRKNT PYSGKNQLET-GIVAFS EASSSQP KNTP CLKSDLG GDRRDVLKQFFEGSQLSERTAGLTPEQLVIGI PDKGSGPDSIQSEVQGKE 1139
Platy RREEPAPSRDGLAPGR-SP PCSLRPRASPRAGLAFP EAGLPPA KPAP CFKSRLR GDVDSVPEQILDPDPPVAGNDGPAPGDLAVVV PERDPGPVGIR----GDP 1011
Frog  SSNNHDNIQSSRGKSSDSV PCT-----SKPSYEQNS EYPYAFP KKQ- CSY---R GDADSYLPPSQD-ESISLKKRFLASEN--VYM PLANTPEPDLPDRRIKDD  975

Human SERQQQRPSNILHLP CFGSKLAKHHSSTTGTPSSDGRQSPFDGDSITPTENPNTLVE LATEEQFKSINVDPLD-ADEHSPFEFLQRGTNVQDQVQD CLLLQA 1103
Pig   SERQQQRQSSILQLP CFGSKLANYHTSSIGTPSSLGRQDSFDGDPIMPTETPNSLAG LATGAQFQNINVDPLN-EDEHTPFDSLQIGTNPQDQVQD CLLLQA 1104
Mouse GEMQQQRPPTIMKLP CFGSN-SKFHSSTTGPPINNRRPTLLNGALSTPTESPNTLVG LATREQLKSINVDKLN-ADEHTTLESFQ-GTSPQDQG-- CLLLQA 1236
Platy EPGPEAGAPGFQWVP CFGSETQNHYLAWTGAPPGNEKPDPSEPVSTAPAETLDAVSG LPTGVPSEGPSLPRSSELSPPFKTLQWEVADGPEQQGAD CSLLQN 1113
Frog  GKVKKGIGKLLEILT CPQDQEIHTNKKAINIAKTRPTASLLNHDKLS----ADAIPV LNTE---QSDAEKPIN-----------AIGNLP-----D CLILKK 1054
```

Figure 3: Alignment of enamelin protein sequences from Human (*Homo sapiens*; NM_031889.2), Pig (*Sus scrofa*; NM_214241.1), Mouse (*Mus musculus*; U82698.1), Platypus (*Ornithorhynchus anatinus*; XM_001512246.1), and Frog (*Xenopus laevis*; NM_001145743.1). Amino acids conserved in all five sequences are in bold. Dots mark post-translational modification sites that have been characterized in pig, including serines phosphorylated by Golgi casein kinase phosphorylation at (human) Ser^{15}, Ser^{152}, and Ser^{177}, N-glycosylations and Asn^{206}, Asn^{213}, and Asn^{226}, and a hydroxyproline at Pro^{514}

Enamelin Defects Cause Enamel Malformations

Enamelin is essential for proper dental enamel formation and is not essential for any other process. Mutations in a single copy of the enamelin gene (*ENAM*, 4q13) cause autosomal dominant AI, with localized hypoplastic (thin) enamel. In its mildest form there are well-circumscribed enamel pits on the tooth surface [72]. In modest cases horizontal bands of thin enamel are observed, particularly in the cervical third of the crown. When both alleles are defective, there is virtually no enamel. The human enamelin gene structure is shown in Figure 4. A standardized nomenclature is used to described *ENAM* mutations [73]. This system numbers nucleotides and amino acids starting from translation initiation (not from the N-terminus of the secreted protein). The ten disease-causing *ENAM* mutations that have been reported to date are: p.K53X [60,74]; p.M71-Q157del [75]; p.A158-Q178del [76], pR179M [77]; p.N197fsX277 [73, 75 78, 79]; p.S216L [80]; p.S246X [81]; p.V340_M341insSQYQYCV [81]; and p.P422fsX448 [72, 79-82] and p.P998fsX1062 [82].

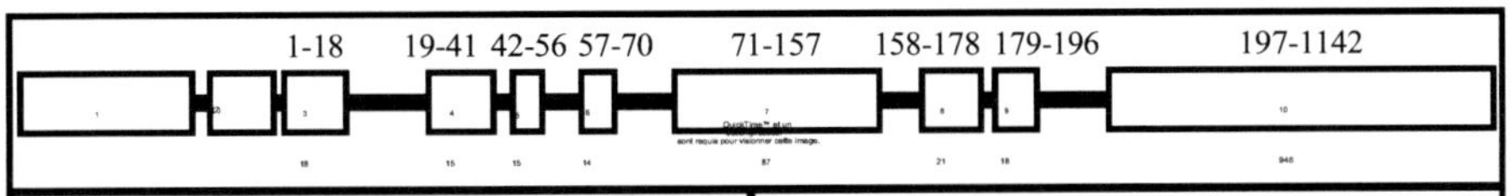

Ex/Int	Nucleotides	Amino Acids	Ex/Int	Nucleotides	Amino Acids
Exon 1	**221: 2-222**	**Non-coding**	–	—	--
Intron 1	320: 223-542				
(Exon 2)	**61: 543-603**	**Non-coding**	—	—	
Intron 2	—		**Exon 7**	**261: 5566-5826**	**87: Met^{71}-Gln^{157}**
Exon 3	**114: 699-812**	**18: Met^{1}-Leu^{18}**	Intron 7	1263: 5827-7089	
Intron 3	3603: 813-2927		**Exon 8**	**63: 7090-7152**	**21: Ala^{158}-Gln^{178}**
Exon 4	**69: 2928-2996**	**15: Val^{19}-Gln^{41}**	Intron 8	135: 10555-10689	
Intron 4	110: 2997-3106		**Exon 9**	**54: 9048-9101**	**18: Arg^{179}-Gly^{196}**
Exon 5	**45: 3107-3151**	**15: Met^{42}-Glu^{56}**	Intron 9	4171: 9102-13272	
Intron 5	757: 3152-3908		**Exon 10**	**4804: 13273-18076**	**946: Asn^{197}-Ala^{1142}**

Ex/Int	Protein	Gene	References
Exon 5	p.K53X	g.2382A>T	Mårdh et al (2002) Hum Mol Genet 11:1069-74 Kim *et al.* (2006)Eur. J. Oral Sci. 114 Suppl 1:3-
Intron 6	p.M71-Q157del	g.4806A>C	Kim et al (2005) J. Dent. Res. 84:278-82
Intron 8	p.A158-Q178del	g.6395G>A	Rajpar*et al.* (2001)Hum Mol Genet 10:1673-7
Exon 9	p.R179M	c.G817T	Gutierrez*et al.* (2007)Arch Oral Biol 52:503-6
Intron 9	p.N197fsX277	g.8344delG	Kida *et al.* (2002)J Dent Res 81:738-42 Hart *et al.* (2003)Arch Oral Biol 48:589-96 Kim *et al.* (2005)J. Dent. Res. 84:278-82 Pavlic*et al.* (2007)Arch Oral Biol 52:209-17
Exon 10	p.S216L	g.12573C>T	Chan*et al.* (in press)J Dent Res
Exon 10	p.S246X	g.12663C>A	Ozdemir*et al.* (2005)J Dent Res 84:1036-41
Exon 10	p.V340-M341insSQYQYCV		Ozdemir et al (2005) J Dent Res 84:1036-41
Exon 10	p.P422fsX448	g.13185/6insAG	Hart*et al.* (2003)J Med Genet 40:900-6 Ozdemir*et al.* (2005)J Dent Res 84:1036-41 Pavlic*et al.* (2007)Arch Oral Biol 52:209-17 Kang *et al.* (2009)J Dent Res. 88:266-9 Chan*et al.* (in press)J Dent Res
Exon 10	p.P998fsX1062	g.14917delT	Kang *et al.* (2009)J Dent Res. 88:266-9

Figure 4: *ENAM* Gene Structure (ref seqs: cDNA, NM_031889.2; and gene, NG_013024.1). The human enamelin gene on chromosome 4q21 is 18076 bp in length. Exons are indicated by numbered boxes. The number of amino acids encoded by each exon is shown below the box. The range of amino acids is shown above. The gene is divided into 10 exons, eight of which are coding. Exon 2 is a non-coding exon that is used in mice, but might not be used in humans (although it retains the appropriate intron/exon junctions). *ENAM* does not undergo alternative splicing. In the gene structure table, the numbers to the left of colons are the total numbers of nucleotides or amino acids in an exon or intron. The numbers to the right of the colons correspond to the range of nucleotides or amino acids in each exon or intron according to the numbering used in the *ENAM* genomic reference sequence. The lower box shows the 10 known disease associated mutations in *ENAM.* For referencing polymorphisms and disease associated mutations, amino acids are numbered starting with the assigned translation initation site. The human enamelin signal peptide is cleaved after Ala^{39}, so the secreted protein is 39 amino acids shorter than the amino acid sequence deduced from the reference sequence.

Enam mutations in mice [83] and targeted *Enam* knockout mice all exhibit defective enamel [20]. Multiple tissue Northern blots [68], *in situ* hybridization [69, 84], and ß-galactosidase expression in the enamelin knockout/lacZ knock-in mice [20, 85] all show enamelin expression is limited to developing teeth. No phenotype besides defective enamel has been observed in AI patients that cannot express enamelin. Not only is enamelin essential for enamel formation, but evolutionary studies suggest that enamelin is not essential for any other processes. Most placental mammals have teeth crowned with enamel, but there are lineages that during evolution stopped developing teeth (anteaters, pangolins, baleen whales) or evolved to make enamel-less teeth (armadillos, sloths, aardvarks, pygmy and dwarf sperm whales). *Enam* frameshift mutations and/or premature stop codons have now been documented in *all* toothless and enamel-less taxa [58, 86]. This is strong evidence that enamelin is only critical for dental enamel formation, otherwise selective pressure for enamelin functions in other tissues would have preserved the integrity of *ENAM* in enamel-less species. Along a similar line, the tooth specificity of amelogenin is supported by the absence of the amelogenin gene in birds [87] . Other chapters in this book claim an important role for amelogenin or specific amelogenin isoforms in other tissues besides teeth, but no deficits in brain, bone, or dentin are observed in patients with defects in *AMELX*.

Enamelin Cleavage Products

The 32 kDa enamelin is the most abundant enamelin cleavage product in developing enamel, comprising 1% of total enamel protein [64]. The porcine 32 kDa enamelin has only 105 amino acids, but it has two phosphorylated serines (Ser^{153} and Ser^{178}) and three glycosylated asparagines (Asn^{207}, Asn^{214}, and Asn^{226}). The 32 kDa enamelin was digested and glycopeptides containing each of the three glycosylation sites were isolated and characterized separately [88, 89] Eight different oligosaccharide structures were observed, five biantennary and three triantennary types (top). Asn^{207} can have any of five biantennary complexes. Asn^{214} uses two of the biantennary complexes, while Asn^{226} uses any of the three triantennary complexes [90].

Analysis of Enam Heterozygous and Null Mice

The *Enam* null (-/-) mice make no true enamel, which is due to a complete failure to deposit mineral at the mineralization front that is associated with the ameloblast distal membrane [20]. Normally the secretion of organic matrix and mineralization of the matrix occur together. In the null mice the organic matrix lacking enamelin is secreted, but mineralization occurs later within the accumulated organic matrix. The *Enam* heterozygous (+/-) mice deposit enamel that looks normal, but reveals important differences upon closer examination. Mandibular incisors from each of the *Enam* genotypes (+/+, +/-, -/-) were sliced at 1 mm increments by sequential strip micro-dissections and analyzed to quantify the mineral weight of each strip [21]. A clear finding was a progressive decrease in mineral content in the enamel deposited with reduced or no *Enam* expression. While the amount of mineral in the enamel layer in the *Enam* heterozygotes was less than the wildtype, the rod organization and the thickness of the enamel layer as a whole were nearly normal.

Mineral is not normally found *within* the ameloblast cell layer, but mineral is found in the cell layer in increasing amounts across the length of incisors in *Enam* null mice. Sometimes focal areas of calcified material covering these teeth adhere tightly to the cells and are lifted off with them [21]. An effect of a lack of enamelin in the *Enam* null mice is that the ameloblast layer becomes increasingly disorganized as enamel formation progresses and some secretory stage ameloblasts undergo apoptosis. The disorganization of ameloblasts and apoptosis is evident in the *Enam* null mice, but not the wildtype or $Enam^{+/-}$ mice (Jan Hu, manuscript in preparation).

Enamelin Function

The "classical" theory of amelogenesis holds that the enamel matrix of developing teeth is comprised of two classes of proteins: amelogenins and non-amelogenins [91]. According to this school of thought, enamel crystals are nucleated at the DEJ and achieve their extremely high aspect ratio (crystal length: crystal width) because enamel matrix proteins selectively bind to the sides of crystals to inhibit their growth in width and thickness, so the crystals only grow in length [1]. This theory does not require a mineralization front and cannot explain how enamelin could dictate the shape of ribbons if they are comprised of amorphous calcium phosphate [18]. Still, the results of *in vitro* studies are interpreted to suggest that the 32 kDa enamelin, which has three large glycosylations on a peptide of 105 amino acids, adopts a beta sheet secondary structure in the presence of calcium to potentially regulate crystal habit

[92] . While the classical theory falls far short of explaining how enamel crystals form, it has not been replaced with a theory that does. In short, at the present time we do not know how enamel crystals form. However, the restricted localization of uncleaved enamelin containing the cysteine-rich C-terminal domain to the mineralization front and the absence of a functioning mineralization front in *Enam* null mice strongly supports the view that enamelin's primary function is as a necessary component of the mineralization front that establishes the mineral ribbons during the secretory stage. We propose that this is the primary function of both enamelin and ameloblastin.

Feedback Mechanisms

The obvious and severe ameloblast cell pathology in the *Enam* and *Ambn* null mice might be directly caused by the loss of protein function, but given the lack of enamel layer upon which the cells normally function, it seems to us that the observed cell pathology is more likely to be a secondary effect. Ameloblasts bind to and reabsorb enamel proteins and their cleavage products throughout the secretory stage. Such activities could be providing feedback to the ameloblasts that help them adjuste their activities to the changing needs of a mineralizing matrix [93]. The "cell signaling" properties of amelogenin [94] and ameloblastin [45, 95] are not likely to induce the differentiation of odontoblasts, osteoblasts or any other type of cell (as differentiation of these cells readily occurs in persons with defective *AMELX*), but might be part of a feedback system that is a normal part of the mechanism of dental enamel formation.

Summary

AMBN and *ENAM* are SCPP genes on chromosome 4q that are part of the proline and glutamine rich group. Both genes are specific for tooth formation. These genes have been shown to degenerate in mammals that have lost the ability to make dental enamel during evolution. In mice that cannot express functional enamelin or ameloblastin the mineralization front along the secretory portion of the ameloblast plasma membrane fails to generate enamel mineral ribbons. A non-functional mineral crust forms over dentin that readily abrades away during function. Ameloblasts undergo pathological changes, such as mineralization of the cell layer, disorganization, and apoptosis. We conclude that enamelin and ameloblastin are critical for the formation of enamel mineral ribbons during the secretory stage of amelogenesis and that their primary function is at the mineralization front.

ACKNOWLEDGEMENTS

This investigation was supported in part by USPHS Program project grants DE011301 and and DE15846 from the National Institute of Dental and Craniofacial Research, National Institutes of Health, Bethesda, MD 29892.

REFERENCES

[1] Simmer JP, Fincham AG. Molecular mechanisms of dental enamel formation. Crit Rev Oral Biol Med 1995; 6: 84-108.

[2] Ronnholm E. The amelogenesis of human teeth as revealed by electron mircoscopy I. The fine structure of the ameloblasts. J Ultrastructure Res 1962; 6: 229-48.

[3] Reith EJ. The stages of amelogenesis as observed in molar teeth of young rats. J Ultrastruct Res 1970; 30: 111-51.

[4] Sasaki T. Cell Biology of Tooth Enamel Formation. Functional Electron Microscopic Monographs. Monogr Oral Sci 1990; 14: 1-204.

[5] Nanci A. Enamel: Composition, Formation, and Structure. In: Nanci A, editor. Ten Cate's Oral Histology Development, Structure, and Function. 6th ed. St. Louis, MO, USA: Mosby, 2008; pp. 141-90.

[6] Daculsi G, Kerebel B. High-resolution electron microscope study of human enamel crystallites: size, shape, and growth. J Ultrastruct Res 1978; 65: 163-72.

[7] Daculsi G, Menanteau J, Kerebel LM, *et al.* Length and shape of enamel crystals. Calcif Tissue Int 1984; 36: 550-5.

[8] Buchroithner B, Klausegger A, Ebschner U, *et al.* Analysis of the LAMB3 gene in a junctional epidermolysis bullosa patient reveals exonic splicing and allele-specific nonsense-mediated mRNA decay. Lab Invest 2004; 84: 1279-88.

[9] Inai T, Kukita T, Ohsaki Y, *et al.* Immunohistochemical demonstration of amelogenin penetration toward the dental pulp in the early stages of ameloblast development in rat molar tooth germs. Anat Rec 1991; 229: 259-70.

[10] Delgado S, Casane D, Bonnaud L, *et al.* Molecular evidence for precambrian origin of amelogenin, the major protein of vertebrate enamel. Mol Biol Evol 2001; 18: 2146-53.

[11] Kawasaki K, Suzuki T, Weiss KM. Genetic basis for the evolution of vertebrate mineralized tissue. Proc Natl Acad Sci U S A 2004; 101: 11356-61.

[12] Kawasaki K, Weiss KM. SCPP gene evolution and the dental mineralization continuum. J Dent Res 2008; 87: 520-31.

[13] Chun Y-HP, Yamakoshi Y, Kim J-W, *et al.* Porcine SPARC: isolation from dentin, cDNA sequence, and computer model. Eur J Oral Sci 2006; 114: 78-85.

[14] Brunati AM, Contri A, Muenchbach M, *et al.* GRP94 (endoplasmin) co-purifies with and is phosphorylated by Golgi apparatus casein kinase. FEBS Lett 2000; 471: 151-5.

[15] Fisher LW, Torchia DA, Fohr B, *et al.* Flexible structures of SIBLING proteins, bone sialoprotein, and osteopontin. Biochem Biophys Res Commun 2001; 280: 460-5.

[16] Moffatt P, Smith CE, St-Arnaud R, *et al.* Characterization of Apin, a secreted protein highly expressed in tooth-associated epithelia. J Cell Biochem 2008; 103: 941-56.

[17] Moffatt P, Smith CE, St-Arnaud R, *et al.* Cloning of rat amelotin and localization of the protein to the basal lamina of maturation stage ameloblasts and junctional epithelium. Biochem J 2006; 399: 37-46.

[18] Beniash E, Metzler RA, Lam RS, *et al.* Transient amorphous calcium phosphate in forming enamel. J Struct Biol 2009; 166: 133-43.

[19] Fukumoto S, Kiba T, Hall B, *et al.* Ameloblastin is a cell adhesion molecule required for maintaining the differentiation state of ameloblasts. J Cell Biol 2004; 167: 973-83.

[20] Hu JC, Hu Y, Smith CE, *et al.* Enamel defects and ameloblast-specific expression in Enam knock-out/lacz knock-in mice. J Biol Chem 2008; 283: 10858-71.

[21] Smith CE, Wazen R, Hu Y, *et al.* Consequences for enamel development and mineralization resulting from loss of function of ameloblastin or enamelin. Eur J Oral Sci 2009; 117: 485-97.

[22] Shimizu M. Investigation of highly aggregative components in porcine enamel proteins. In: Fearnhead RW, Suga S, Eds Tooth Enamel IV. New York: Elsevier Science Publishers, 1984; pp. 156-60.

[23] Fukae M, Tanabe T. Separation of non-amelogenin component from purified amelogenin preparation of immature porcine enamel. Jpn J Oral Biol 1985; 27: 1249-51.

[24] Fukae M, Tanabe T. Nonamelogenin components of porcine enamel in the protein fraction free from the enamel crystals. Calcif Tissue Int 1987; 40: 286-93.

[25] Fukae M, Tanabe T. ^{45}Ca-labeled proteins found in porcine developing dental enamel at an early stage of development. Adv Dent Res 1987; 1: 261-6.

[26] Uchida T, Tanabe T, Fukae M, *et al.* Immunochemical and immunohistochemical studies, using antisera against porcine 25 kDa amelogenin, 89 kDa enamelin and the 13-17 kDa nonamelogenins, on immature enamel of the pig and rat. Histochem 1991; 96: 129-38.

[27] Uchida T, Fukae M, Tanabe T, *et al.* Immunochemical and immunocytochemical study of a 15 kDa non-amelogenin and related proteins in the porcine immature enamel: proposal of a new group of enamel proteins sheath proteins. Biomed Res 1995; 16: 131-40.

[28] Krebsbach PH, Lee SK, Matsuki Y, *et al.* Full-length sequence, localization, and chromosomal mapping of ameloblastin: a novel tooth-specific gene. J Biol Chem 1996; 271: 4431-5.

[29] Cerny R, Slaby I, Hammarstrom L, *et al.* A novel gene expressed in rat ameloblasts codes for proteins with cell binding domains. J Bone Min Res 1996; 11: 883-91.

[30] Hu C-C, Fukae M, Uchida T, *et al.* Sheathlin: cloning, cDNA/polypeptide sequences, and immunolocalization of porcine enamel proteins concentrated in the sheath space. J Dent Res 1997; 76: 648-57.

[31] Simmons D, Gu TT, Krebsbach PH, *et al.* Identification and characterization of a cDNA for mouse ameloblastin. Connect Tissue Res 1998; 39: 3-12.

[32] Simmer JP, Snead ML. Molecular biology of the amelogenin gene. In: Robinson C, Kirkham J, Shore R, Eds. Dental Enamel: Formation to Destruction: CRC Press, 1995; pp. 59-84.

[33] MacDougall M, Simmons D, Gu TT, *et al.* Cloning, characterization and immunolocalization of human ameloblastin. Eur J Oral Sci 2000; 108: 303-10.

[34] Toyosawa S, Fujiwara T, Ooshima T, *et al.* Cloning and characterization of the human ameloblastin gene. Gene 2000; 256: 1-11.

[35] Shintani S, Kobata M, Toyosawa S, *et al.* Identification and characterization of ameloblastin gene in a reptile. Gene 2002; 283: 245-54.

[36] Shintani S, Kobata M, Toyosawa S, *et al.* Identification and characterization of ameloblastin gene in an amphibian, Xenopus laevis. Gene 2003; 318: 125-36.

[37] Shintani S, Kobata M, Toyosawa S, *et al.* Expression of ameloblastin during enamel formation in a crocodile. J Exp Zoolog B Mol Dev Evol 2006; 306: 126-33.

[38] Kobayashi K, Yamakoshi Y, Hu JC, *et al.* Splicing determines the glycosylation state of ameloblastin. J Dent Res 2007; 86: 962-7.

[39] Yamakoshi Y, Tanabe T, Oida S, *et al.* Calcium binding of enamel proteins and their derivatives with emphasis on the calcium-binding domain of porcine sheathlin. Arch Oral Biol 2001; 46: 1005-14.

[40] Iwata T, Yamakoshi Y, Hu JC, *et al.* Processing of ameloblastin by MMP-20. J Dent Res 2007; 86: 153-7.

[41] Bartlett JD, Simmer JP, Xue J, *et al.* Molecular cloning and mRNA tissue distribution of a novel matrix metalloproteinase isolated from porcine enamel organ. Gene 1996; 183: 123-8.

[42] Ryu OH, Fincham AG, Hu CC, *et al.* Characterization of recombinant pig enamelysin activity and cleavage of recombinant pig and mouse amelogenins. J Dent Res 1999; 78: 743-50.

[43] Caterina JJ, Skobe Z, Shi J, *et al.* Enamelysin (matrix metalloproteinase 20)-deficient mice display an amelogenesis imperfecta phenotype. J Biol Chem 2002; 277: 49598-604.

[44] Bartlett JD, Beniash E, Lee DH, *et al.* Decreased mineral content in MMP-20 null mouse enamel is prominent during the maturation stage. J Dent Res 2004; 83: 909-13.

[45] Fukae M, Kanazashi M, Nagano T, *et al.* Porcine sheath proteins show periodontal ligament regeneration activity. Eur J Oral Sci 2006; 114 Suppl 1: 212-8.

[46] Murakami C, Dohi N, Fukae M, *et al.* Immunochemical and immunohistochemical study of 27 and 29 kDa calcium binding proteins and related proteins in the porcine tooth germ. Histochem Cell Biol 1997; 107: 485-94.

[47] Akita H, Fukae M, Shimoda S, *et al.* Localization of glycosylated matrix proteins in secretory porcine enamel and their possible functional roles in enamel mineralization. Arch Oral Biol 1992; 37: 953-62.

[48] Uchida T, Murakami C, Wakida K, *et al.* Sheath Proteins: synthesis, secretion, degradation and fate in forming enamel. Eur J Oral Sci 1998; 106: 308-14.

[49] Vymetal J, Slaby I, Spahr A, *et al.* Bioinformatic analysis and molecular modelling of human ameloblastin suggest a two-domain intrinsically unstructured calcium-binding protein. Eur J Oral Sci 2008; 116: 124-34.

[50] Kozak M. Compilation and analysis of sequences upstream from the translational start site in eukaryotic mRNAs. Nucl Acids Res 1984; 12: 857-72.

[51] Fong CD, Hammarstrom L, Lundmark C, *et al.* Expression patterns of RNAs for amelin and amelogenin in developing rat molars and incisors. Adv Dent Res 1996; 10: 195-200.

[52] Fong CD, Slaby I, Hammarstrom L. Amelin: an enamel-related protein, transcribed in the cells of epithelial root sheath. J Bone Miner Res 1996; 11: 892-8.

[53] Lee SK, Krebsbach PH, Matsuki Y, *et al.* Ameloblastin expression in rat incisors and human tooth germs. Int J Dev Biol 1996; 40: 1141-50.

[54] Uchida T, Murakami C, Dohi N, *et al.* Synthesis, secretion, degradation and fate of ameloblastin during the matrix formation stage of the rat incisor as shown by immunocytochemistry and immunochemistry using region-specific antibodies. J Histochem Cytochem 1997; 45: 1329-40.

[55] Begue-Kirn C, Krebsbach PH, Bartlett JD, *et al.* Dentin sialoprotein, dentin phosphoprotein, enamelysin and ameloblastin: tooth-specific molecules that are distinctively expressed during murine dental differentiation. Eur J Oral Sci 1998; 106: 963-70.

[56] Fong CD, Cerny R, Hammarstrom L, *et al.* Sequential expression of an amelin gene in mesenchymal and epithelial cells during odontogenesis in rats. Eur J Oral Sci 1998; 106 Suppl 1: 324-30.

[57] Fong CD, Hammarstrom L. Expression of amelin and amelogenin in epithelial root sheath remnants of fully formed rat molars. Oral Surgery, Oral Medicine, Oral Pathology, Oral Radiology, & Endodontics 2000; 90: 218-23.

[58] Demere TA, McGowen MR, Berta A, *et al.* Morphological and molecular evidence for a stepwise evolutionary transition from teeth to baleen in mysticete whales. Syst Biol 2008; 57: 15-37.

[59] MacDougall M, DuPont BR, Simmons D, *et al.* Ameloblastin gene (AMBN) maps within the critical region for autosomal dominant amelogenesis imperfecta at chromosome 4q21. Genomics 1997; 41: 115-8.

[60] Kim JW, Simmer JP, Lin BP, *et al.* Mutational analysis of candidate genes in 24 amelogenesis imperfecta families. Eur J Oral Sci 2006; 114 Suppl 1: 3-12.

[61] Wazen RM, Moffatt P, Zalzal SF, *et al.* A mouse model expressing a truncated form of ameloblastin exhibits dental and junctional epithelium defects. Matrix Biol 2009; 28: 292-303.

[62] Sonoda A, Iwamoto T, Nakamura T, *et al.* Critical role of heparin binding domains of ameloblastin for dental epithelium cell adhesion and ameloblastoma proliferation. J Biol Chem 2009; 284: 27176-84.

[63] Fukae M. Discussion of poster 38. In: Fearnhead RW, editor. Tooth Enamel V. Tokyo: Florence Publishers, 1989; pp. 313.

[64] Tanabe T, Aoba T, Moreno EC, *et al.* Properties of phosphorylated 32 kd nonamelogenin proteins isolated from porcine secretory enamel. Calcif Tissue Int 1990; 46: 205-15.

[65] Uchida T, Tanabe T, Fukae M, *et al.* Immunocytochemical and immunochemical detection of a 32 kDa nonamelogenin and related proteins in porcine tooth germs. Arch Histol Cytol 1991; 54: 527-38.

[66] Fukae M, Tanabe T, Murakami C, *et al.* Primary structure of the porcine 89-kDa enamelin. Adv Dent Res 1996; 10: 111-8.

[67] Hu C-C, Fukae M, Uchida T, *et al.* Cloning and characterization of porcine enamelin mRNAs. J Dent Res 1997; 76: 1720-9.

[68] Hu C-C, Simmer JP, Bartlett JD, *et al.* Murine enamelin: cDNA and derived protein sequences. Connect Tissue Res 1998; 39: 47-61.

[69] Hu CC, Hart TC, Dupont BR, *et al.* Cloning human enamelin cDNA, chromosomal localization, and analysis of expression during tooth development. J Dent Res 2000; 79: 912-9.

[70] Sire JY, Al-Hashimi N, Delgado S. Evolutionary analysis of mammalian enamelin, the largest enamel protein, supports a crucial role for the 32 kDa peptide and reveals selective adaptation in rodents and primates. J Mol Evol in press.

[71] Kawasaki K. The SCPP gene repertoire in bony vertebrates and graded differences in mineralized tissues. Dev Genes Evol 2009; 3: 3.

[72] Hart TC, Hart PS, Gorry MC, *et al.* Novel ENAM mutation responsible for autosomal recessive amelogenesis imperfecta and localised enamel defects. J Med Genet 2003; 40: 900-6.

[73] Hart PS, Michalec MD, Seow WK, *et al.* Identification of the enamelin (g.8344delG) mutation in a new kindred and presentation of a standardized ENAM nomenclature. Arch Oral Biol 2003; 48: 589-96.

[74] Mårdh CK, Backman B, Holmgren G, *et al.* A nonsense mutation in the enamelin gene causes local hypoplastic autosomal dominant amelogenesis imperfecta (AIH2). Hum Mol Genet 2002; 11: 1069-74.

[75] Kim JW, Seymen F, Lin BP, *et al.* ENAM mutations in autosomal-dominant amelogenesis imperfecta. J Dent Res 2005; 84: 278-82.

[76] Rajpar MH, Harley K, Laing C, *et al.* Mutation of the gene encoding the enamel-specific protein, enamelin, causes autosomal-dominant amelogenesis imperfecta. Hum Mol Genet 2001; 10: 1673-7.

[77] Gutierrez SJ, Chaves M, Torres DM, *et al.* Identification of a novel mutation in the enamalin gene in a family with autosomal-dominant amelogenesis imperfecta. Arch Oral Biol 2007; 52: 503-6.

[78] Kida M, Ariga T, Shirakawa T, *et al.* Autosomal-dominant hypoplastic form of amelogenesis imperfecta caused by an enamelin gene mutation at the exon-intron boundary. J Dent Res 2002; 81: 738-42.

[79] Pavlic A, Petelin M, Battelino T. Phenotype and enamel ultrastructure characteristics in patients with ENAM gene mutations g.13185-13186insAG and 8344delG. Arch Oral Biol 2007; 52: 209-17.

[80] Chan H-C, Mai L, Oikonomopoulou A, *et al.* Altered enamelin phosphorylation site causes AI. J Dent Res submitted.

[81] Ozdemir D, Hart PS, Firatli E, *et al.* Phenotype of ENAM Mutations is Dosage-dependent. J Dent Res 2005; 84: 1036-41.

[82] Kang HY, Seymen F, Lee SK, *et al.* Candidate gene strategy reveals ENAM mutations. J Dent Res 2009; 88: 266-9.

[83] Masuya H, Shimizu K, Sezutsu H, *et al.* Enamelin (Enam) is essential for amelogenesis: ENU-induced mouse mutants as models for different clinical subtypes of human amelogenesis imperfecta (AI). Hum Mol Genet 2005; 14: 575-83.

[84] Hu JC, Sun X, Zhang C, Simmer JP. A comparison of enamelin and amelogenin expression in developing mouse molars. Eur J Oral Sci 2001; 109: 125-32.

[85] Seedorf H, Klaften M, Eke F, *et al.* A mutation in the enamelin gene in a mouse model. J Dent Res 2007; 86: 764-8.
[86] Meredith RW, Gatesy J, Murphy WJ, *et al.* Molecular decay of the tooth gene Enamelin (ENAM) mirrors the loss of enamel in the fossil record of placental mammals. PLoS Genet 2009; 5: e1000634.
[87] Sire JY, Delgado SC, Girondot M. Hen's teeth with enamel cap: from dream to impossibility. BMC Evol Biol 2008; 8: 246.
[88] Yamakoshi Y. Carbohydrate moieties of porcine 32 kDa enamelin. Calcif Tissue Int 1995; 56: 323-30.
[89] Yamakoshi Y, Pinheiro FH, Tanabe T, *et al.* Sites of asparagine-linked oligosaccharides in porcine 32 kDa enamelin. Connect Tissue Res 1998; 39: 39-46; discussion 63-7.
[90] Hu JC, Yamakoshi Y. Enamelin and autosomal-dominant amelogenesis imperfecta. Crit Rev Oral Biol Med 2003; 14: 387-98.
[91] Termine JD, Belcourt AB, Christner PJ, *et al.* Properties of dissociatively extracted fetal tooth matrix proteins. J Biol Chem 1980; 20: 9760-8.
[92] Fan D, Lakshminarayanan R, Moradian-Oldak J. The 32kDa enamelin undergoes conformational transitions upon calcium binding. J Struct Biol 2008; 163: 109-15.
[93] Smith CE, Nanci A. Secretory activity as a function of the development and maturation of ameloblasts. Connect Tissue Res 1989; 22: 147-56.
[94] Nebgen DR, Inoue H, Sabsay B, *et al.* Identification of the chondrogenic inducing activity from bovine dentin (bCIA) as a low molecular mass amelogenin polypeptide. J Dent Res 1999; 78: 1484-94.
[95] Kanazashi M, Gomi K, Nagano T, *et al.* The 17-kDa sheath protein in enamel proteins induces cementum regeneration in experimental cavities created in a buccal dehiscence model of dogs. J Periodontal Res 2006; 41: 193-9.

CHAPTER 6

Potential Role of Adaptor Protein Complex-3 (Ap-3) In Amelogenesis

Jason L. Shapiro[1], Rodrigo S. Lacruz[1], Steven J. Brookes[2], S. Petter Lyngstadaas[3] and Michael L. Paine[1,*]

[1] *University of Southern California School of Dentistry, Center for Craniofacial Molecular Biology, 2250 Alcazar Street, CSA room 103, Los Angeles, CA 90033, USA;* [2] *Department of Oral Biology, Leeds Dental Institute, University of Leeds, Clarendon Way, Leeds, LS2 9LU, United Kingdom and* [3] *Department of Biomaterials, Faculty of Dentistry, University of Oslo, P.O. Box 1109 Blindern, N-0317 Oslo, Norway*

Abstract: As identified using *in vitro* methodologies, the enamel matrix proteins (EMPs) bind a class of proteins called lysosomal associated membrane proteins (LAMPs), whose members are LAMP1, LAMP2 and CD63/LAMP3. LAMPs are transmembrane proteins present in the plasma membrane, and all three directly interact with the AP-3 complex to initiate receptor-mediated endocytosis. In yeast, AP-3 associated endocytosis is clathrin-independent, while in higher organisms the requirement of clathrin is unclear. AP-3 is a protein complex with four subunits referred to as β, δ, μ and σ. Three other adaptor protein complexes (AP-1, AP-2 and AP-4), each having four similar but unique subunits, are also involved with endocytosis and are either clathrin-dependent (AP-1 and AP-2) or clathrin-independent (AP-4). Only AP-3 interacts directly with plasma membrane-bound LAMPs. It is likely that endocytosis of the degraded EMPs plays a significant role in enamel maturation, and if so, AP-3 dysfunction may result in enamel abnormalities. We have initiated *in vivo* studies to better define the dental phenotype in a strain of mice null for the β subunit of AP-3 (coded by the *AP3B1* gene), which results in the loss of AP-3 function. The driving hypothesis of future studies is that *"failure of normal ameloblast endocytosis of the degraded EMPs during enamel maturation results in functionally inferior enamel more prone to dental disease"*. The question we expect to answer from these mice studies is whether the receptor-mediated AP-3 endocytotic pathway is a prominent feature of amelogenesis. This chapter discusses the potential role of AP-3 mediated endocytosis in amelogenesis and describes animal experimental models that could be used to examine such a relationship.

Key Words: Adaptor Protein Complex; Amelogenesis; Enamel Formation; Endocytosis; Hermansky-Pudlak Syndrome; Pearl Mice

ENAMEL PROTEINS AND ENAMEL MATRIX ASSEMBLY

Enamel organic matrix assembly, and the subsequent process of biomineralization, occurs outside of the cell in the extracellular space. Enamel matrix assembly follows the paradigm of basement membrane assembly, however, unlike the basement membrane, enamel does not remodel, nor does it remain in close contact with the cells that synthesize the enamel matrix proteins. Rather, cells that produce enamel (ameloblasts) migrate away from the preformed dentine surface depositing enamel matrix in their wake. This matrix is composed predominantly of amelogenin protein [1, 2], with traces (<10%) of ameloblastin [3, 4] and enamelin [5] proteins. The matrix undergoes partial mineralization almost immediately after secretion [6]. Prior to the final phase of enamel maturation, during which the mineral content increases dramatically, the matrix proteins are degraded by extracellular proteases and the debris removed from the tissue. Once enamel has matured, the ameloblasts remain dormant until the tooth erupts, and at this time these cell are shed from the enamel surface. Many genetic factors clearly impact on amelogenesis. Amelogenin, ameloblastin and enamelin represent those structural proteins whose expression remains relatively unique to the mineralized tooth structure [7-9]. It is apparent that the developmental timing in which these gene products are presented to the enamel matrix must be finely controlled and regulated [10]. Because of the limited tissue expression of these enamel proteins, it appears that their removal from the enamel matrix during enamel maturation has required specific proteases whose spatiotemporal expression must also be exquisitely regulated. Proteases relatively unique to the developing enamel organ are the serine protease kallikrein-4 (KLK4) [11-13] and the matrix metalloproteinase (MMP20) [14, 15].

***Correspondence Author:** Dr. Michael Paine, University of Southern California School of Dentistry, Center for Craniofacial Molecular Biology, 2250 Alcazar Street, CSA room 103, Los Angeles, CA 90033, USA; E-mail: paine@usc.edu

Michel Goldberg (ED)

BRIEF HISTORICAL BACKGROUND OF LITERATURE ON ENAMEL MATRIX PROTEIN REMOVAL DURING ENAMEL MATURATION

Much of our understanding of the removal of the organic enamel matrix during the events of amelogenesis is derived from rodent studies using a radiolabel amino acid "pulse" administered to the animal and studied at various time intervals following administration [16-19]. The pathways discussed to explain the removal of the enamel proteins favor a passive diffusion (resorptive) process such as pinocytosis into ameloblasts [20], or, as described for rodents, pinocytosis of the enamel proteins into odontogenic processes [21, 22]. In general, theories regarding the final removal of the proteins have excluded ameloblast-directed endocytosis. This is because: 1) the levels of clathrin protein within the cytoplasm of secretory ameloblasts is negligible [23], and the presence of clathrin has historically been the hallmark of receptor-mediated endocytosis [24]; and 2) it is hard to reconcile that the apical face of polarized ameloblasts could simultaneously manage both an extreme secretory, and a resorptive, activity [19]. However, the possibility that endocytosis occurs has not completely ruled out. The ultrastructural arrangement of ameloblasts, most notably the presence of multivesicular bodies, and the quantities of proteins cycling through the lysosomes, which are in keeping with endocytotic processing in other cell types, is consistent with this model [25].

In the past decade the concept of passive diffusion (pinocytosis) has been challenged with the discoveries of four unique adaptor protein complexes, and the acknowledgment that receptor-mediated, clathrin-independent endocytotic pathways exist [24, 26-29]. Today it is well-known that receptor-mediate clathrin-independent endocytosis does occur [24, 30-34], and our previous understanding of pinocytosis, or the "passive" cellular uptake of degraded matrix proteins is over simplistic or just simply not correct [35, 36].

Much of our current knowledge of amelogenesis has been derived from rodent models and there must also be caution when equating the events of amelogenesis in rodents to other animal species. Amelogenesis in rodent teeth differs from amelogenesis in primate teeth in a number of ways. In rats, the linear thickness of the lower incisor enamel, which in the unworn enamel near the incisal edge is generally ~100 μm thick, is produced in a 7.5-day period [37]. The half-life of enamel proteins *in vivo* is estimated at 8.9-days [17]. Thus, in rodents this would suggest that the enamel most proximal to the dentin-enamel junction (DEJ) is still very immature or unmineralized at the onset of the maturation stage, and could allow for passage of degraded enamel proteins into odontoblastic processes as previously suggested [21, 22]. In human lower central incisors for instance, at a similar anatomical region of the rat incisor, the linear enamel thickness measures on average ~600 μm, and takes about 150 days to form [38]. If we assume the same half-life for the enamel proteins, we must then assume the DEJ is fully mineralized/mature weeks after it is initiated. Thus in primates the only options for removal of the enamel organic matrix, days after the initiation of amelogenesis, are either directly through the apical face of ameloblasts (pinocytosis or endocytosis), or intercellular movement (either passive or orchestrated) along the basolateral surfaces of ameloblasts. While a passive diffusion (pinocytosis) of the enamel matrix debris into secretory or maturation-stage ameloblasts may explain enamel matrix removal, alternative explanations are also reasonable. One alternative explanation would be that as ameloblasts secrete enamel proteins into the enamel matrix they simultaneously employ a "receptor-mediated" endocytotic pathway to allow for the removal of organic enamel debris that results from enzymatic degradation. This explanation is feasible with recent *in vitro* data that has demonstrated that enamel matrix proteins interact directly with a class of ubiquitously expressed integral membrane-bound proteins [39, 40]. The members of this protein class are called lysosomal-associated membrane protein (LAMP)-1, LAMP2 and CD63/LAMP3 [40-42].

A POTENTIAL PATHWAY FOR EMP REMOVAL DURING AMELOGENESIS

The realization that amelogenin and other EMPs bind LAMP1 [41, 42], LAMP2 [42] and CD63 [40, 42, 43], lead us to hypothesize that amelogenin may be rapidly taken up by the ameloblast cell through receptor-mediated endocytosis [44]. LAMP1, LAMP2 and CD63 are ubiquitously expressed and localize to the plasma membrane. They are also present in the membranes of the endosome/late endosome and lysosome [45, 46]. A lysosomal targeting motif is present at the carboxyl-terminals of LAMP1, LAMP2 and CD63 [47], suggesting that they all may employ a similar mechanism in their trafficking from the plasma membrane to the lysosome. Although LAMP1 and CD63 are expressed by ameloblasts at all stages of amelogenesis, LAMP1 is more highly expressed in the early secretory stage while CD63 is more highly expressed in late-secretory and post-secretory stages [44]. Protein interactions between the secreted enamel matrix proteins [such as amelogenin, ameloblastin and enamelin) and membrane-bound proteins (such as LAMP1, LAMP2 and CD63) likely occur at the ameloblast Tomes' processes [43]. Such interactions may be required to establish short-term order of the forming matrix [43], and/or to mediate feedback signals to the transcriptional machinery of ameloblasts [41, 48-51], and/or to quickly endocytose matrix protein debris during enamel biomineralization [42, 44]. It is the last theme of endocytosis that has been a focus of our attention in recent years.

LAMPS & ADAPTOR PROTEIN COMPLEXES & ENDOCYTOSIS: AP-3 MEDIATED ENDOCYTOSIS AS A POTENTIAL PATHWAY FOR EMP REMOVAL DURING AMELOGENESIS

Adaptor protein (AP) complexes are heterotetramers that cycle between the cell cytosol and membranes, and they mediate the sorting of membrane proteins in the secretory and endocytic pathways. AP complexes frequently, but not always, involve in the formation of clathrin-coated vesicles. Four distinct AP complexes have been identified; these are AP-1, AP-2, AP-3 and AP-4. Widely accepted has been the notion that AP-2 and AP-3 mediate endocytosis from the plasma membrane, and AP-1, AP-3 and AP-4 each play a role in the endosomal/lysosomal sorting pathways [24, 29]. AP-1 and AP-2 mediated endocytosis and have an absolute requirement for clathrin, while AP-4 mediated endocytosis is clathrin-independent [24, 26-29]. In yeast, AP-3 associated endocytosis is clathrin-independent, while in higher organisms the requirement of clathrin is unclear. Over the past decade the molecular mechanisms of non-clathrin associated endocytotic pathways have been investigated [24, 30-36]. Using RNA isolated from ameloblast-like (LS8 cells) [44, 52] we have identified, by RT-PCR, RNA transcripts representing all four AP complexes (unpublished data).

The intracellular trafficking of plasma membrane-bound LAMP1, LAMP2 and CD63 involves the recruiting of, and binding to, the AP-3 complex [32, 34, 47, 53]. Data suggest that AP-3 related intracellular trafficking may proceed independently of any association with clathrin, or alternatively have minimal clathrin requirements (Figure 1, panel A). Although in mammals a clathrin consensus-binding motif is part of the AP-3 β subunit (coded by the *AP3B1* gene), there is little or no physiological evidence to support the association of clathrin and AP-3 *in vivo* [30-32, 34, 54, 55]. For example, while significant amounts of AP-1 and AP-2 are a feature of biochemically purified clathrin-coated vesicles, only trace amounts of AP-3 can be characterized in these same vesicles [30, 32, 34]. This lack of association between AP-3 and clathrin-coated vesicles is also supported by the fact that in yeast AP3B1 has no clathrin consensus-binding motif, and yeast AP-3 related trafficking is clathrin-independent [32].

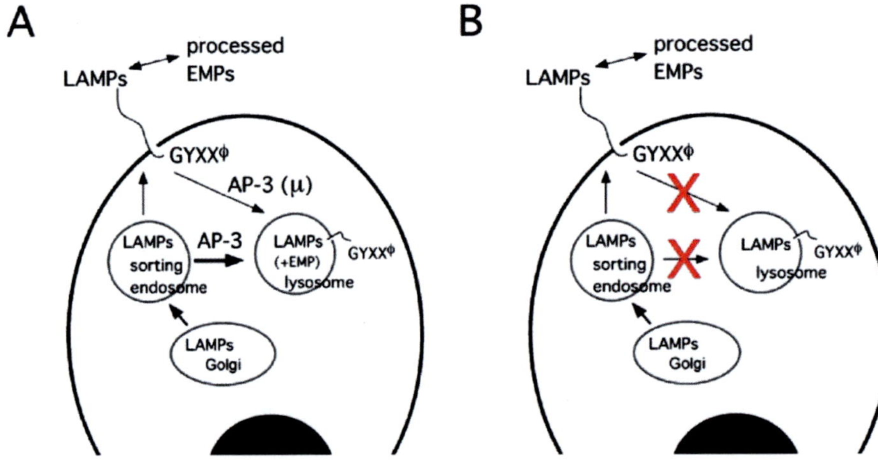

Figure 1: Intracellular Trafficking of LAMPs. Following LAMP1, LAMP2 and CD63 (LAMPs) synthesis they are sorted and packaged in Golgi bodies, and sorted to endosomes. From the endosome, LAMPs are either directly transported to lysosomes (major pathway), or transported to the plasma membrane (minor pathway). Mutations to any of the AP-3 subunits, impacting on AP-3 activity (panel B) results in the accumulation of LAMPs in the plasma membrane. The schematic shows how processed enamel matrix proteins (EMPs), through a direct protein-protein interaction with the LAMPs, could result in their movement into lysosomes for complete proteolysis (panel A), and a block in AP-3 activity would result in the accumulation of EMPs in the extracellular matrix (panel B).

Plasma membrane-bound CD63 trafficking to the late endosome/lysosome is mediated through a direct interaction with μ subunit (coded by the *AP3M1* gene) of AP-3 [32, 56]. AP-3 facilitates the budding of vesicles from the Golgi membrane and may be directly involved in protein sorting to the endosomal/lysosomal system. The trafficking of CD63 from the cell membrane to the lysosome is initiated by a direct protein-protein interaction between CD63, through a lysosomal targeting motif (GYXX∅; where X is any amino acid and ∅ is a bulky hydrophobic amino acid) located at the C'terminus, and AP3M1 [47, 57]. This signature AP3M1-binding motif is also present at the C'-termini of LAMP1 and LAMP2 [47], suggesting that CD63, LAMP1 and LAMP2 all employ the same mechanism in their trafficking from the plasma membrane to the lysosome [42] (Figure 1, panel A).

HUMAN PHENOTYPES ASSOCIATED WITH MUTATIONS IN THE AP-3 βSUBUNIT

Hermansky-Pudlak Syndrome (HPS) is an autosomal recessive disease linked to the following gene loci: *HPS1, AP3B1/HPS2, HPS3, HPS4, HPS5, HPS6, DTNBP1/HPS7 and BLOC1S3/HPS8,* also referred to as HPS types 1-8, and gene products from all 8 loci are involved with some aspect of endosome-lysosome biosynthesis [58, 59]. AP3B1 is involved in protein trafficking to lysosomes or specialized endosomal-lysosomal organelles. Patients with HPS have albinism, bleeding problems, inflammatory bowel disease, and defects in many cytoplasmic organelles including melanosomes, platelet-dense granules and lysosomes [59]. Although a rare disease worldwide, HPS is not uncommon in Puerto Rico with a frequency of approximately 1:800 (or ~ 3,700 affected individuals), giving a carrier frequency of 1:21. Significant populations of HPS sufferers are documented in the Switzerland and also Japan. The Medical Genetics Branch of the NIH estimates that one in every 400-2,000 people worldwide are carriers of a mutation causing HPS, and it is currently estimated that 1 in every 500,000-1,000,000 people worldwide are sufferers of HPS [60-63]. The biggest dental concern is periodontal disease, often left untreated because of the excessive gingival bleeding, and medical support and management is needed in patients for dental surgeries [64, 65]. There is a report in the literature noting "severe dental decay" in addition to "aggressive periodontitis" in two related individuals (consanguineous pedegree) with type 2 HPS resulting from a mutation to the *AP3B1* gene [64, 66]. In addition, there is a reference from the "emedicine" website [67] describing HPS patients as having abnormal enamel (a description that is unreferenced). To the best of our knowledge there are no other reports in literature describing the tooth enamel and dentin phenotypes in HPS patients.

Thus, in humans, mutations in the β subunit (AP3B1) of AP-3 have been associated with a high caries rate [64, 66] which can be associated with mechanically weak or hypomineralized enamel [68]. It is clear therefore that further studies are needed to define the enamel phenotype in all HPS types, as all eight types/genes have endosome-lysosome biosynthesis deficiencies.

ANIMAL PHENOTYPES ASSOCIATED WITH MUTATIONS IN AP-3 SUBUNITS

Two animal models have been described that resemble HPS, and these are the pearl mice with mutations to the *AP3B1* gene (β subunit) [69], and also the mocha mice that have mutations to the *AP3D1* gene (δ subunit) [70]. Multiple pearl animal lines, and one mocha line, each with unique gene mutations, are commercially available to study through The Jackson Laboratory (http://www.jax.org/) [69, 71]. The homozygous pearl phenotype includes hypopigmentation of hair and eyes, and a prolonged bleeding time associated with platelet storage pool deficiencies (Figure 2). Compared to the mandibular incisor of a wild-type control animal, the pearl mice mandibular incisor teeth exhibit a hypoplastic-like enamel with a yellowish appearance (Figure 2). Mocha mice are recognizable at birth by the absence of visible pigment in the eyes, and their hair has considerably smaller and fewer melanin granules than normal [72]. The behavior of the mocha animal is abnormal, characterized by hyperactivity and a characteristically tilted head [72]. Both the pearl and mocha animals have a considerably shortened lifespan. To date, the enamel morphology of pearl and mocha mice has not been described, and there is no available literature to suggest that the dentitions of either animal model have been examined. A thorough examination of the dental enamel of these pearl and mocha mice, along with an examination of the dentitions of individuals with HPS type 2, should give definitive data related to the requirements of AP-3 endocytotic activity during amelogenesis. A working hypothesis for future studies is *"failure of normal ameloblast endocytosis of the degraded EMPs during enamel maturation results in functionally inferior enamel more prone to dental disease"*, and this can be visualized in Figure 1 with the inclusion of the LAMP-processed EMP interaction, and how this then feeds into the AP-3 endocytotic pathway (Figure 1, panel B).

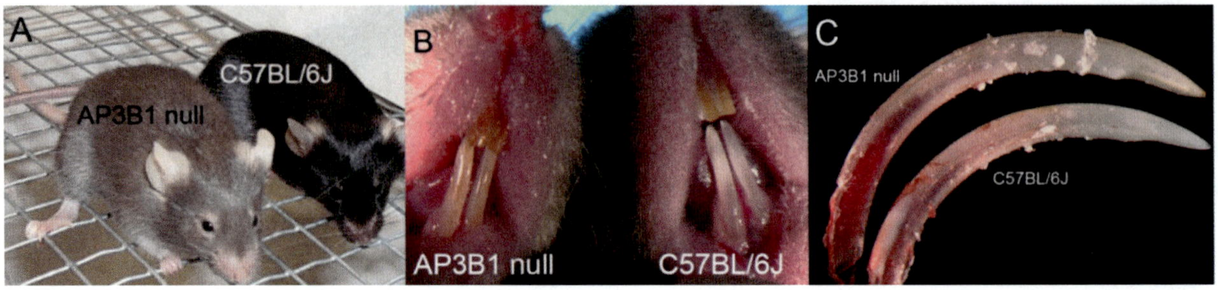

Figure 2: Dentition of 12-month AP3B1 null (pearl) animals compared to age-matched wild-type (C57BL/6J) animals. Panel A shows the pearl coat color vs the wild-type animal. Panel B; mandibular incisor teeth of the pearl mice is a yellow color as compared to wild-type. Incisor teeth (panel C) are noticeably larger in the pearl mice when compared to wild-type, however, a larger sample size is needed to confirm these observations.

CONCLUSION

Hermansky-Pudlak Syndrome (HPS) is an autosomal recessive disease linked to multiple gene loci, and each gene loci codes for a protein that is involved with endosome-lysosome biosynthesis. Mouse models for HPS are available to study, and these include "pearl" mice with mutations to the *AP3B1* gene locus. The *AP3B1* gene locus codes for a protein contained within the adaptor protein-3 (AP-3) complex, a protein complex mediating receptor-mediated endocytosis. A few case reports note enamel anomalies in the dentition of HPS individuals [67, 73], and our initial gross observations of pearl mice mandibular incisor teeth show enamel with a hypoplastic-like appearance (Figure 2). More detailed studies are needed to establish a direct relationship between AP-3 directed endocytosis and amelogenesis.

REFERENCES

[1] Snead ML, Zeichner-David M, Chandra T, *et al.* Construction and identification of mouse amelogenin cDNA clones. Proc Natl Acad Sci USA 1983; 80: 7254-8.

[2] Du C, Falini G, Fermani S, *et al.* Supramolecular assembly of amelogenin nanospheres into birefringent microribbons. Science 2005; 307: 1450-4.

[3] Fong CD, Slaby I, Hammarstrom L. Amelin, an enamel related protein, transcribed in cells of the epithelial root sheath. J Bone Min Res 1996; 11: 892-8.

[4] Lee SK, Krebsbach P, Matsuki Y, *et al.* Ameloblastin expression in rat incisors and human tooth germs. Int J Dev Biol 1996; 40: 1141-50.

[5] Hu C-C, Fukae M, Uchida T, *et al.* Cloning and characterization of porcine enamelin mRNAs. J Dent Res 1997; 76: 1720-9.

[6] Simmer JP, Fincham AG. Molecular mechanisms of dental enamel formation. Crit Rev Oral Biol Med 1995; 6 :84-108.

[7] Begue-Kirn C, Krebsbach PH, Bartlett JD, *et al.* Dentin sialoprotein, dentin phosphoprotein, enamelysin and ameloblastin: tooth-specific molecules that are distinctively expressed during murine dental differentiation. Eur J Oral Sci 1998; 106: 963-70.

[8] Nanci A, Zalzal S, Lavoie P, *et al.* Comparative immunochemical analyses of the developmental expression and distribution of ameloblastin and amelogenin in rat incisors. J Histochem Cytochem 1998; 46: 911-34.

[9] Lee SK, Kim SM, Lee YJ, *et al.* The structure of the rat ameloblastin gene and its expression in amelogenesis. Mol Cells 2003; 15: 216-25.

[10] Paine ML, White SN, Luo W, *et al.* Regulated gene expression dictates enamel structure and tooth function. Matrix Biol 2001; 20: 273-92.

[11] Nelson PS, Gan L, Ferguson C, *et al.* Molecular cloning and characterization of prostase, an androgen-regulated serine protease with prostate-restricted expression. Proc Natl Acad Sci USA 1999; 96: 3114-9.

[12] Hu JC, Zhang C, Sun X, Yang Y, *et al.* Characterization of the mouse and human PRSS17 genes, their relationship to other serine proteases, and the expression of PRSS17 in developing mouse incisors. Gene 2000; 251: 1-8.

[13] Ryu O, Hu JC, Yamakoshi Y, *et al.* Porcine kallikrein-4 activation, glycosylation, activity, and expression in prokaryotic and eukaryotic hosts. Eur J Oral Sci 2002; 110: 358-65.

[14] Caterina JJ, Skobe Z, Shi J, *et al.* Enamelysin (MMP-20) deficient mice display an amelogenesis imperfecta phenotype. J Biol Chem 2002; 277: 49598-604.

[15] Bartlett JD, Simmer JP. Proteinases in developing dental enamel. Crit Rev Oral Biol Med 1999; 10: 425-41.

[16] Smith CE. Ameloblasts: secretory and resorptive functions. J Dent Res 1979; 58(Spec. Issue B): 695-707.

[17] Smith CE, Dahan S, Fazel A, *et al.* Correlated biochemical and radioautographic studies of protein turnover in developing rat incisor enamel following pulse-chase labeling with L-[35S]- and L-[methyl-3H]-methionine. Anat Rec 1992; 232: 1-14.

[18] Smith CE, Pompura JR, Borenstein S, *et al.* Degradation and loss of matrix proteins from developing enamel. Anat Rec 1989; 224: 292-316.

[19] Smith CE. Cellular and chemical events during enamel maturation. Crit Rev Oral Biol Med 1998; 9: 128-61.

[20] Reith EJ, Cotty VF. The absorptive activity of ameloblasts during the maturation of enamel. Anat Rec 1967; 157: 577-88.

[21] Warshawsky H, Josephsen K. The behavior of substances labeled with 3H-proline and 3H-fucose in the cellular processes of odontoblasts and ameloblasts. Anat Rec 1981; 200: 1-10.

[22] Josephsen K, Warshawsky H. Radioautography of rat incisor dentin as a continuous record of the incorporation of a single dose of 3H-labeled proline and tyrosine. Am J Anat 1982;164: 45-56.

[23] Nakamura M, Bringas P, Nanci A, *et al.* Translocation of enamel proteins from inner enamel epithelia to odontoblasts during mouse tooth development. Anat Rec 1994; 238: 383-96.

[24] Robinson MS. Adaptable adaptors for coated vesicles. Trends Cell Biol 2004; 14: 167-74.

[25] Nanci A, Smith CE. Development and calcification of enamel. In: Bonucci E, Ed Calcification in Biological Systems. Boca Raton, FL: CRC Press; 1992; pp. 313-43.

[26] Ohno H. Clathrin-associated adaptor protein complexes. J Cell Sci 2006; 119(Pt 18): 3719-21.

[27] Ohno H. Physiological roles of clathrin adaptor AP complexes: lessons from mutant animals. J Biochem 2006;139: 943-8.

[28] Ohno H. Overview: membrane traffic in multicellular systems: more than just a housekeeper. J Biochem 2006;139: 941-2.

[29] Janvier K, Bonifacino JS. Role of the endocytic machinery in the sorting of lysosome-associated membrane proteins. Mol Biol Cell 2005;16: 4231-42.

[30] Simpson F, Bright NA, West MA, *et al.* A novel adaptor-related protein complex. J Cell Biol 1996;133: 749-60.

[31] Dell'Angelica EC, Klumperman J, Stoorvogel W, *et al.* Association of the AP-3 adaptor complex with clathrin. Science 1998; 280: 431-4.

[32] Robinson MS, Bonifacino JS. Adaptor-related proteins. Curr Opin Cell Biol 2001; 13: 444-53.

[33] Johannes L, Lamaze C. Clathrin-dependent or not: is it still the question? Traffic 2002; 3: 443-51.

[34] Peden AA, Oorschot V, Hesser BA, *et al.* Localization of the AP-3 adaptor complex defines a novel endosomal exit site for lysosomal membrane proteins. J Cell Biol 2004; 164: 1065-76.

[35] Le Roy C, Wrana JL. Clathrin- and non-clathrin-mediated endocytic regulation of cell signalling. Nat Rev Mol Cell Biol 2005; 6: 112-26.

[36] Nichols BJ, Lippincott-Schwartz J. Endocytosis without clathrin coats. Trends Cell Biol 2001; 11: 406-12.

[37] Smith CE, Nanci A. Protein dynamics of amelogenesis. Anat Rec 1996; 245: 186-207.

[38] Reid DJ, Dean MC. Variation in modern human enamel formation times. J Human Evolution 2006; 50: 329-46.

[39] Paine CT, Paine ML, Snead ML. Identification of tuftelin- and amelogenin-interacting proteins using the yeast two-hybrid system. Connect Tissue Res 1998; 38(1-4): 257-67.

[40] Wang HJ, Tannukit S, Zhu DH, *et al.* Enamel matrix protein interactions. J Bone Mineral Res 2005; 20: 1032-40.

[41] Tompkins K, George A, Veis A. Characterization of a mouse amelogenin [A-4]/M59 cell surface receptor. Bone 2006; 38: 172-80.

[42] Zou Y, Wang H, Shapiro JL, *et al.* Determination of protein regions responsible for interactions of amelogenin with CD63 and LAMP1. Biochem J 2007; 408: 347-54.

[43] Zhu D, Paine ML, Luo W, *et al.* Altering biomineralization by protein design. J Biol Chem 2006; 281: 21173-82.

[44] Shapiro JL, Wen X, Okamoto CT, *et al.* Cellular uptake of amelogenin, and its localization to CD63, and Lamp1-positive vesicles. Cell Mol Life Sci 2007;64:244-56.
[45] Duffield A, Kamsteeg EJ, Brown AN, *et al.* The tetraspanin CD63 enhances the internalization of the H,K-ATPase beta-subunit. Proc Natl Acad Sci USA 2003; 100: 15560-5.
[46] Cook NR, Row PE, Davidson HW. Lysosome associated membrane protein 1 (Lamp1) traffics directly from the TGN to early endosomes. Traffic 2004; 5: 685-99.
[47] Rous BA, Reaves BJ, Ihrke G, *et al.* Role of adaptor complex AP-3 in targeting wild-type and mutated CD63 to lysosomes. Mol Biol Cell 2002; 13: 1071-82.
[48] Veis A, Tompkins K, Alvares K, *et al.* Specific amelogenin gene splice products have signaling effects on cells in culture and in implants in vivo. J Biol Chem 2000; 275: 41263-72.
[49] Xu L, Harada H, Taniguchi A. The Exon 6ABC Region of Amelogenin mRNA Contribute to Increased Levels of Amelogenin mRNA through Amelogenin Protein-enhanced mRNA Stabilization. J Biol Chem 2006; 281: 32439-44.
[50] Xu L, Harada H, Taniguchi A. The Effects of LAMP1 and LAMP3 on M180 Amelogenin Uptake, Localization and Amelogenin mRNA Induction by Amelogenin Protein. J Biochem 2008; 144: 531-7.
[51] Xu L, Harada H, Yokohama-Tamaki T, *et al.* Reuptake of extracellular amelogenin by dental epithelial cells results in increased levels of amelogenin mRNA through enhanced mRNA stabilization. J Biol Chem 2006; 281: 2257-62.
[52] Shapiro JL, Wang H, Wen X, *et al.* An amelogenin minigene to study alternative splicing. DNA Cell Bio. 2006; 25: 1-5.
[53] Berditchevski F, Odintsova E. Tetraspanins as Regulators of Protein Trafficking. Traffic 2007; 8: 89-96.
[54] Shi G, Faundez V, Roos J, *et al.* Neuroendocrine synaptic vesicles are formed in vitro by both clathrin-dependent and clathrin-independent pathways. J Cell Biol 1998; 143: 947-55.
[55] Peden AA, Rudge RE, Lui WW, *et al.* Assembly and function of AP-3 complexes in cells expressing mutant subunits. J Cell Biol 2002; 156: 327-36.
[56] Nakatsu F, Ohno H. Adaptor protein complexes as the key regulators of protein sorting in the post-Golgi network. Cell Struct Funct 2003; 28: 419-29.
[57] Di Pietro SM, Dell'Angelica EC. The cell biology of Hermansky-Pudlak syndrome: recent advances. Traffic 2005; 6: 525-33.
[58] Huizing M, Boissy RE, Gahl WA. Hermansky-Pudlak syndrome: vesicle formation from yeast to man. Pigment Cell Res 2002; 15: 405-19.
[59] Wei ML. Hermansky-Pudlak syndrome: a disease of protein trafficking and organelle function. Pigment Cell Res 2006; 19: 19-42.
[60] Markello TC. Rare type of albinism linked to deadly lung disease. February 4, 2008. Available from: FOXNews.com. [http://www.foxnews.com/story/0,2933,328029,00.html].
[61] Gahl WA. Hermansky-Pudlack syndrome. 2007. Available from: [http://www.ncbi.nlm.nih.gov/bookshelf/br.fcgi?book=gene&part=hps].
[62] Witkop CJ, Almadovar C, Pineiro B, *et al.* Hermansky-Pudlak syndrome (HPS). An epidemiologic study. Ophthalmic Paediatr Genet 1990; 11: 245-50.
[63] Witkop CJ, Nunez Babcock M, Rao GH, *et al.* Albinism and Hermansky-Pudlak syndrome in Puerto Rico. Bol Asoc Med P R 1990; 82: 333-9.
[64] Jung J, Bohn G, Allroth A, *et al.* Identification of a homozygous deletion in the AP3B1 gene causing Hermansky-Pudlak syndrome, type 2. Blood 2006; 108: 362-9.
[65] Feliciano NZ, Rivera E, Agrait E, *et al.* Hermansky-Pudlak syndrome: dental management considerations. J Dent Child (Chic) 2006; 73: 51-6.
[66] Kotzot D, Richter K, Gierth-Fiebig K. Oculocutaneous albinism, immunodeficiency, hematological disorders, and minor anomalies: a new autosomal recessive syndrome? Am J Med Genet 1994; 50: 224-7.
[67] Izquierdo NJ. Hermansky-Pudlak syndrome. 2008. Available from: [http://emedicine.medscape.com/article/1200277-overview].
[68] White SN, Paine ML, Ngan AY, *et al.* Ectopic expression of dentin sialoprotein during amelogenesis hardens bulk enamel. J Biol Chem 2007; 282: 5340-5.
[69] Yang W, Li C, Ward DM, *et al.* Defective organellar membrane protein trafficking in Ap3b1-deficient cells. J Cell Sci 2000; 113: 4077-86.

[70] Kantheti P, Qiao X, Diaz ME, *et al.* Mutation in AP-3 delta in the mocha mouse links endosomal transport to storage deficiency in platelets, melanosomes, and synaptic vesicles. Neuron 1998; 21: 111-22.

[71] Feng L, Seymour AB, Jiang S, *et al.* The beta3A subunit gene (Ap3b1) of the AP-3 adaptor complex is altered in the mouse hypopigmentation mutant pearl, a model for Hermansky-Pudlak syndrome and night blindness. Hum Mol Genet 1999; 8: 323-30.

[72] Drasbek KR, Holm MM, Delenclos M, *et al.* Mapping of the spontaneous deletion in the Ap3d1 gene of mocha mice: fast and reliable genotyping. BMC Res Notes 2008; 1: 119.

[73] Jung KK, Liu XW, Chirco R, *et al.* Identification of CD63 as a tissue inhibitor of metalloproteinase-1 interacting cell surface protein. Embo J 2006; 25: 3934-42.

CHAPTER 7

Amelogenin: Possible Roles in Regeneration of Tooth Supporting Tissues, in Long Bone and During Embryonic Craniofacial Complex Development

Dan Deutsch*, Amir Haze, Yael Gruenbaum-Cohen, Shay Sharon, Dekel Shilo, Nechama C. Silverstein and Anat Blumenfeld

Dental Research Laboratory, Institute of Dental Sciences, Faculty of Dental Medicine, Hebrew University - Hadassah, Jerusalem, Israel; Tel: +972-2-6758565, Fax: +972-2-6757307, Zip Code 91120; Email: dddan@cc.huji.ac.il

Abstract: For decades, the amelogenins which comprise 90% of the developing extracellular enamel matrix proteins were known to be exclusively expressed in ectodermal enamel and play a major role in its structural organization and biomineralization. In more recent years other roles for amelogenin have been discovered. This manuscript focuses on amelogenins possible roles during regeneration of tooth supporting tissues, in normal long bone, and during development of the embryonic craniofacial complex; A single recombinant human amelogenin protein ($rHAM^+$), induced *in-vivo* regeneration of all tooth-supporting (periodontal) tissues after creation of experimental periodontitis. Amelogenin recruited (directly or indirectly) mesenchymal stem cells during periodontal regeneration. Amelogenin beads applied on developing embryonic mesenchyme and tooth germ recruited mesenchymal cells. Amelogenin was expressed in normal and regenerating alveolar bone cells (osteocytes, osteoblasts and osteoclasts), periodontal ligament, cementum and bone marrow stromal cells. Amelogenin was also expressed in long bone, periosteum, articular cartilage and differentially in ephyphysial growth plate cells. Amelogenin expression was highest in areas of high bone turnover and remodeling in normal and regenerating tissues. Spatio-temporal expression of amelogenin during embryonic craniofacial development is dynamic. These results and accumulating reports suggest that amelogenin participates in regulation of some developmental processes, acts as a signaling molecule affecting both normal and regenerating tissues, and is involved in maintaining the balance between bone formation and resorption. The pattern of amelogenin expression and the induction of periodontal regeneration, possibly offer future treatment to some widespread periodontal, bone, ligament and joint diseases, which are of major clinical, scientific and financial challenges.

Key Words: Amelogenin, Periodontal Regeneration, Long Bone, Soft Tissues, Alveolar Bone, Recruitment, Mesenchymal Stem Cells, Craniofacial Embryonic Development

For over four decades amelogenin was considered as a specific enamel protein. Enamel, is an ectodermal tissue covering vertebrate teeth. Mature enamel is composed of highly organized tightly packed hydroxy-apatite crystallites. The major enamel proteins produced during enamel development by the ameloblast cells (a specialized cell layer of the enamel organ) are the amelogenins. They comprise 90% of the developing extracellular enamel matrix proteins [1] and play a major role in the biomineralization and structural organization of enamel. Amelogenins are hydrophobic molecules that self-assemble *in vitro* and *in vivo* into nanospheric structures which regulate the oriented and elongated growth, shape and size of the enamel mineral crystal [2] [3] [4] [5] [6]. During enamel development and mineralization, the abundant secreted amelogenins in the extracellular enamel are sequentially and discretely degraded by specific proteases, the metalloprotease MMP20 (Enamelysin) [7] [8] [9] and the serine protease KLK4 (EMSP1) [10] [8] [9]. Other enamel extracellular matrix proteins include: ameloblastin, enamelin, tuftelin, dentin phosphoprotein (DPP) and amelotin. These proteins have been implicated in various steps of enamel formation.

The enamel matrix proteins undergo post-translational modifications and post-secretory processing [11] [12]. These factors, as well as alternative mRNA splicing [13], give rise to the heterogeneous mixture of polypeptides in the enamel extracellular matrix. The amelogenins are eventually, together with other enamel matrix proteins, replaced by mineral ions, calcium and phosphorus, the enamel finally becoming hard, fully mineralized (96%) and mature [14].

While the role of amelogenin in ectodermal enamel has become clearer, with the accumulating data over the past 40 years, its role(s) in cells of other mesenchymal mineralizing tissues and in soft tissues, is still to be established.

The amelogenin sequence is highly conserved throughout species and evolution [15]. The human amelogenin gene has been mapped to Xp22.1-p22.3 and Yp11.2, with 90% of the transcripts expressed from the X chromosome [16]. However, in some species, such as mouse, the amelogenin gene maps only to the X chromosome [17] [18]. The gene was known for years to contain 7 exons, which undergo extensive alternative mRNA splicing [19] [20] [21]. Later, two additional exons downstream of exon 7 (exons 8 and 9) have been identified in rare, alternatively spliced RNA transcripts of mouse amelogenin [22] [23] [24]. In mouse, for example, 16 different mRNA isoforms have been identified [13]. The most abundant isoform of the native protein secreted into the enamel matrix lacks the internal region encoded by exon 4, and [16]. This isoform is termed M180 in the mouse and HX175 in humans. The relatively large number of amelogenin alternatively spliced mRNA isoforms, code for several proteins which undergo post-translational modifications and post-secretory processing. These amelogenins have different structures and characteristics, which possibly reflect different functions of amelogenin [20] [25] [26] [27].

In human, mutations in the X-chromosomal copy of the amelogenin gene *AMELX* have been associated with the hereditary disease Amelogenesis Imperfecta [28]the most common genetic disorder affecting enamel [29] [30]. Defective enamel formation has also been demonstrated by knock-down of amelogenin expression using antisense oligonucleotides [31], ribozymes [32] and in amelogenin knock-out and transgenic mice, which resulted in enamel characteristic of hypoplastic amelogenesis imperfecta, with reduced enamel thickness [33]. A single amelogenin protein, M180, as well as the small amelogenin isoform LRAP, each was able to cause a significant rescue of the amelogenin null dental enamel phenotype [34] [35].

In 2001, the only phenotype described for the amelogenin KO mouse was of abnormal enamel formation. As often happens, additional, different phenotypes of the amelogenin null mouse were later described. A progressive deterioration of cementum (a mineralized tissue covering the tooth root surface) was observed in the amelogenin null mouse. The defects in cementum were characterized by increased presence of osteoclasts, and were also associated with an increased expression of receptor activator of nuclear factor-κB ligand (RANKL) near the cementum. RANKL is produced by osteoblasts and bone marrow stromal cells and interacts by cell-to-cell contact with its receptor RANK on the osteoclast precursors, promoting osteocalstogenesis [36]. This result suggests that amelogenin is a negative regulator of osteoclastogenesis through the RANKL/RANK mediated pathway [36] [37] [38]. Interestingly, *in vivo* application of amelogenin suppresses root resorption [39]. In 2006, an additional phenotypic defect was published: the weight of the null mouse was significantly reduced compared to the wild type; at birth the wild type and null mice were of equal weight, thereafter, from day 1 to 21, the wild type mice weighed significantly more at each time point than the null mice of the same age [24]. Detailed changes in other tissues such as long bone, and tissues of the cranio-facial complex, have not been reported, perhaps because the focus of studies was mainly on the tooth. These findings in the amelogenin knockout mice and accumulating mutations in AMELX, causing amelogenesis imperfecta, illustrates the importance of amelogenin in developing enamel and the surrounding tooth supporting tissues.

In the past decades many studies in the field of molecular biology and biochemistry, have described the function of amelogenin in structural organization and biomineralization of enamel; in controlling the size, shape and direction of formation of the enamel mineral crystallites [3] [5]. However, in the last 10 years, amelogenin has also been implicated in dentinogenesis; several specific amelogenin isoforms have been found in dentin matrix [40] and in odontoblasts [41] [42]. In cementogenesis, several reports suggest the expression of amelogenin in remnants of Hertwig's epithelial root sheath and in the periodontal ligament (PDL) cells [36] [43] [37] [44] [45] [46] [47].

Cell signaling functions have been attributed to amelogenin low-mass isoforms such as LRAP (leucine-rich amelogenin protein, composed of exons 1,2,3,5,6d,7, also termed [A-4] and M59), [A+4] (composed of exons 1,2,3,4,6d,7, also termed M73), and to the amelogenin degradation product TRAP (Tyrosine rich amelogenin peptide), [40] [20] [44] [42] [48] [49]. LRAP and [A+4] have signaling activity mainly related to osteo-chondrogenesis *in vitro* and *in vivo*. When LRAP and [A+4] were implanted into mouse oral mucosa they recruited, among inflammatory cells, mesenchymal progenitors that eventually differentiated into osteo-chondrogenic cells. The *in vivo* implants were infiltrated by cells, became vascularized, and formed islands of extracellular matrix [50]. LRAP and [A+4] were shown to have different signaling effects on ameloblast and odontoblast differentiation in a developing tooth culture model [42] [46] and when implanted in the pulp [44]. LRAP was shown to induce ectopic bone formation, possibly by cell signaling [20]. It induced osteogenesis in various cell types including rat muscle fibroblasts [50], mouse cementoblasts [51] mouse oral mucosa cells [42] and mouse embryonic stem cells [47]. Properties related to intracellular signaling have been reported for LRAP, as gene expression changes were observed when it was added to organ or cell culture or injected into tissues [52] [51] [53] [49] [46] [54] [55].

The first cell surface receptor for LRAP was identified as LAMP-1 [56] [54]. Later, the most abundant full length amelogenin isoform lacking exon 4 (M180) and LRAP were found to bind to LAMP-1, as well as LAMP-2 and CD63, also called LAMP-3 [57]. LAMP-1 and LAMP-2 are ubiquitously expressed lysosomal integral membrane proteins which are also localized to the plasma membrane and function in the endocytic system. CD63 is a member of the tetraspanin superfamily. Tetraspanins mediate signal transduction events that play a role in the regulation of cell development, growth, mobility and activation. LAMP-3 localizes to late endosomes, lysosomes and secretary vesicles, and is also expressed in the plasma membrane of most cell types. The exact binding regions of these 3 proteins for specific amelogenin (LRAP and M180) sequences were reported [57]. Exogenously added M180 amelogenin moves rapidly into established CD63 positive vesicles that subsequently localize to the perinuclear region of the cell. Also, amelogenins included in Emdogain^{R} and are recognized by antibodies against M180, move into LAMP-1 established positive vesicles that subsequently localize to the perinuclear region of the cell [58]. More recently, [59], showed that LAMP-1, which is the receptor for LRAP, does not affect M180 amelogenin uptake. M180 binds to CD63/LAMP-3 and concentrates in vesicles at the perinuclear region of the cell. Overexpression of CD63 resulted in significantly greater uptake of amelogenin, which also concentrates at the perinuclear region, while blocking CD63 by anti-LAMP-3 antibody decreased M180 amelogenin uptake, but did not affect amelogenin mRNA induction by the exogenously added amelogenin protein, a phenomenon previously shown by the same group [60]. Hence, Xu et al. 2008, concluded that LAMP3 is probably related to amelogenin M180 degradation, and as yet unknown receptor is involved with amelogenin protein-mediated amelogenin mRNA induction. Xu et al. 2008, also proposed that LAMP1 may function as a specific, endocytosing ligand binding receptor for LRAP, that may also be involved in the trafficking of LRAP to late endosomes or lysosomes. We still don't know what is the reason and function for amelogenin concentration at the perinuclear region, and how amelogenin (LRAP and M180) exert their signaling activity.

Regeneration of mesenchymal mineralizing tissues affected by chronic diseases comprises major scientific and clinical challenges. Periodontal diseases are prevalent diseases and are substantial public health burden world wide. They involve the chronic and progressive destruction of the tooth supporting tissues, mainly the alveolar bone, periodontal ligament (PDL) and cementum, which attaches the tooth to the alveolar bone of the jaw. These diseases often lead to tooth loss.

A major discovery was made, when in 1997, Hammarstrom *et al.,* showed for the first time that application of acidic extract of enamel matrix proteins (mainly hydrophobic proteins), extracted from porcine developing teeth, can induce regeneration of the periodontal tissues. This was the basis for the development of the FDA approved medical device termed Emdogain^{R}.

The novel idea that enamel matrix proteins could induce periodontal regeneration emerged from observations on normal and pathologic tooth development. Before its breakdown, the HERS secretes enamel matrix proteins, which induce the formation of cementum, followed by periodontal ligament and alveolar bone formation. Cementum is a normal constituent of the dental crown in herbivorous, where it covers the enamel. Some of these animals have continuously growing teeth or very long crowns and short roots. In these situations, the cementum assists both in the attachment of the tooth and as a forming part of the grinding occlusal surface. The coronal cementum is formed shortly after the completion of the secretory stage of the ameloblasts. The sequence of events seems to break the continuity of the covering epithelium through an apoptotic process, resulting in exposure of the enamel matrix to the cells of the dental sac (follicle). These mesenchymal cells then differentiate into cementoblasts and start forming the cementum. Studies on developing rat molars, which normally have no coronal cementum, have shown that pathological and artificial removal of the maturing enamel organ and exposure of the enamel matrix to the follicular cells resulted in the formation of a cementum-like tissue on the surface of the enamel matrix [61] [62]. Hammarstrom *et al.* suggested that application of acidic extract of enamel matrix proteins has the ability to regenerate the periodontal tissues by mimicking the normal periodontal development process.

The enamel matrix proteins (EMPs) are comprised of a heterogeneous mixture of many polypeptides encoded by several genes [63] [64]. It was not clear, however, which of the enamel matrix proteins comprising the acidic extract used for induction of the periodontal regeneration is the active component, since this extract contains also several non-amelogenin proteins. Also, the molecular mechanisms involved in the regeneration process were not clear [65].

The heterogeneity of the enamel matrix makes isolation and purification of sufficiently large quantities of any one of the proteins from this tissue, extremely challenging, since trace amount of other proteins will always exist in the enriched, purified fraction. In the past, expression of recombinant amelogenin proteins has been reported in prokaryotic system [66] [67] [68]. These recombinant amelogenin proteins have been used in various structural and functional studies [69] [70]. We expressed, for the first time, a recombinant human amelogenin protein in eukaryotic (not bacterial) cells using a recombinant baculovirus, containing only the human amelogenin cDNA (no use of other cDNAs, or amelogenin protein or any other enamel matrix protein). The baculovirus expression system has a number of potential benefits, including high levels of expression, correct folding and post-translational modification, and production of biologically active proteins for analysis. In addition, since one of our main reasons for producing the recombinant amelogenin protein was for *in vivo* studies, we preferred to use the baculovirus system, to avoid the necessity for testing and removal of endotoxin that may contaminate prokaryotic (*E. coli*) products.

As described above, we produced, expressed and characterized the recombinant human amelogenin protein (HX175, $rHAM^+$), which corresponds to M180 in mouse (both lacking exon 4), in the eukaryotic baculovirus system in quantities sufficient for structural, functional and regenerative studies. $rHAM^+$ was characterized by SDS–PAGE, Western blot, ESI-TOF spectrometry, peptide mapping, and MS/MS sequencing. Production of pure, full-length amelogenin opened up the possibility to investigate novel functions of amelogenin [71].

We tested the possibility that a single application of $rHAM^+$ alone, could bring about the regeneration of the tooth supporting tissues (periodontium) after induction of experimental periodontitis in the dog [27]. The results showed (Figure 1) that application of $rHAM^+$ alone, brought about significant and progressive (up to 8 weeks – the end of the study) regeneration of all three periodontal tissues; alveolar bone, PDL and cementum (Figures 1, 2) [27]. The regeneration process mimics the normal pattern of periodontal development: in which the cementum is first produced, in the youngest regenerated tissue, followed by the PDL and alveolar bone, producing a functional periodontium (Figure 2). Electron micrographs of the regenerated cementum and PDL showed that the structure of the PDL Sharpey's fibers, penetrated into the regenerated cementum, as in normal functional periodontium (Figure 2D). The single application of $rHAM^+$ caused massive recruitment of MSCs into the regenerating site, already at two weeks, when the regeneration process was detectable. The expression of two markers of MSCs - CD105 and STRO-1 was significantly higher in the granulation tissue, PDL, bone and bone marrow at the regenerated regions as compared to control (Figure 3, Haze et al. 2009). The regeneration process progressively increased up to the end of the experiment (8 weeks). By that time, some of the MSCs already differentiated to form the periodontal tissues, and their count was reduced. We also noticed increased vascularization of the regenerating bone and elevated amelogenin expression in cells surrounding blood vessels, as compared to control (Figure 4). We therefore, identified the human amelogenin protein HX175, that corresponds to mouse M180, as an active component of the EMP which is responsible, directly or indirectly, for the regeneration of the tooth-supporting tissues. This does not exclude the possibility that other components of the EMPs also contribute to the regeneration process.

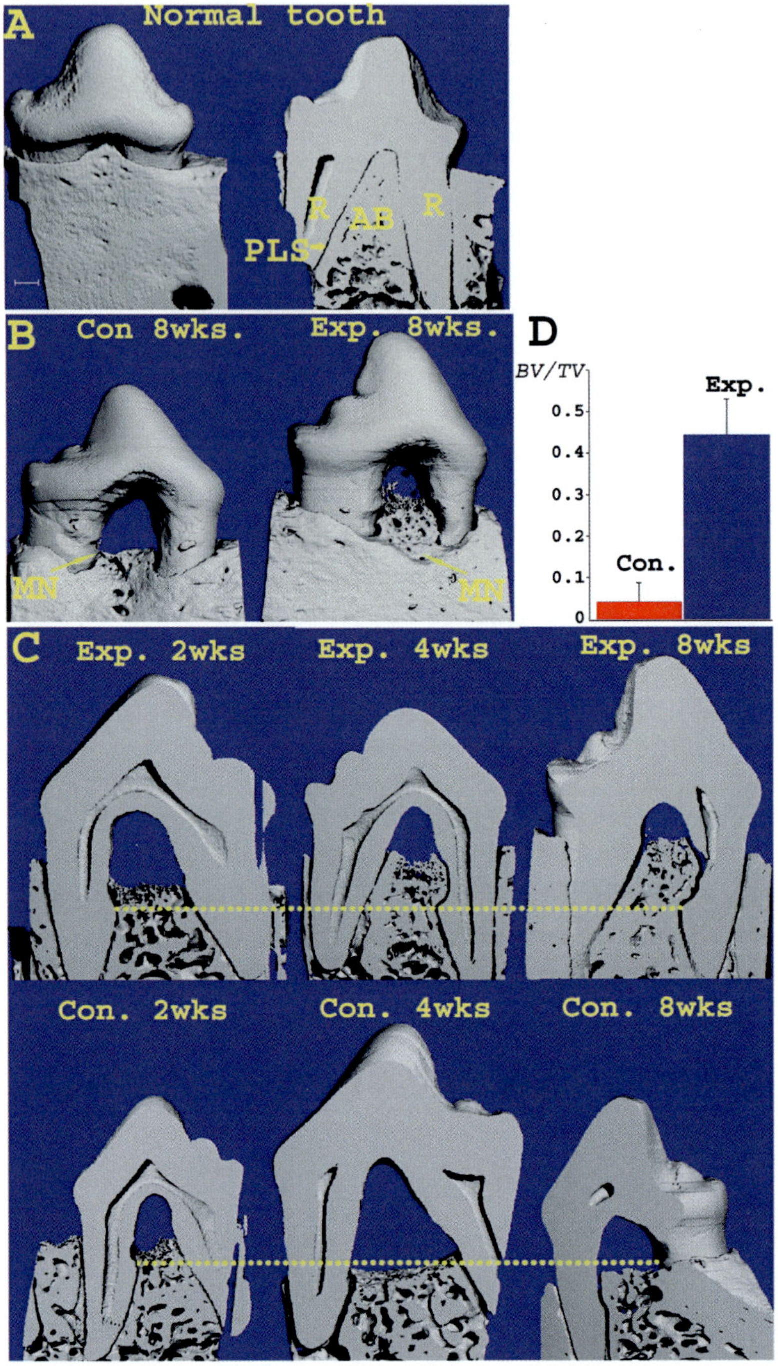

Figure 1: A: 3-dimensional reconstruction of micro-CT scans of normal dog tooth, without any treatment, and a micro-CT cross section of the tooth. (R-root, PLS-periodontal ligament space, AB- alveolar bone) (bar = 1mm). B: 3-dimensional reconstruction of micro-CT scans, 8 weeks after application of rHAM+ in PGA carrier (Exp.) or PGA carrier only (Con.). The yellow arrows points to the marking notches, indicating the bone height at the time of application of rHAM+ or PGA, respectively. C: Coronal micro-CT cross-sections of the 3D image of the experimental and control teeth 2, 4 and 8 weeks after treatment. The yellow line connects the marking notches. In the experimental tissues the regeneration started at 2 weeks, after 4 and 8 weeks there is significant and progressive regeneration. In the control almost no regeneration is seen. D: Statistical analysis of regenerated Bone-Volume (BV) divided by Total-Volume of the furcation (TV) (above the marking notch and between the tooth roots) 4 and 8 weeks (pooled results) after treatment with rHAM+ in PGA carrier (Exp.) or PGA carrier alone (Con.), P-value<0.002. Reproduced from Haze et al. 2009.

Formation, remodeling and regeneration of tissues generally require recruitment of different types of multipotent cells. Stem cells of all types are characterized by their self-renewal ability through asymmetric division, and the ability to give rise to differentiating cells, both *in vivo* and *in vitro*. In response to specific factors and signals, adult MSCs from different sources have the potential to differentiate into multiple phenotypes including muscle, bone, cementum, cartilage, fat, tendon, ligament and nerve [72] [73] Lee *at al.* 2008 meaning that cells derived from one tissue could be used to form a different tissue.

The origin of the mesenchymal stem / progenitor cells recruited during periodontal tissues regeneration could be the adjacent, native periodontal tissues or bone marrow cells. King and Hughes [74] demonstrated, in the periodontal regeneration model, migration of cells from the adjacent unwounded PDL into the wounded area. Kawaguchi [75] showed that bone marrow stromal cells have the potential to regenerate the periodontium.

Interesting in this respect, our preliminary results indicate that application of rHAM$^+$ to critical size calvarial defect, also a membranous bone, brought about regeneration of the defect (unpublished)

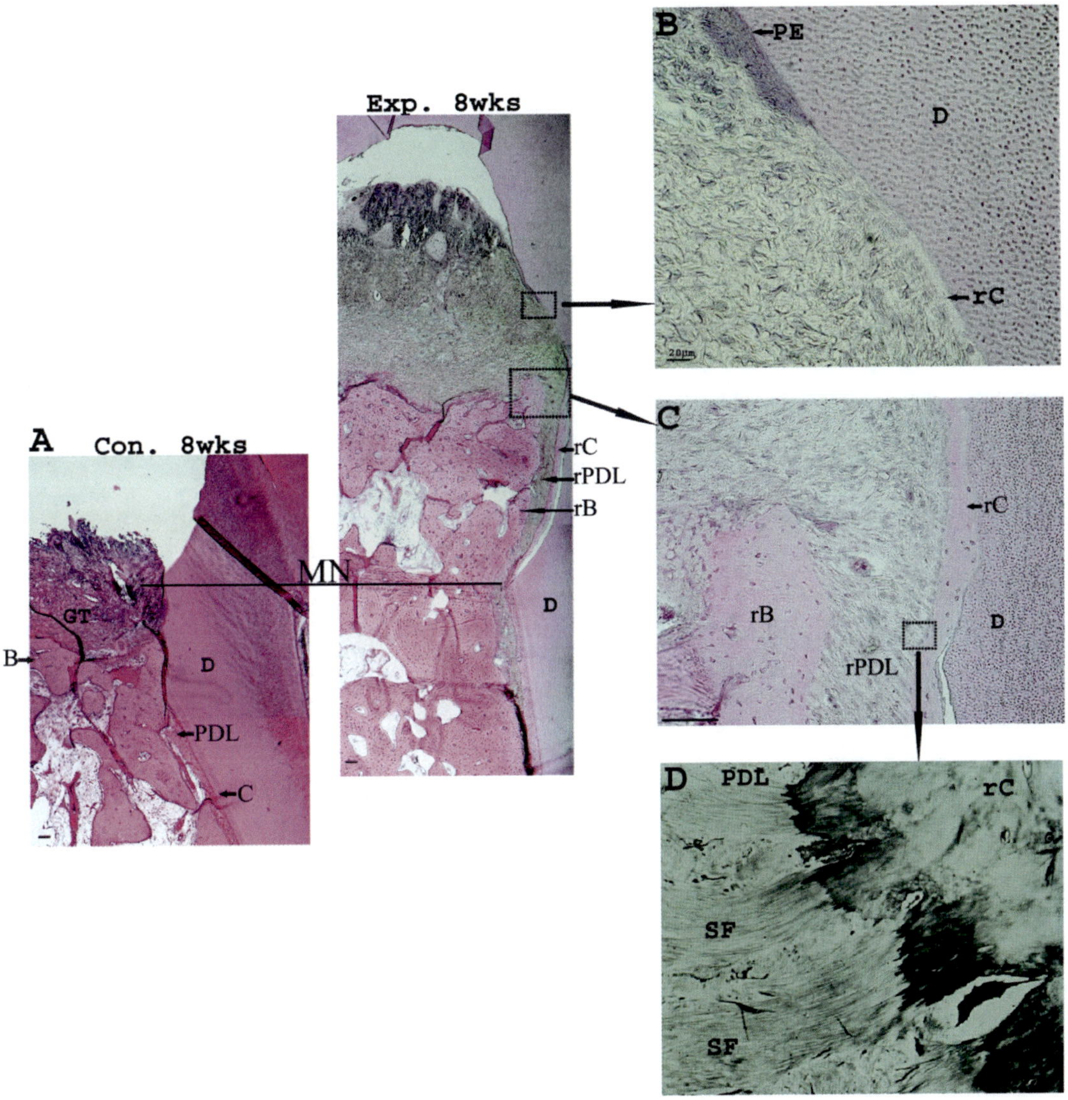

Figure 2: A: Histological pictures of the dog experimental tooth and dog control tooth 8 weeks after treatment with rHAM$^+$ in PGA carrier (Exp.) or PGA carrier alone (Con.) (PDL = Periodontal ligament, D = Dentin, GT = Granulation tissue, MN = Marking Notch, r = regenerated, B = Bone, C = Cementum, bar = 100μm). B: Higher magnification (bar = 20μm) of the regenerating front showing the penetrating oral epithelium (PE) from above and the ascending regenerating cementum from below. Organized PDL and bone are not apparent yet. C: Enlargement of the regenerated area (bar = 100μm) showing newly regenerated cementum, PDL and bone (lower part – C2). In the younger regenerating area (upper part – C1), only organized regenerating cementum and PDL are apparent. D: Electron microscopy micrograph of the experimental tooth after treatment with rHAM$^+$ shows regenerated Sharpey's fibers anchoring the regenerated PDL to the newly regenerated cementum (Zimmermann B., Bernimoulin J.P. Haegewald S. and Deutsch D.). Modified from Haze et al. 2009.

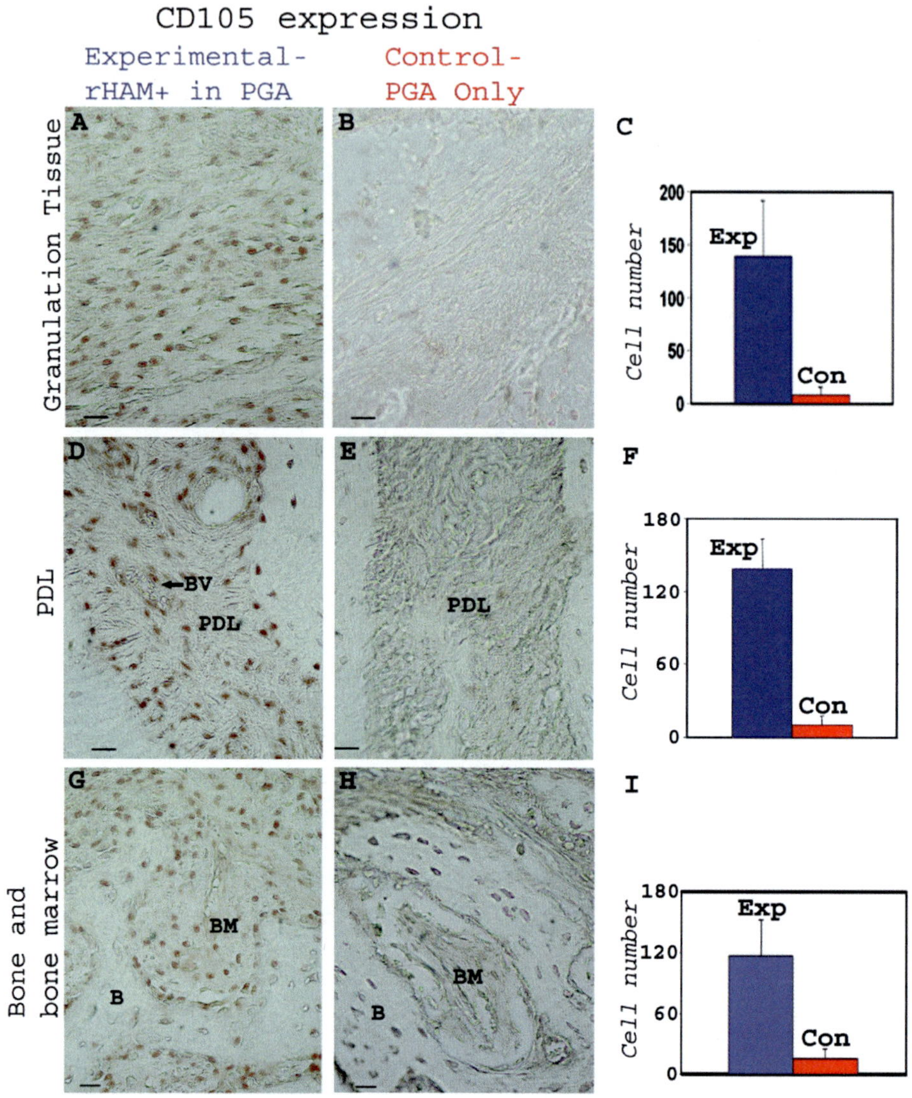

Figure 3: Immunohistochemical analysis of dog periodontal tissues comparing the number of cells expressing CD105 (Endoglin) in teeth two weeks after treatment with $rHAM^{+}$ dissolved in PGA, with the control, two weeks after treatment with PGA carrier only. CD105 expression, using polyclonal antibody, in the A: granulation tissue, D: PDL, G: alveolar bone (B) and bone marrow (BM) of the experimental tooth. CD105 expression in the B: granulation tissue, E: PDL, H: alveolar bone (B) and bone marrow (BM) of the control tooth. Statistical analysis comparing the average number of cells expressing CD105 in the C: granulation tissue, F: PDL, I: bone and bone marrow cells of the experiment tooth with the control tooth, two weeks after the treatment. Many more cells expressing CD105 were observed in the experimental tooth; in the granulation tissue, periodontal ligament, and in bone and bone marrow cells as compared to control. BV = blood vessel. Reproduced from Haze et al. 2009.

CD105 (also termed Endoglin) is a cell membrane glycoprotein (TGFβ receptor) and is considered as a marker for bone marrow mesenchymal stem cells (MSCs) [76] [77] [78] [79] [80] [81] [82]. Aslan *et al.* [82] immunoisolated CD105 positive MSCs and demonstrated that they can differentiate into osteogenic, chondrogenic, and adipogenic lineages. CD105 positive cells are also detected within the vascular system, and CD105 is also one of the markers for neovascularization [83] [84]. Several studies have also used STRO-1 as a marker for bone marrow stromal stem cells [76] [85] [86] [87] [88] [89]. Dennis *et al.* showed that STRO-1 positive cells have the ability to differentiate into myofibroblasts with a vascular smooth muscle phenotype, adipocytes, osteoblasts and chondrocytes [86]. The over-expression of CD105 and STRO-1 in the regenerating tissues, suggests that amelogenin promotes the regeneration not only by local mesenchymal stem / progenitor cells recruitment, but also perhaps by inducing, directly or indirectly, angiogenesis for metabolic support of the developing tissues. These findings correlate with the observations of rich vascularization of the regenerating tissues, and amelogenin expression in cells normally surrounding blood vessels (Figure 4, Haze, et al. 2009). The cells surrounding regenerated blood vessels might be pericytes, which are involved in regulating angiogenesis and can differentiate, along several lineages including osteogenic and chondrogenic phenotypes [75]. The finding that amelogenin promotes angiogenesis in the regenerating tissues explains Collett [90] and Yuan *et al.* [91] *in-vivo* and *in-vitro* findings demonstrating chemotaxis of endothelial cells and induction of blood vessel formation by enamel matrix proteins. As discussed above, ectopic application of LRAP to rat muscle induced mesenchymal cells in-growth into the implants followed by vascularization [20]. Recently, the use of amelogenin protein (Xelma, Mölnlycke Health Care) in the treatment of hard to heal wounds such as venous leg ulcers in elder and diabetic patients was described [92] [93].

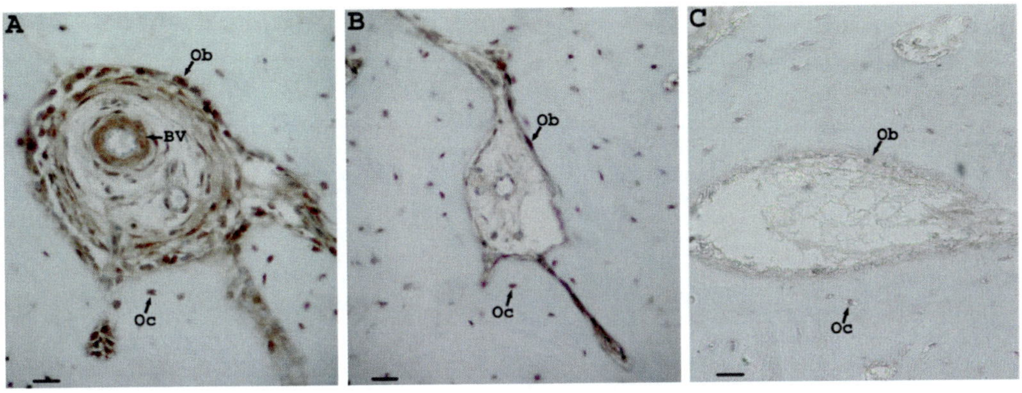

Figure 4: Comparison between amelogenin expression 8 weeks after treatment with $rHAM^+$, using a polyclonal amelogenin antibody. A: in dog bone cells in the regenerating area, and B: distal to the regenerating area (under the marking notch), in the same section. C: control- non-immune rabbit serum replacing the first antibody (Bar = 20µm, Ob = osteoblast, Oc = osteocyte, BV = blood vessel). Reproduced from Haze et al. 2009.

A hint on amelogenin function in the early stages of tooth and mandible development emerges from the application of amelogenin ($rHAM^+$) beads on E13.5 mouse embryonic mandibular mesenchyme, which brought about recruitment and cell movement towards the beads [94]. This observation was strengthened by the application of $rHAM^+$ beads, in combination with DiI application, on E13.5 and E14.5 embryonic incisor tooth germs mesenchymal tissue, respectively. Agarose beads containing $rHAM^+$ or PBS (control) were placed on the mesenchymal region of the incisor tooth germ of 250µm frontal sections of E14.5 mandibles. The DiI, which binds to cell membranes, revealed movement of mesenchymal cells towards the amelogenin beads, partially covering the beads after 2 and 3 days (Figure 5). No such recruitment of mesenchymal cells was detected towards the control PBS bead. Since amelogenin is endogenously expressed in these mesenchymal and tooth germ tissues at the days $rHAM^+$ beads were applied (Figure 16b), these experiments represent over-expression and not ectopic expression. The observed cell recruitment suggests a signaling function for amelogenin. This is in line with the accumulating data on the signaling function, directly or indirectly, of amelogenin ($rHAM^+$, HX175) in the regeneration of the periodontal tissues after experimental periodontitis [27]. As we described above, a cell surface receptor for amelogenin M180 (equivalent to HX175) was recently identified as CD63 (LAMP-3), [58] [57] [59] CD63 is a member of the tetraspanin superfamily which mediate signal transduction events that play a role in the regulation of cell development, growth, mobility and activation.

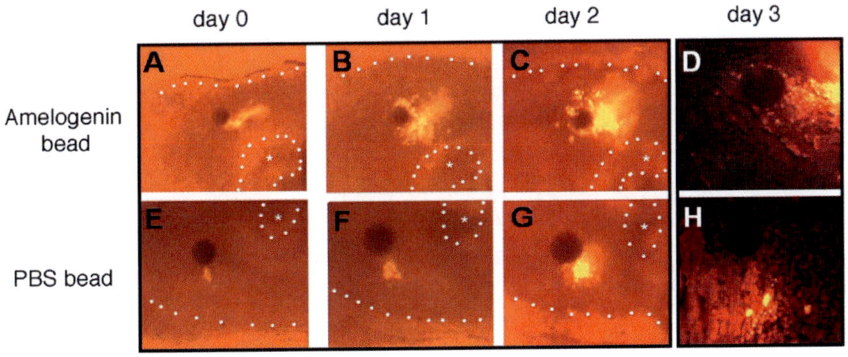

Figure 5: Movement (recruitment) of DiI – labeled mesenchymal cells in the incisor tooth germ region, towards amelogenin ($rHAM^+$) beads but not towards control PBS bead. Frontal slices through the incisor region of E14.5 mandibles cultured for three days after addition of beads. Oral and incisor epithelium are outlined in white. The mesenchyme around the incisor cap stage

tooth germs (outlined and marked by *) was labeled with DiI (orange). A-D: rHAM$^+$ bead at day 0 (A), day 1 (B), day 2 (C), day 3 (D). A-C: Merged light/dark field image of cultured slice showing DiI label moving towards and around the rHAM$^+$ bead. D: Section showing DiI cells associated with the rHAM$^+$ bead. E-H: Similar slice with a PBS (control) bead at day 0 (E), day 1 (F), day 2 (G), day 3 (H). E-G: Merged light/dark field image of cultured slice showing DiI label remaining distinct from the PBS bead. H: Section showing DiI cells not associated with the PBS bead. Reproduced from Gruenbaum-Cohen et al. 2009.

Having established the involvement of amelogenin in the regeneration of the tooth supporting tissues after induction of experimental periodontitis, we first studied the detailed expression of amelogenin in normal tissues of the periodontium, to decipher the basic mechanisms associated with the regeneration process. Amelogenin expression was detected in the cells of all tooth supporting tissues: cementum, PDL and alveolar bone, in dog, rat and human [25] [27], suggesting that application of the recombinant amelogenin protein represents over-expression rather than ectopic expression.

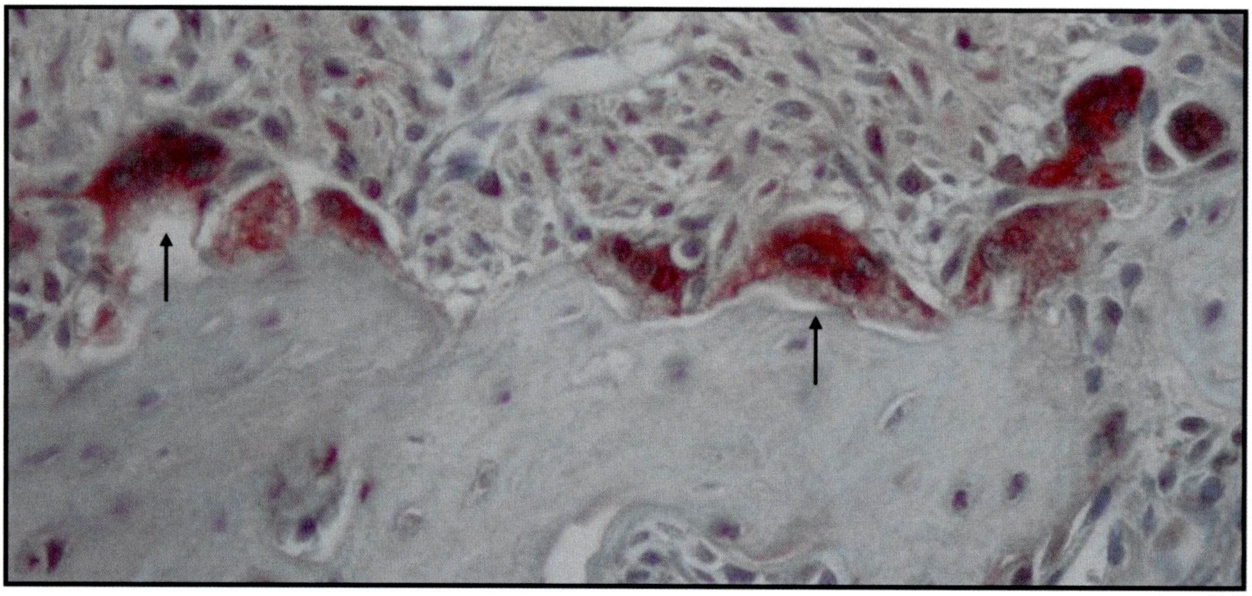

Figure 6: Amelogenin expression in rat alveolar bone ostoeclasts (Ocl) using a polyclonal amelogenin antibody.

In addition to the expression of amelogenin in the ectodermal ameloblasts and developing enamel, we found that amelogenin was also expressed in the mesenchymal cells of the alveolar bone; in osteocytes, in osteoblasts lining the alveolar bone trabecules, in cells surrounding blood vessels, in osteoclasts (Figure 6), and in few distinct bone marrow cells [27]. As was previously reported [95] [96], amelogenin expression was also detected in PDL cells and in clusters of cementoblasts along the root. The expression of amelogenin in the epithelial ameloblast cells was much higher as compared to the mesenchymal, periodontal tissues, cells [27]. The large difference in amelogenin expression could explain why the presence of amelogenin in bone and bone marrow cells was overlooked in the past. This difference in expression level might represent different role(s) for amelogenin in these tissues; in the forming (ectodermal) enamel, amelogenin serves mainly as an extracellular structural protein, while in mesenchymal cells amelogenin might be involved in signaling.

While studying amelogenin mRNA and protein expression in normal rat and dog periodontal tissues, we noticed that amelogenin expression is highest in bone cells adjacent to the PDL and in the periosteal cells, as compared to bone cells distal to the PDL and the periosteum (Figure 7, Haze et al. 2009). The bone adjacent to the PDL absorbs all the mastication forces and bone turnover and remodeling is much higher in this area, as compared to bone remote to the PDL region. In addition, the periosteum covers the actively growing bone of the jaw. It is the main site of bone growth and remodeling, and it contains mainly progenitor cells. These findings suggest that in the normal uninjured animal, amelogenin expression is increased at sites of high bone activity and remodeling. A similar phenomenon was seen in the regenerated alveolar dog bone; amelogenin was highly expressed in endosteal progenitor cells, osteoblasts, and cells surrounding blood vessels in the regenerated area, and to a much lesser extent in bone cells distal to the regenerated area [27]. Veis [50] demonstrated that amelogenin splice products, implanted ectopically into rat muscle, induced mesenchymal cells in-growth into the implants followed by vascularization, extracellular matrix production, and mineralization. These accumulating data suggest that amelogenin serves as an inducer of bone formation.

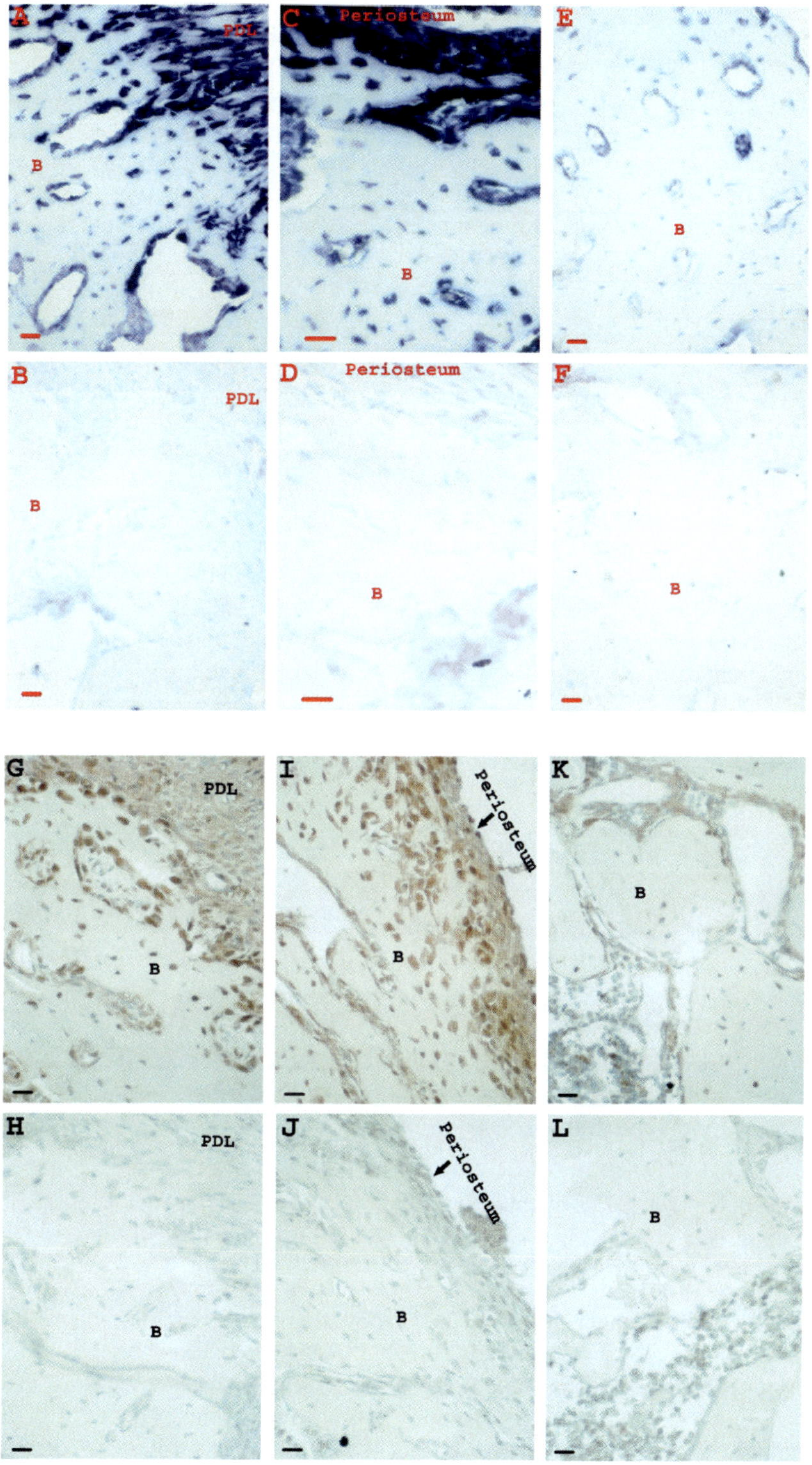

Figure 7: A-F: In situ hybridization of rat periodontal tissues using rat amelogenin probe. In the same slide, a much higher amelogenin mRNA expression was detected in bone cells adjacent to the PDL (A) and in periosteal cells (C) compared to bone cells distal to the PDL and periosteum (E). Figures B, D and F are the corresponding sense probe (controls). G-L:

Immunohistochemistry analysis using the amelogenin polyclonal antibody. Similar to the in-situ hybridization results, a much higher amelogenin protein expression was detected in bone cells adjacent to the PDL (G) and in periosteal cells (I) as compared with bone cells distal to the PDL and periosteum (K) (in the same slide). Figures H, J and L are the corresponding controls, PBS replacing the first antibody. (Bar = 20μm, B = bone). Reproduced from Haze et al. 2009.

The accumulating data indicate that amelogenin stimulates a cascade of events enhancing remodeling and regeneration of periodontal tissues. The observed regeneration of all periodontal tissues using the externally applied amelogenin, probably reflects enhancement of its normal endogenous activity in local remodeling of tissues. Amelogenin induces, directly or indirectly, mesenchymal stem / progenitor cell recruitment at the site of the injury. Application of amelogenin induces local neovascularization to support the developing tissues [27], and possibly might change the fine balance between osteoclast and osteoblast activity, favoring regeneration over the natural process of degeneration after induction of chronic periodontitis. This degeneration process is characterized by connective tissue and epithelial proliferation into the injured area, an event thought to prevent proper regeneration of the periodontal tissues [61].

We assumed that since amelogenin is expressed in tooth supporting tissue cells (cementoblasts and PDL cells) of mesenchymal origin, it might also be expressed in long bones cells, though they differ in embryonic origin and pattern of development; Long bone tissues originate from the embryonic mesoderm and not from embryonic neural crest cells, which gives rise to the mesenchymal tissues of the calvaria and tooth attachment apparatus - cementum, periodontal ligament, and alveolar bone.

Amelogenin mRNA and protein were found to be expressed in rat and dog articular cartilage chondrocytes, epiphyseal bone cells, and differentially in specific cell layers of the epiphyseal growth plate (Figure 8, Haze, et al. 2007). The epiphyseal growth plate is responsible for elongation and growth of long bones through endochondral ossification. Veis [20] showed that LRAP, a specific amelogenin splice product, induced Cbfa1 and collagen type II expression (chondrogenic and osteogenic differentiation markers) in rat muscle fibroblasts *in vitro*, indicating a possible role for amelogenin in cartilage formation and/or in its transition into bone.

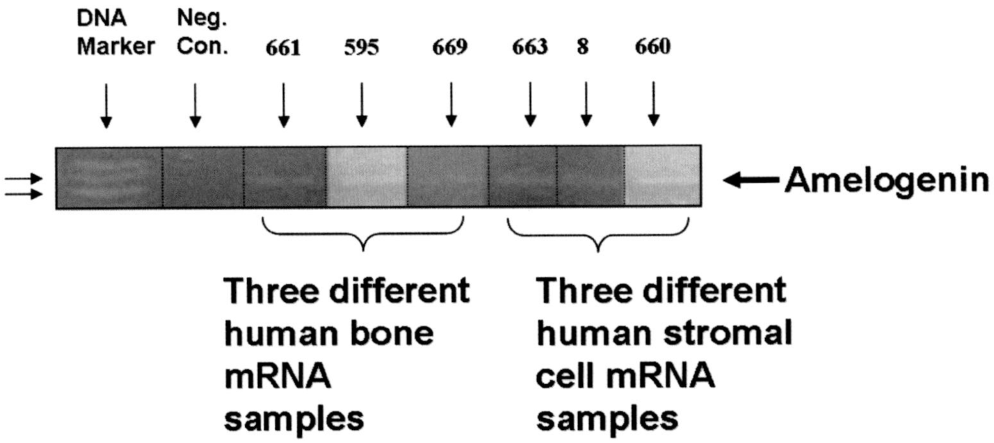

Figure 8: Amleogenin mRNA is expressed in cultured human bone cells and bone marrow stromal cells (kindly provided by M.Young, NIDCR, NIH, USA). RT-PCR and PCR amplification were performed using primers designed according to the published human amelogenin HX175 sequence (gi: 178528). The actual sequence can be seen in Haze et al. 2007.

Amelogenin mRNA (Figure 9) and protein (Figures 10-13) were also expressed in long bone periosteum (Figure 10, which is composed of progenitor cells), in rat and dog osteoblasts and osteoclasts lining the bone trabecules (Figures 10, 11) and by some osteocytes. Some of these bone cells co-express proteins specific to formation of mesenchymal mineralized tissues, such as bone sialoprotein (Figure 12 left) and osteocalcin (Figure 13). In long bone marrow (Figure 11), amelogenin was found to be expressed by distinct cells, some of them co-express CD105 (Figure 12 right), suggesting these might be mesenchymal stem cells. Amelogenin expression in osteocytes, osteoblasts, osteoclasts, bone marrow cells, and cartilage cells, together with the accumulating data indicating amelogenin induction of osteogenesis [50] and inhibition of osteoclastogenesis [36] [37], suggest that amelogenins may be essential in regulating the critical balance between osteoblastic and osteoclastic activity in bone development and remodeling, possibly through the RANKL/RANK mediated pathway [36] [37]. During alveolar bone regeneration after induced inflammation, amelogenin might act by increasing bone formation over the resorption process.

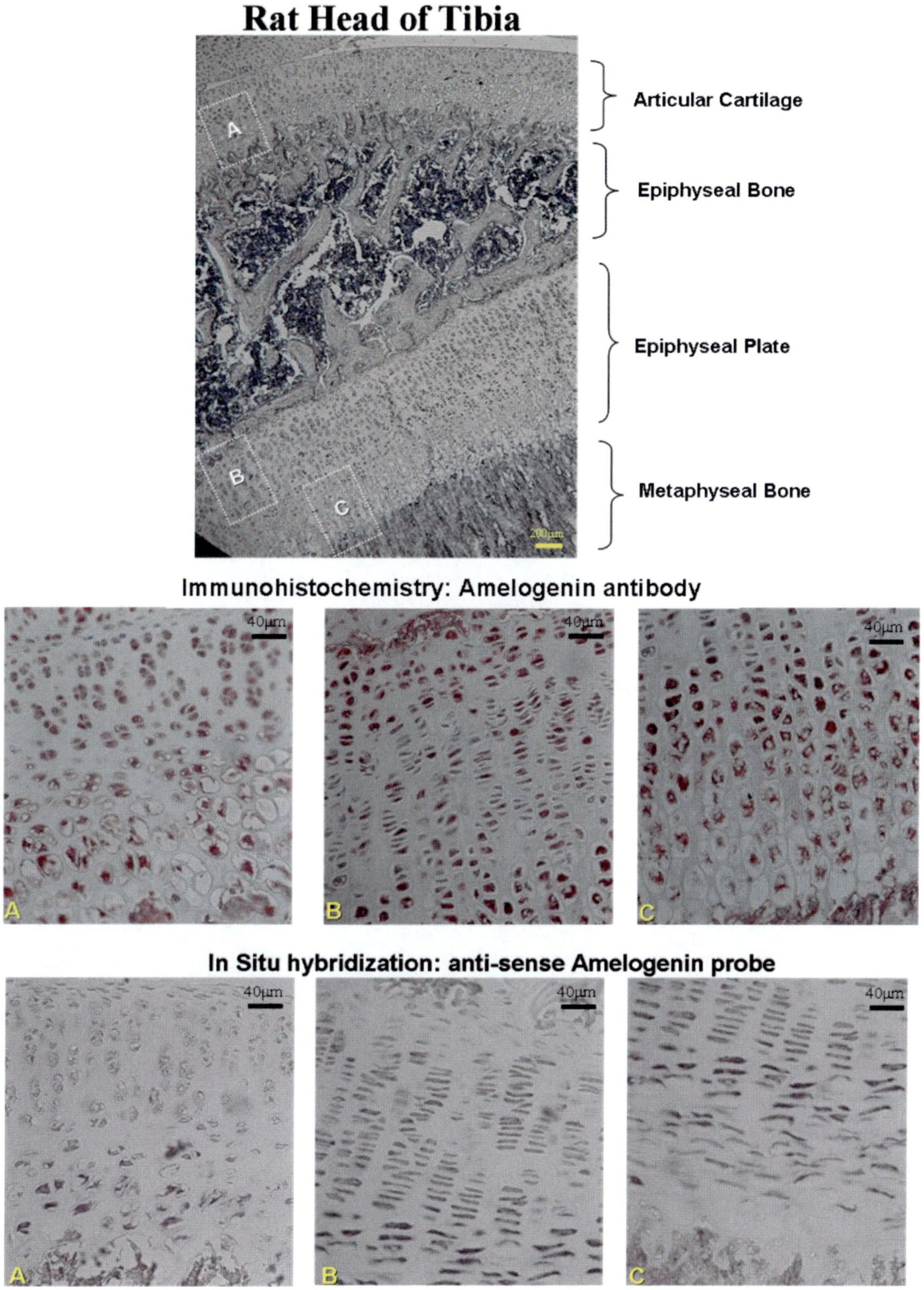

Figure 9: Amelogenin expression in the rat head of tibia, using an amelogenin monoclonal antibody. Up: the histology of the head of tibia, demonstrating the articular cartilage, epiphyseal bone, epiphyseal plate and metaphyseal bone. Amelogenin protein

expression (red) and mRNA expression (blue) is demonstrated in articular cartilage chondrocytes(A), in cells lining bone trabecules, and differentially in epiphyseal growth plate cells (B – upper part of epiphyseal growth plate and C – lower part). No staining was observed in the corresponding controls (not shown).

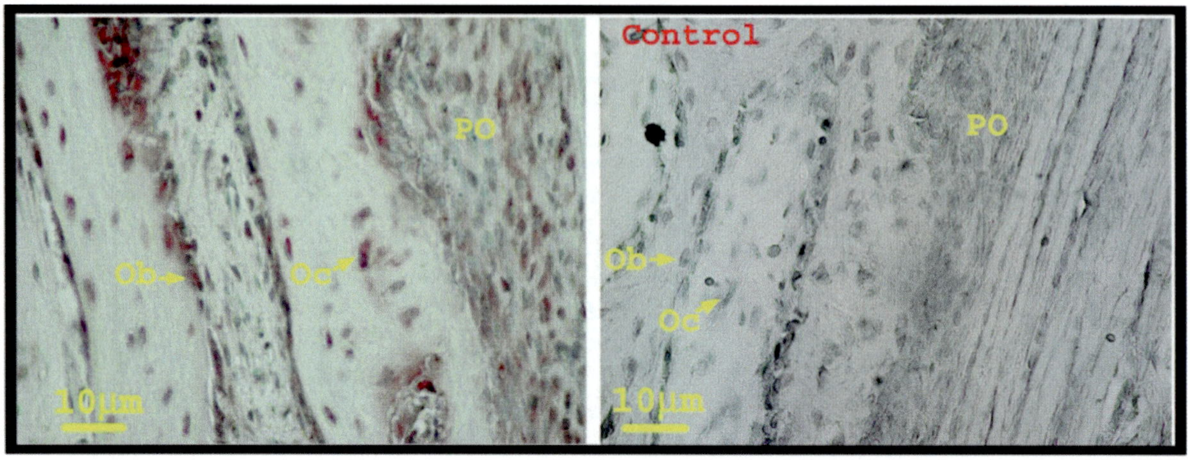

Figure 10: Immunohistochemical analysis of periosteum and bone, using amelogenin polyclonal antibody. Amelogenin expression was detected in periosteum cells, osteoblsts and osteocytes. No staining was observed in the control, non-immune serum replacing the first antibody (Bar = 10μm, periosteum cells=PO, osteoblsts=Ob, osteocytes=Oc). Reproduced from Haze et al. 2007.

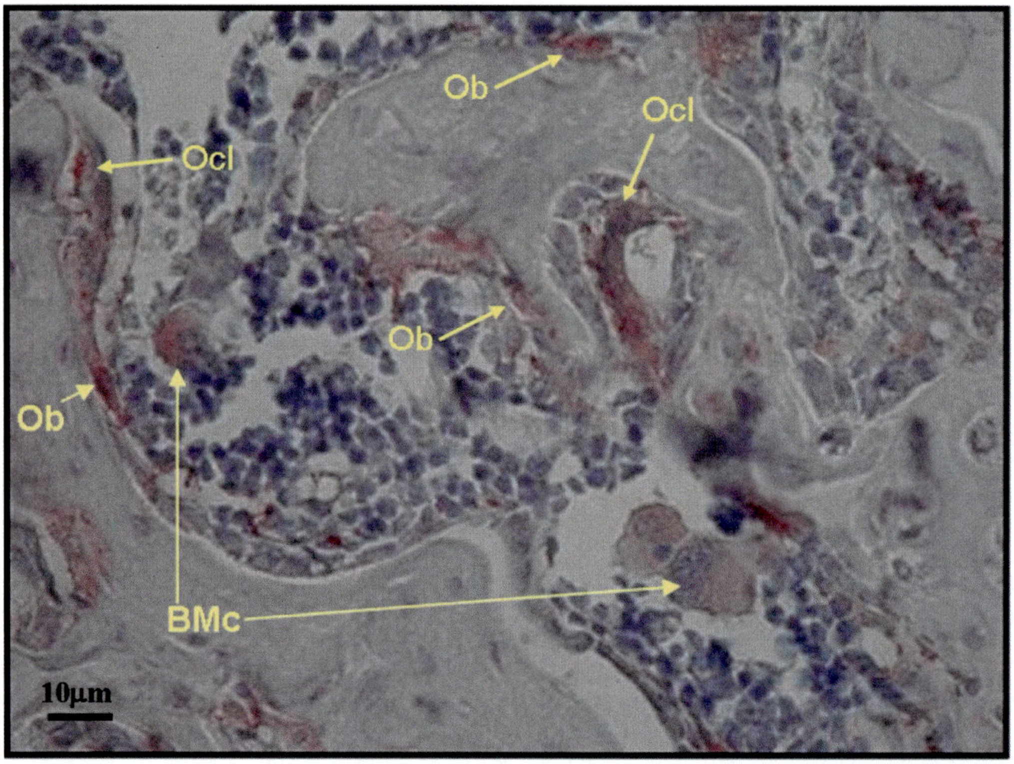

Figure 11: Amelogenin expression in rat epiphyseal bone marrow cells, using amelogenin polyclonal antibody. Amelogenin protein expression was detected in specific bone marrow cells, in osteoblasts and in osteoclasts. No staining was observed in the control, non-immune serum replacing the first antibody (not shown). (Bar = 10μm, bone marrow cells=BMc, osteoblasts=Ob, osteoclasts=Ocl). Reproduced from Haze et al. 2007.

We have identified amelogenin expression in long bone marrow cells (Figures 9, 11, 12 right), some of which are mesenchymal stem cells, and in cells surrounding blood vessels [97]. We show that some of the bone marrow cells expressing amelogenin are megakaryocytes, and hematopoietic stem cells [25]. The expression of amelogenin in macrophages and in bone osteoclasts, which both share a common monocytic progenitor cell, suggests that the common progenitor cell might also express amelogenin. Amelogenin might have a regulatory effect on the recruitment and differentiation of the monocytic cells from the bone marrow towards becoming mineralized tissue-resorbing cells (bone and cementum osteoclasts).

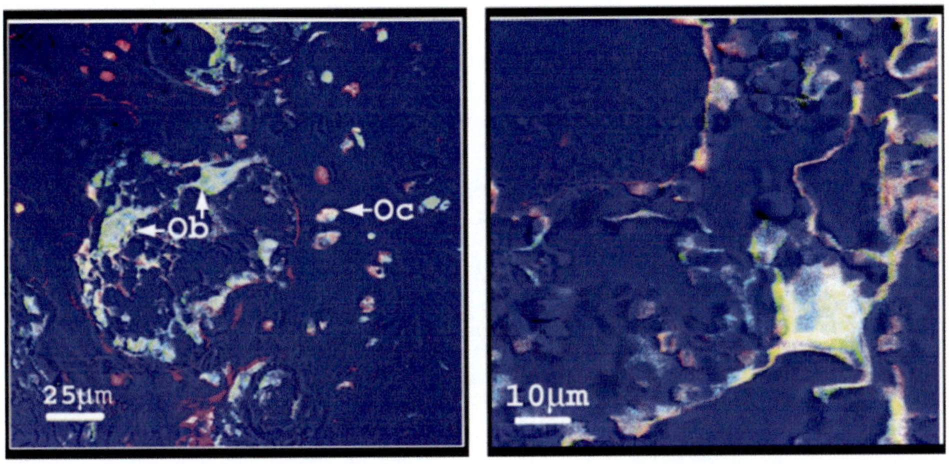

Figure 12: Left: Co-localization (yellow) of amelogenin (green) and bone sialoprotein (BSP, red), which is a mesencymal mineralized tissues cell marker, in epiphyseal trabecules (Bar = 25μm, osteoblsts=Ob, osteocytes=Oc). Right: Co-localization (yellow) of amelogenin (green) and CD105 (red) in bone marrow (Bar = 25μm). Reproduced from Haze et al. 2007.

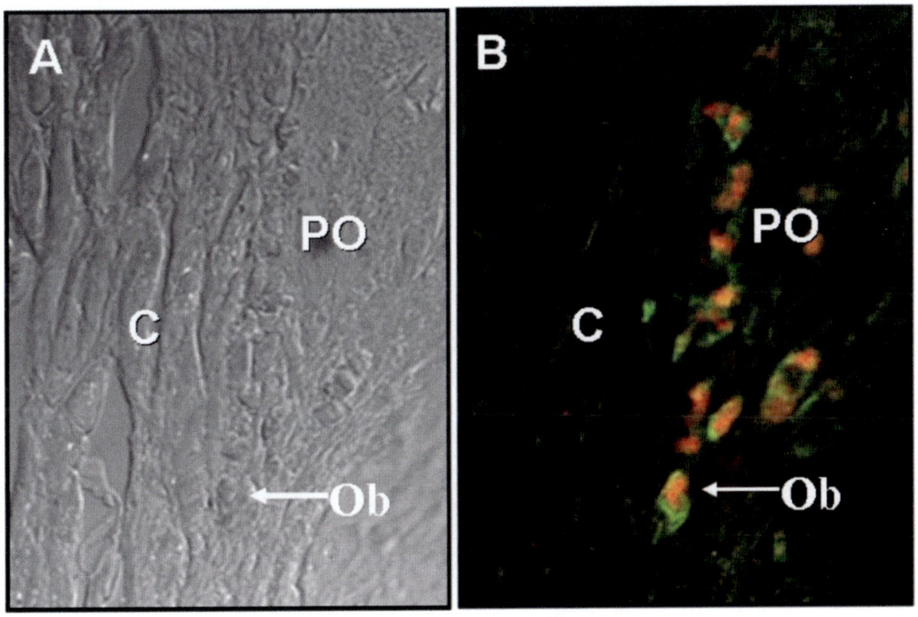

Figure 13: Co-localization (yellow) of amelogenin (green) and Osteocalcin (red) a marker for mineralizing cells in rat long bone diaphysis (C=Cortical bone, PO=Periosteum, Ob=Osteoblast).

The sequence of the full length dog amelogenin (excluding exon 4, which is equivalent to mouse M180) was identified in dog bone marrow cells, and sequence of the LRAP splice product was identified in rat bone marrow cells. Amelogenin sequences were also identified in human bone and stromal cells, which are mostly comprised of MSCs [97].

Amelogenin expression in long bone cells, long bone stromal cells, and its differential expression in the epiphyseal growth plate cells, articular cartilage cells and cells of the periosteal bone [97], suggest that long bone phenotypes should be investigated in details in families affected by X-linked Amelogenesis Imperfecta (AI) and in the amelogenin knock-out mouse.

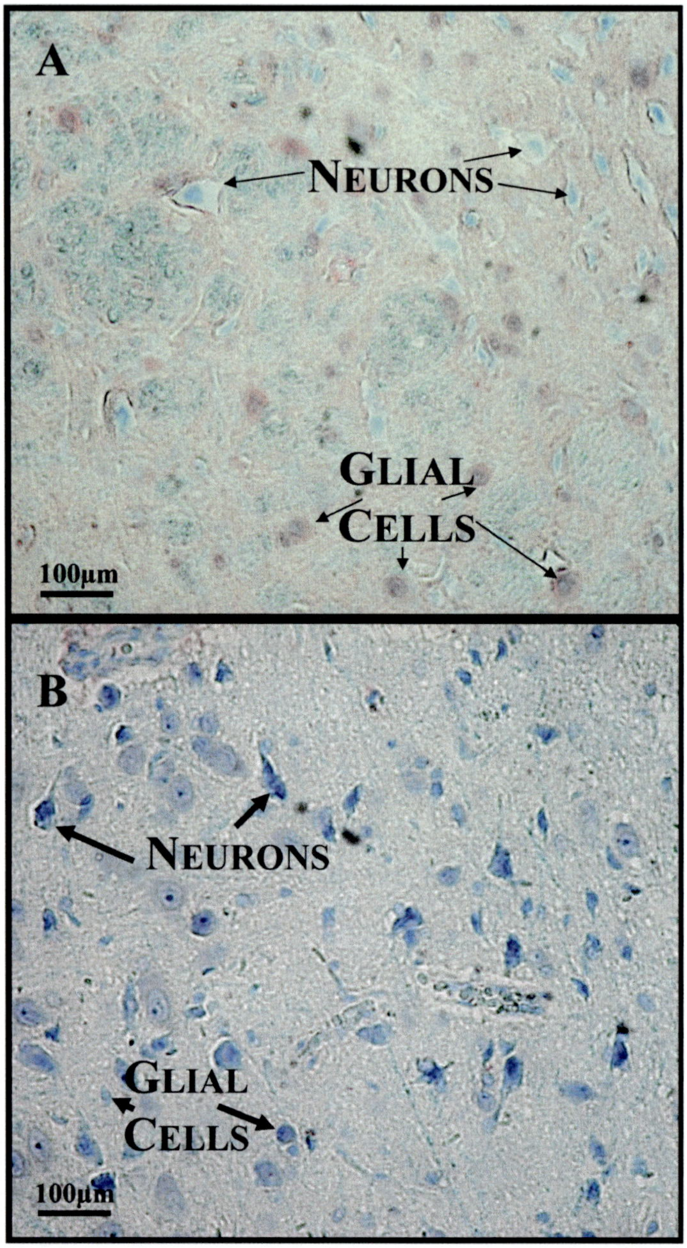

Figure 14: Immunohistochemistry of rat midbrain (transversal section) with A: rat amelogenin antibody B: control - pre-immune serum. Specific staining was observed in glial cells, while no staining of neurons was detected. (Bar = 100µm). Reproduced from Deutsch et al. 2006.

Amelogenin is also expressed in cells of non-mineralizing tissues such as the brain, specifically in the supportive, non-neuronal cells of glial origin (Figure 14). Two amelogenin transcripts were identified in the mouse midbrain (Figure 15), corresponding to the prevalent isoform M180 (full-length transcript lacking exon 4) and the rare isoform M194 (full-length transcript including exon 4). It is not clear yet what is the role of amelogenin M180 in mouse brain glial cells: it might be involved in the hydrophobic coating of neuronal axons by glial cells, functions in brain signaling, or might has a yet unknown function. The amelogenin isoform M194, which includes exon 4, is a less prevalent transcript, and might exert a different function.

M180 was identified as an EST in mouse brain pituitary gland, and amelogenin protein was also identified in salivary gland ductal cells and myoepithelial cells.

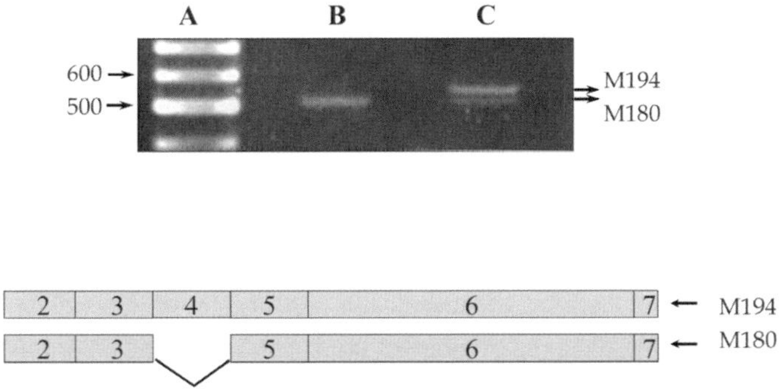

Figure 15: Amelogenin expression in brain and macrophages. RT-PCR was followed by separation a 2% agarose gel, and cDNA sequencing. (Lane B) The single cDNA band product in macrophage cell line RAW 264.7 corresponded to the mouse amelogenin M180 transcript. (Lane C) The two cDNA bands in mouse brain pons and medulla corresponded to the mouse amelogenin isoforms M180 and M194. Reproduced from Deutsch et al. 2006.

The expression of amelogenin in many different types of cells of ectodermal and mesenchymal mineralizing tissues and soft tissues [98] [1] [2] [16] [3] [14] [99] [100] [101] [102] [63] [103] [22] [40] [104] [95] [50] [4] [105] [23] [106] [36] [107] [108] [43] [20] [109] [5] [96] [41] [25] [24] [97] [27], which have distinct functions, and the striking difference in the levels of amelogenin expressed in the ameloblast cells as compared with the other mineralizing mesenchymal cell types (≈ 1000-fold higher in the ameloblast cells) [22] and other soft tissues, suggest that amelogenin has a multifunctional role.

Very few detailed studies were carried out on amelogenin expression in the cranio-facial complex during prenatal development, and these studies focused mainly on the late stages of prenatal development, just before birth, when ameloblasts and odontoblasts had already differentiated, and begun to produce developing enamel and the underlying dentin [110] [42]. This is in contrast to the vast information in the literature on other genes, their corresponding proteins and the pathways associated with embryonic cranio-facial and specifically with tooth development, morphogenesis and differentiation [111] [112] [113] [114].

Having studied the postnatal expression of amelogenin in various craniofacial tissues including tooth supporting tissues, and brain, and in long bone, we focused on the detailed dynamic spatio-temporal expression of amelogenin in different tissues and organs of the developing embryonic mouse craniofacial complex during E10.5 to E18.5 [94]. We were interested in the changes in the dynamic expression of amelogenin, since these changes in expression pattern reflect the role of amelogenin during embryonic development. The major tissues studied were: brain, eye, peripheral nerve, ganglia, tooth germ, cartilage and bone (Figure 16). We showed that the most abundant amelogenin isoform, M180 and the amelogenin protein are expressed in the craniofacial complex from early stages of development (E10.5), up to the late stages.

The amelogenin protein is expressed in some tissues of the cranio-facial complex long before the initiation of tooth formation. In the developing brain, positive staining for amelogenin was already detected at E10.5 in the cranial part of the neural tube at the external limiting membrane, and in the eye - at the outer peripheral area of the inner part of the optic cup, which gives rise to the photoreceptors (Figure 16a). The amelogenin protein was mainly identified in glial cells, in neural-crest derived cells and possibly (but it is still not clear yet) in neurons, as it was detected in the brain, the retina of the eye, peripheral ganglia and the peripheral nerve trunks (Figure 16a,b). Several lines of evidence indicate that amelogenin is mainly expressed by the glial cells; (i) virtually no staining for amelogenin was detected in the cortex, which is mainly composed of neuroblasts, while the sub-cortical regions, where many more glial cells exist, was positively stained for amelogenin. (ii) As was described above, amelogenin was detected in postnatal glial cells surrounding brain neurons but not in the neurons themselves [25].

Figure 16: Spatio-temporal distribution of amelogenin expression in tissues of E10.5 to E18.5 mouse embryonic cranio-facial complex. (Amelogenin expression - brown-red staining, hematoxylin – blue staining). (A) In the eye, brain and peripheral nerve trunk at E10.5, E11.5, E12.5, E13.5, E14.5, E15.5, E16.5 and E18.5. (B) In the tooth germ, cartilage, bone and ganglion at E12.5, E13.5, E14.5, E15.5, E16.5 and E18.5.

Eye: Ch=choroidal blood vessels; Cr=cornea; EI=sub-epithelial region; GC=ganglion layer; LF=lens fibers; OC=optic cup; Pr=photoreceptors; Re=retina; Sc=sclera; Vi=vitreous. Brain: C=cortex; CP=cortical plate; ELM=external limiting membrane; LV=lateral ventricle; MB=midbrain; P=pons; Tc=telencephalon; TCr= temporal cortex; TL=temporal lobe. Peripheral nerve trunk: NF=peripheral nerve fibers. Tooth germ: Ab= ameloblasts; Av=alveolar bone trabecules; C=cervical loop; D=dentin; DL=dental lamina; DP=dental papilla; EM=extracellular enamel matrix; IEE=inner enamel epithelium; Od=odontoblasts; OEE=outer enamel epithelium; PD=pre-dentin; SI=stratum intermedium; SR=stellate reticulum; TG=tooth germ. Cartilage: DC= differentiated chondrocytes; HC=Hypertrophic cartilage; Pc=Pre-chondrocytes; WDC=well developed chondrocytes. Bone: BT=bone trabecules. No amelogenin staining was detected in the corresponding control (PBS) sections (not shown). Reproduced from Gruenbaum-Cohen et al. 2009.

Figure 16A

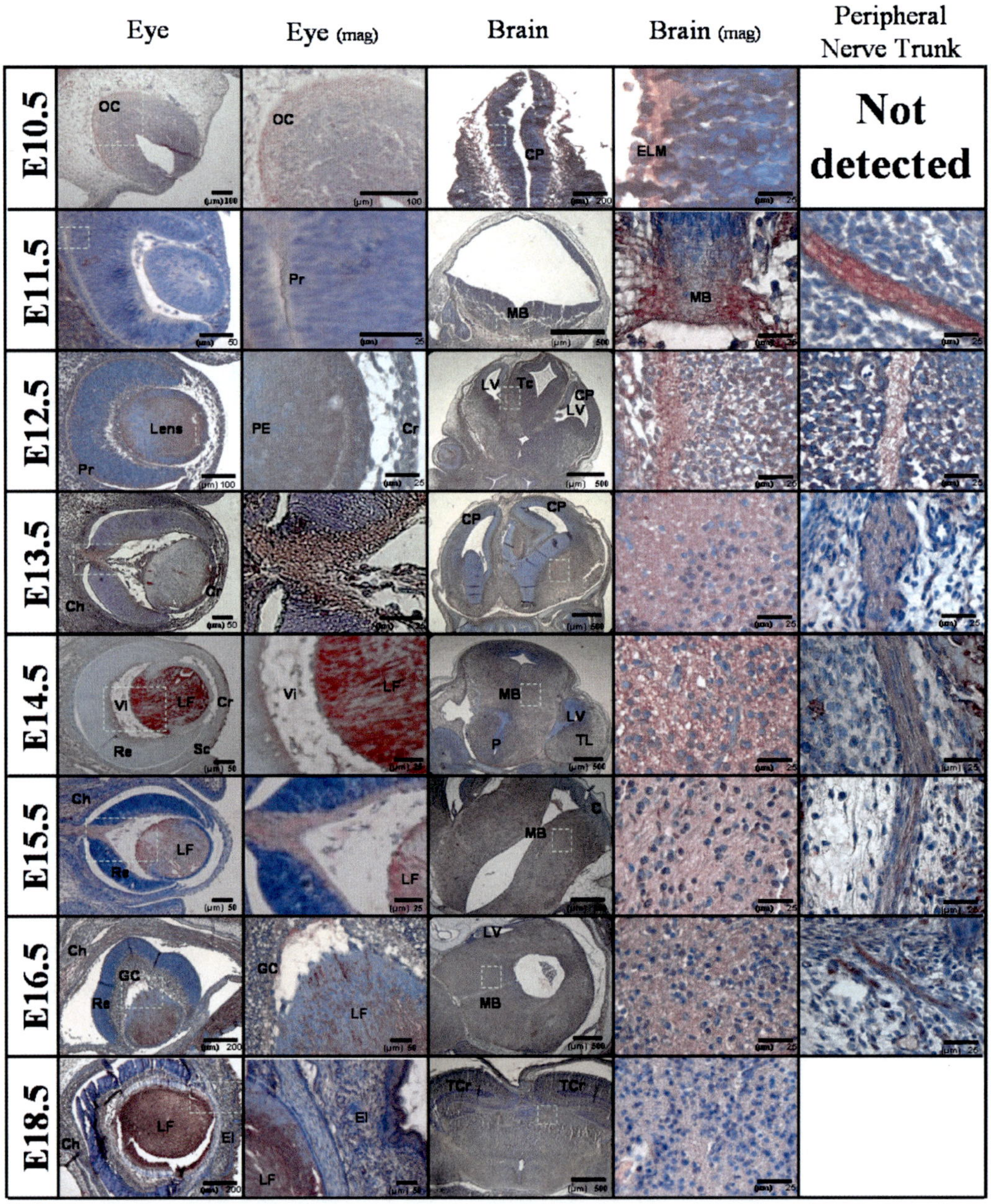

Figure 16B

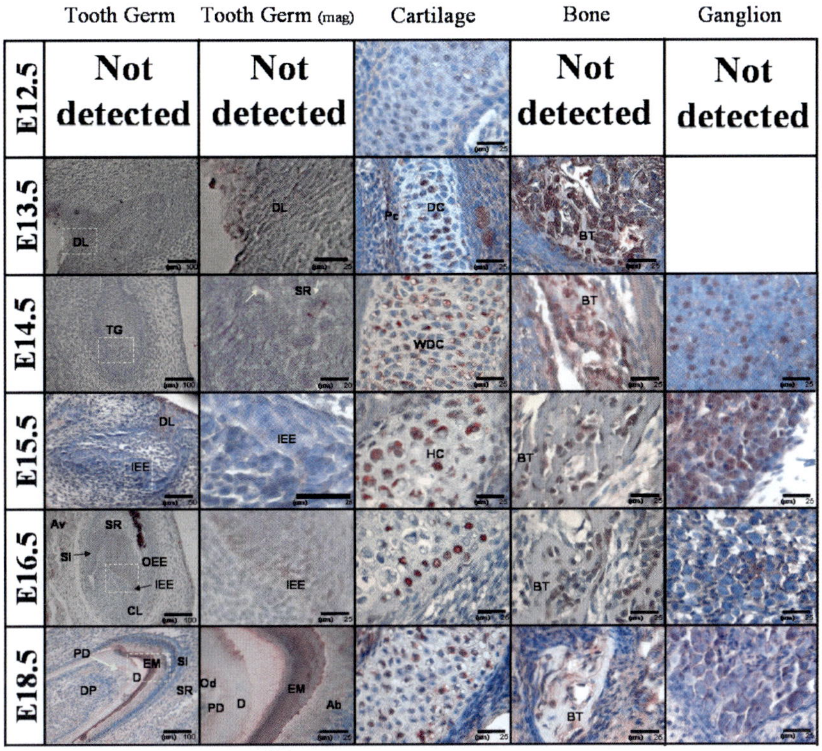

As was previously described, amelogenin is a structural protein during enamel bio-mineralization that regulates the shape, size and direction of mineral crystal growth. The patterns of amelogenin expression in lens fibers, in brain fibers and in nerve trunk fibers suggest a possible role for amelogenin in elongating structures within some developing cells. It is tempting to speculate that the model of elongated amelogenin nanospheres [5] might be somehow relevant to its role in developing fibers, but other mechanisms are also feasible. In the eye, amelogenin is mainly expressed in the posterior lens epithelium cells which elongate up to several hundred times during the process of differentiation into fiber cells. Interestingly, the strongest staining for amelogenin was detected in the ameloblasts, extracellular enamel matrix, and the eye lens, possibly indicating a similar role for amelogenin in these tissues. In the nervous tissues; brain, optic nerve and nerve trunks, amelogenin expression was mostly localized to fiber like structures. Glial and mesenchymal cells are known to surround nerve fibers, whether they are axons or dendrites, and a major role of glial cells during development is to support and direct the growth and elongation of neurons.

Amelogenin protein expression was seen already at E13.5 in the dental lamina, and continued through embryonic tooth development to E18.5 (Figure 16b). From E13.5 up to E16.5 (E17.5 was not analyzed), no extracellular enamel or dentin are yet formed, and no biomineralization of enamel or dentin takes place. Amelogenin, therefore, has different function(s) at these stages than that of regulating the size, shape and direction of mineral crystal growth. Late in development and close to birth (E18.5), amelogenin expression was mainly seen in the mineralizing extracellular enamel matrix and in the secreting ameloblasts, and also in the stratum intermedium, pre-dentin and dentin, and some expression in the dental papilla. The latter expression pattern, observed by us at E18.5, has been extensively described, mainly in postnatal mice.

In the craniofacial complex, neural crest cells also give rise to non-neuronal ecto-mesenchymal tissues such as bone, cartilage and mesenchymal regions of the teeth [115] that were all positive for amelogenin (Figure 16b). During palate development, amelogenin staining was detected in the region of both, yet vertical, palatine shelves at E11.5. The palate continued to be positive at least until E15.5. In prechondrocytes that will eventually develop into cartilage, at the base of the skull amelogenin expression was already detected at E11.5, and during cartilage formation amelogenin was detected mainly in prehypertrophic and hypertrophic chondrocytes. In the bone amelogenin was first detected in periosteal osteoblasts, at the beginning of bone organization, at E13.5. At later stages most bone cell types and not just osteoblasts in the cranial bones (mainly membranous bone which does not develop from cartilage), were positively stained. Cells surrounding blood vessels in various cranio-facial regions were stained positively for amelogenin since E12.5, this is in-line with the strong staining for amelogenin in the regenerating periodontal tissues (see above).

The accumulating results indicate possible signaling and various structural roles for amelogenin during early stages of embryonic craniofacial development, in addition to its known function during enamel biomineralization, which occurs very late during embryonic development and also postnataly. The expression of amelogenin in different tissues is dynamic and depends on the embryonic stage of development, perhaps indicating that amelogenin participates in the regulation of some developmental processes, as well as postnatal regeneration processes. The recruitment of mesenchymal cells in the tooth germ and mandible, at early stages of embryonic development, and the recruitment of mesenchymal stem cells during regeneration of tooth supporting tissues, combined with the relatively high expression specifically in bone regions with high turnover and remodeling (bone cells adjacent to the PDL and in the periosteal cells), points to the functional significance of amelogenin in these tissues. The process of bone regeneration requires recruitment of mesenchymal stem cells to the injured area and tight control over osteogenic and osteoclastogenic activity. Amelogenin might serve (directly or indirectly) as one of the key proteins in mesenchymal stem cell recruitment from the periodontal tissues and from the alveolar bone marrow, and/or in the differentiation of these cells *in-vivo*, which brings about the regeneration of the periodontal tissues. Amelogenin expression in the periosteum and differentially in cells of the epiphyseal growth plate also implies a role for amelogenin in long bone formation. The accumulating results indicate that the amelogenins have multifunctional roles.

The results described in this chapter open new horizons as to the function(s) of amelogenin in different tissues during embryonic development, postnatal development and regeneration processes. Naturally, there are numerous questions that can be asked and many studies that can be conducted to reveal the molecular mechanisms and pathways with which amelogenin is associated.

The significant progressive induction of periodontal regeneration by the recombinant amelogenin protein, and amelogenin expression in long bone cells, bone marrow and cartilage cells, may possibly offer, in the future, treatment to some of the widespread periodontal, bone, ligament and joint diseases, which are of major clinical, scientific and financial challenges.

ACKNOWLEDGEMENTS

This work was partially supported by Deutsche Forschungsgemeinschaft (DFG) grant no. Be 1142/4-1, Israel Science Foundation (ISF) grant no. 597/02, and USA-Israel Binational Grant Foundation (BSF) grant no. 2003-239.

REFERENCES

[1] Termine, JD, Belcourt AB. Miyamoto MS, *et al.* Properties of dissociatively extracted fetal tooth matrix proteins. I. Principal molecular species in developing bovine enamel. J Biol Chem 1980; 255(20): 9760-8.
[2] Robinson C, Fuchs P, Weatherell JA. The appearance of developing rat incisor enamel using a freeze fracturing technique. Cryst Growth 1981. 53: 160-5.
[3] Fincham AG, Moradian-Oldak J, Simmer JP *et al.*, Self-assembly of a recombinant amelogenin protein generates supramolecular structures. J Struct Biol 1994; 112(2): 103-9.
[4] Moradian-Oldak J. Amelogenins: assembly, processing and control of crystal morphology. Matrix Biol 2001. 20(5-6): 293-305.
[5] Du C, Falini G, Fermani S *et al.* Supramolecular assembly of amelogenin nanospheres into birefringent microribbons. Science 2005; 307(5714): 1450-4.
[6] Veis A. Materials science. A window on biomineralization. Science 2005; 307(5714): 1419-20.
[7] Bartlett JD, Simmer JP, Xue J *et al.* Molecular cloning and mRNA tissue distribution of a novel matrix metalloproteinase isolated from porcine enamel organ. Gene 1996; 183(1-2): 123-8.

[8] Lu Y, Papagerakis P, Yamakoshi Y *et al.* Functions of KLK4 and MMP-20 in dental enamel formation. Biol Chem 2008. 389(6): 695-700.
[9] Nagano T, Kakegawa A, Yamakoshi Y, *et al.* Mmp-20 and Klk4 cleavage site preferences for amelogenin sequences. J Dent Res 2009. 88(9): 823-8.
[10] Simmer J, Fukae M, Tanabe T *et al.* Purification, characterization, and cloning of enamel matrix serine proteinase 1. J Dent Res 1998; 77(2): 377-86.
[11] Brookes SJ, Robinson C, Kirkham J, *et al.* Biochemistry and molecular biology of amelogenin proteins of developing dental enamel. Arch Oral Biol, 1995; 40(1): 1-14.
[12] Fincham AG, Moradian-Oldak J. Recent advances in amelogenin biochemistry. Connect Tissue Res, 1995; 32(1-4): 119-24.
[13] Bartlett JD, Ball RL, Kawai T, *et al.,* Origin, splicing, and expression of rodent amelogenin exon 8. J Dent Res, 2006. 85(10): 894-9.
[14] Deutsch D, Catalano-Sherman I, Dafni L, *et al.,* Enamel matrix proteins and ameloblast biology. Connect Tissue Res, 1995; 32(1-4): 97-107.
[15] Sire JY, Delgado S, Fromentin D, *et al.,* Amelogenin: lessons from evolution. Arch Oral Biol 2005; 50(2): 205-12.
[16] Salido EC, Yen PH, Koprivinkar K, *et al.,* The human enamel protein gene amelogenin is expressed from both the X and the Y chromosomes Am J Hum Genet 1992; 50(2): 303-16.
[17] Lau EC, Mohandas TK, Shapiro LJ, *et al.* Human and mouse amelogenin gene loci are on the sex chromosomes Genomics 1989; **4**(2): 162-8.
[18] Sasaki S, Shimokawa H The amelogenin gene. Int J Dev Biol 1995; 39(1): 127-33.
[19] Simmer JP, Fincham AG Molecular mechanisms of dental enamel formation. Crit Rev Oral Biol Med, 1995; 6(2): 84-108.
[20] Veis A. Amelogenin gene splice products: potential signaling molecules. Cell Mol Life Sci 2003; 60(1): 38-55.
[21] Papagerakis P, Ibarra JM, Inozentsva N, *et al.*, Mouse amelogenin exons 8 and 9: sequence analysis and protein distribution. J Dent Res 2005; 84(7): 613-7.
[22] Li W, Mathews C, Gao C, *et al.,* Identification of two additional exons at the 3' end of the amelogenin gene. Arch Oral Biol 1998; 43(6): 497-504.
[23] Baba O,Takahashi N, Terashima T, *et al.* Expression of alternatively spliced RNA transcripts of amelogenin gene exons 8 and 9 and its end products in the rat incisor. J Histochem Cytochem 2002; 50(9): 1229-36.
[24] Li Y, Yuan Z-A, Aragon MA, *et al.,* Comparison of body weight and gene expression in amelogenin null and wild-type mice. Eur J Oral Sci, 2006; 114 Suppl 1: 190-3; discussion 201-2, 381.
[25] Deutsch D, Haze-Filderman A, Blumenfled A, *et al.,* Amelogenin, a major structural protein in mineralizing enamel, is also expressed in soft tissues: brain and cells of the hematopoietic system. Eur J Oral Sci 2006; 114 Suppl 1: p. 183-9; discussion 201-2, 381.
[26] Iacob S, Veis A Identification of temporal and spatial expression patterns of amelogenin isoforms during mouse molar development. Eur J Oral Sci 2006; 114(1): 194-200; 201-2, 381.
[27] Haze A, Taylor AL, Haegenwald S, *et al.*, Regeneration of bone and periodontal ligament induced by recombinant amelogenin after periodontitis. J Cell Mol Med, 2009; PMID :19228267.
[28] Hart PS, Vlaservich AC, Hart JT, *et al.,* Polymorphism (g2035C>T) in the amelogenin gene. Hum Mutat 2000; 15(3): 298.
[29] Wright JT, Hart PS, Aldred MJ, *et al.*, Relationship of phenotype and genotype in X-linked amelogenesis imperfecta. Connect Tissue Res 2003; 44 Suppl 1: 72-8.
[30] Kim JW, Simmer JP, Hu YY, *et al.* Amelogenin p.M1T and p.W4S mutations underlying hypoplastic X-linked amelogenesis imperfecta. J Dent Res 2004; 83(5): 378-83.
[31] Diekwisch T., David S, Bringas P, *et al.*. Antisense inhibition of AMEL translation demonstrates supramolecular controls for enamel HAP crystal growth during embryonic mouse molar development. Development 1993; 117(2): 471-82.
[32] Lyngstadaas SP, Risnes S, Sproat BS, *et al.* A synthetic, chemically modified ribozyme eliminates amelogenin, the major translation product in developing mouse enamel in vivo. Embo J 1995; 14(21): 5224-9.
[33] Gibson CW, Yuan ZA, Hall B, *et al.* Amelogenin-deficient mice display an amelogenesis imperfecta phenotype. J Biol Chem 2001; 276(34): 31871-5.

[34] Li Y, Struggs C, Wright JT, *et al.* Partial rescue of the amelogenin null dental enamel phenotype. J Biol Chem 2008; 283(22): 15056-62.

[35] Gibson CW, Li Y, Daly B, *et al.* The leucine-rich amelogenin peptide alters the amelogenin null enamel phenotype. Cells Tissues Organs 2009; 189(1-4): 169-74.

[36] Hatakeyama J, Sreenath T, Hatakeyama T, *et al.* The receptor activator of nuclear factor-kappa B ligand-mediated osteoclastogenic pathway is elevated in amelogenin-null mice. J Biol Chem 2003; 278(37): 35743-8.

[37] Hatakeyama J, Philip D, Hatakeyama Y *et al.* Amelogenin-mediated Regulation of Osteoclastogenesis, and Periodontal Cell Proliferation and Migration. J Dent Res 2006; 85(2): 144-9.

[38] Nishiguchi M, Yuasa K, Saito K, *et al.* Amelogenin is a negative regulator of osteoclastogenesis via downregulation of RANKL, M-CSF and fibronectin expression in osteoblasts. Arch Oral Biol 2007; 52(3): 237-43.

[39] Yagi Y, Suda N, Yamakoshi Y, *et al.* In vivo application of amelogenin suppresses root resorption. J Dent Res 2009; 88(2): 176-81.

[40] Nebgen DR, Inoue H, Sabsay B, *et al.* Identification of the chondrogenic-inducing activity from bovine dentin (bCIA) as a low-molecular-mass amelogenin polypeptide. J Dent Res 1999; 78(9): 1484-94.

[41] Tompkins K, Alvares K, George A, *et al.* Two related low molecular mass polypeptide isoforms of amelogenin have distinct activities in mouse tooth germ differentiation in vitro. J Bone Miner Res 2005; 20(2): 341-9.

[42] Lacerda-Pinheiro S, Septier D, Tompkins K, *et al.* Amelogenin gene splice products A+4 and A-4 implanted in soft tissue determine the reorientation of CD45-positive cells to an osteo-chondrogenic lineage. J Biomed Mater Res A 2006; 79(4): 1015-22.

[43] Viswanathan HL, Berry JE, Foster BL, *et al.* Amelogenin: a potential regulator of cementum-associated genes. J Periodontol 2003; 74(10): 1423-31.

[44] Lacerda-Pinheiro S, Jegat N, Septier D, *et al.* Early in vivo and in vitro effects of amelogenin gene splice products on pulp cells. Eur J Oral Sci 2006; 114 Suppl 1: 232-8; discussion 254-6, 381-2.

[45] Swanson EC, Fong HK, Foster ML, *et al.* Amelogenins regulate expression of genes associated with cementoblasts in vitro. Eur J Oral Sci 2006**;** 114 Suppl 1: p. 239-43; discussion 254-6, 381-2.

[46] Le TQ, Zhang Y, Li W, *et al.* The effect of LRAP on enamel organ epithelial cell differentiation. J Dent Res 2007; 86(11): 1095-9.

[47] Warotayanont R, Zhu D, Snead ML, et al. Leucine-rich amelogenin peptide induces osteogenesis in mouse embryonic stem cells. Biochem Biophys Res Commun 2008; 367(1): 1-6.

[48] Zeichner-David M, Chen LS, Hsu J, *et al.* Amelogenin and ameloblastin show growth-factor like activity in periodontal ligament cells. Eur J Oral Sci 2006; 114 Suppl 1: 244-53; discussion 254-6, 381-2.

[49] Jegat N, Septier D, Veis A, *et al.* Short-term effects of amelogenin gene splice products A+4 and A-4 implanted in the exposed rat molar pulp. Head Face Med 2007; 3: 40.

[50] Veis A, Tompkin K, Alvares K, *et al.* Specific amelogenin gene splice products have signaling effects on cells in culture and in implants in vivo. J Biol Chem 2000; 275(52): 41263- 72.

[51] Boabaid F, Gibson CW, Kuehl MA, *et al.* Leucine-rich amelogenin peptide: a candidate signaling molecule during cementogenesis. J Periodontol 2004; **75**(8):1126- 36.

[52] Tompkins K, Veis A. Polypeptides translated from alternatively spliced transcripts of the amelogenin gene, devoid of the exon 6a, b, c region, have specific effects on tooth germ development in culture. Connect Tissue Res 2002; 43(2-3): 224- 31.

[53] Tompkins K. Molecular mechanisms of cytodifferentiation in mammalian tooth development. Connect Tissue Res 2006; 47(3): 111- 8.

[54] Iacob S, Veis A. Identification of the functional activity of the [A-4] amelogenin gene splice product in newborn mouse ameloblasts. Bone 2008; 42: 1072- 9.

[55] Goldberg M, Six N, Septier D, *et al.* Dentin extracellular matrix molecules implanted into exposed pulps generate reparative dentin: a novel strategy in regenerative dentistry. J Dent Res 2009; 88(5): 396- 9.

[56] Tompkins K, George A, Veis A. Characterization of a mouse amelogenin [A-4]/M59 cell surface receptor. Bone, 2006; 38(2): 172-80.

[57] Zou Y, Wang HJ, Shapiro JL, *et al.* Determination of protein regions responsible for interactions of amelogenin with CD63 and LAMP1. Biochem J 2007; 408(3): 347-54.

[58] Shapiro JL, Wen X, Okamoto CT, *et al.* Cellular uptake of amelogenin, and its localization to CD63, and Lamp1-positive vesicles. Cell Mol Life Sci 2007; 64(2): 244-56.

[59] Xu L, Harada H, Taniguchi A. The Effects of LAMP1 and LAMP3 on M180 Amelogenin Uptake, Localization and Amelogenin mRNA Induction by Amelogenin Protein. J Biochem 2008; 144(4): 531-7.
[60] Xu L, Harada H, Taniguchi A, *et al.* Reuptake of extracellular amelogenin by dental epithelial cells results in increased levels of amelogenin mRNA through enhanced mRNA stabilization J Biol Chem 2006; 281(4): 2257-62.
[61] Hammarstrom L. Enamel matrix, cementum development and regeneration. J Clin Periodontol 1997; 24(9 Pt 2): 658-68.
[62] Gestrelius S, Lyngstadaas SP, Hammarstrom L. Emdogain--periodontal regeneration based on biomimicry. Clin Oral Investig 2000; 4(2): 120-5.
[63] Hammarstrom L, Heijl L, Gestrelius S. Periodontal regeneration in a buccal dehiscence model in monkeys after application of enamel matrix proteins. J Clin Periodontol 1997; 24(9 Pt 2): 669-77.
[64] Mumulidu A, Hildebrand B, Fabi B, *et al.* Purification and analysis of a 5kDa component of enamel matrix derivative. J Chromatogr B Analyt Technol Biomed Life Sci 2007; 857(2): 210-8.
[65] Saito A, nanbu Y, Nagahata T, *et al.* Treatment of intrabony periodontal defects with enamel matrix derivative in private practice: a long-term retrospective study. Bull Tokyo Dent Coll 2008; 49(2): p. 89-96.
[66] Simmer JP, Lau EC, Hu CC, *et al.* Isolation and characterization of a mouse amelogenin expressed in Escherichia coli. Calcif. Tissue Int 1994; 54: 312–9.
[67] Deutsch D, Chityat E, Hekmati M, *et al.* High Expression of Human Amelogenin in E. coli. Adv Dent Res 1996; 10: 187–194.
[68] Ryu O, Fincham AG, Hu CC, *et al.* Characterization of recombinant pig enamelysin activity and cleavage of recombinant pig and mouse amelogenins. J Dent Res 1999; 78: 743–50.
[69] Fincham AG, Moradian-Oldak J, Sarte PE. Mass-spectrographic analysis of a porcine amelogenin identifies a single phosphorylated locus. Calcif Tissue Int 1994; 55(5): 398-400.
[70] Habelitz S, Kullar A, Marshall SJ, *et al.* Amelogenin-guided crystal growth on fluoroapatite glass-ceramics. J Dent Res 2004; 84: 698–702.
[71] Taylor AL, Haze-Filderman A, Blumenfeld A, *et al.* High yield of biologically active recombinant human amelogenin using the baculovirus expression system. Protein Expr Purif 2006; 45(1): 43-53.
[72] Gafni Y, Turgeman G, Liebergal M, *et al.* Stem cells as vehicles for orthopedic gene therapy. Gene Ther 2004; 11(4): 417-26.
[73] Bluteau G, Luder HU, De Bari C, *et al.* Stem cells for tooth engineering. Eur Cell Mater 2008; 31(16): 1-9.
[74] King GN, Hughes FJ. Bone morphogenetic protein-2 stimulates cell recruitment and cementogenesis during early wound healing. J Clin Periodontol 2001; 28(5): 465-75.
[75] Kawaguchi H, Hirachi A, Hasegawa N, *et al.* Enhancement of periodontal tissue regeneration by transplantation of bone marrow mesenchymal stem cells. J Periodontol 2004; 75: 1281-7.
[76] Simmons PJ, Torok-Storb B. Identification of stromal cell precursors in human bone marrow by a novel monoclonal antibody, STRO-1. Blood 1991; 78(1): 55-62.
[77] Barry FP, Boynton RE, Haynesworth S, *et al.* The monoclonal antibody SH-2, raised against human mesenchymal stem cells, recognizes an epitope on endoglin (CD105). Biochem Biophys Res Commun 1999; 265(1): 134-9.
[78] Pittenger MF, Mackay AM, Beck SC, *et al.* Multilineage potential of adult human mesenchymal stem cells. Science 1999; 284(5411): 143-7.
[79] Tuli R, Tulia S, Nandia S, *et al.* Characterization of multipotential mesenchymal progenitor cells derived from human trabecular bone. Stem Cells 2003; 21(6): 681-93.
[80] Alsalameh S, Amin R, Gemba T. *et al.* Identification of mesenchymal progenitor cells in normal and osteoarthritic human articular cartilage. Arthritis Rheum 2004; 50(5): 1522-32.
[81] Oswald J, Boxberger S, Jorgensen B, *et al.* Mesenchymal stem cells can be differentiated into endothelial cells in vitro. Stem Cells 2004; 22(3): 377-84.
[82] Aslan H, Zilberman Y, Kandel L. Osteogenic differentiation of noncultured immunoisolated bone marrow-derived CD105+ cells. Stem Cells 2006, 24(7): 1728-37.
[83] Duff SE, Li C, Garland JM, *et al.* CD105 is important for angiogenesis: evidence and potential applications. FASEB J 2003; 17(9): 984-92.
[84] Fonsatti E, Sigalotti L, Arslan P, *et al.* Emerging role of endoglin (CD105) as a marker of angiogenesis with clinical potential in human malignancies. Curr Cancer Drug Targets 2003; 3(6): 427-32.

[85] Gronthos S, Simmons PJ, The growth factor requirements of STRO-1-positive human bone marrow stromal precursors under serum-deprived conditions in vitro. Blood 1995; 85(4): 929-40.
[86] Dennis JE, Carbillet JP, Caplan A, *et al.* The STRO-1+ marrow cell population is multipotential. Cells Tissues Organs 2002; 170(2-3): 73-82.
[87] Gronthos S, Zannettino ACW, Hay SJ, *et al.* Molecular and cellular characterisation of highly purified stromal stem cells derived from human bone marrow. J Cell Sci 2003; 116(Pt 9): 1827-35.
[88] Chen SC, Marino V, Gronthos S, *et al.* Location of putative stem cells in human periodontal ligament. J Periodontal Res 2006; 41(6): 547-53.
[89] Nagatomo K, Komaki M, Sekiya I, *et al.* Stem cell properties of human periodontal ligament cells. J Periodont Res 2006; 41(4): p. 303-10.
[90] Collett GD, Canfield AE. Angiogenesis and pericytes in the initiation of ectopic calcification. Circ Res 2005; 96(9): 930-8.
[91] Yuan K, Chen CL, Lin MT. Enamel matrix derivative exhibits angiogenic effect in vitro and in a murine model. J Clin Periodontol 2003; 30(8): 732-8.
[92] Romanelli M, Dini V, Vowden P, *et al.* Amelogenin, an extracellular matrix protein, in the treatment of venous leg ulcers and other hard-to-heal wounds: experimental and clinical evidence. Clin Interv Aging 2008; 3(2): 263-72.
[93] Chadwick P, Acton C. The use of amelogenin protein in the treatment of hard-to-heal wounds. Br J Nurs 2009; 18(6): S22, S24, S26.
[94] Gruenbaum-Cohen Y, Tucker AS, Haze A, *et al.*, Amelogenin in Cranio-facial Development: The Tooth as a Model to Study the Role of Amelogenin During Embryogenesis. J Exp Zool Mol Dev Evol 2009; 312B: 445-57.
[95] Fong CD, Hammarstrom L. Expression of amelin and amelogenin in epithelial root sheath remnants of fully formed rat molars. Oral Surg Oral Med Oral Pathol Oral Radiol Endod 2000; 90(2): 218-23.
[96] Janones DS, Massa LF, Arana-Chavez VE, Immunocytochemical examination of the presence of amelogenin during the root development of rat molars. Arch Oral Biol 2005; 50(5): 527-32.
[97] Haze A, Taylor AL, Blumenfeld A, *et al.* Amelogenin expression in long bone and cartilage cells and in bone marrow progenitor cells. Anat Rec (Hoboken) 2007; 290(5): 455-60.
[98] Eastoe JE Organic matrix of tooth enamel. Nature 1960; 187: 411-2.
[99] Adeleke-Stainback P, Chen E, Collier P, *et al.* Analysis of the regulatory region of the bovine X-chromosomal amelogenin gene. Connect Tissue Res 1995; 32(1-4): 115-8.
[100] Simmer JP. Alternative splicing of amelogenins. Connect Tissue Res 1995. 32(1-4): 131-6.
[101] Hamamoto Y, Nakajima T, Ozawa H, *et al.* Production of amelogenin by enamel epithelium of Hertwig's root sheath. Oral Surg Oral Med Oral Pathol Oral Radiol Endod 1996; 81(6): 703-9.
[102] Fincham AG, Simmer JP. Amelogenin proteins of developing dental enamel. Ciba Found Symp 1997; 205: 118-34.
[103] Robinson C, Brookes SJ, Shore RC, *et al.* The developing enamel matrix: nature and function. Eur J Oral Sci 1998; 106 Suppl 1: 282-91.
[104] Fincham AG, Moradian-Oldak J, Simmer JP. The structural biology of the developing dental enamel matrix. J Struct Biol 1999; 126(3): 270-99.
[105] Fukae M, Tanabe T, Yamakoshi Y, *et al.* Immunoblot detection and expression of enamel proteins at the apical portion of the forming root in porcine permanent incisor tooth germs. J Bone Miner Metab 2001; 19(4): 236-43.
[106] Oida S, Nagano T, Yamakoshi Y, *et al.* Amelogenin gene expression in porcine odontoblasts. J Dent Res 2002; 81(2): 103-8.
[107] Papagerakis P, MacDougall M, Hotton D, *et al.* Expression of amelogenin in odontoblasts. Bone 2003; 32(3): 228-40.
[108] Snead ML. Amelogenin protein exhibits a modular design: implications for form and function. Connect Tissue Res 2003; 44 Suppl 1: 47-51.
[109] Bosshardt DD, Nanci A. Hertwig's epithelial root sheath, enamel matrix proteins, and initiation of cementogenesis in porcine teeth. J Clin Periodontol 2004; 31(3): 184-92.
[110] Zeichner-David M, Vo H, Tan H, *et al.* Timing of the expression of enamel gene products during mouse tooth development. Int J Dev Biol 1997; 41(1): 27-38.

[111] Tucker AS, Sharpe PT. Molecular genetics of tooth morphogenesis and patterning: the right shape in the right place. J Dent Res 1999; 78(4): 826-34.
[112] Jernvall J, Thesleff I. Reiterative signaling and patterning during mammalian tooth morphogenesis. Mech Dev 2000; 92(1): 19-29.
[113] Tucker A, Sharpe P. The cutting-edge of mammalian development; how the embryo makes teeth. Nat Rev Genet 2004; 5(7): 499-508.
[114] Mitsiadis, T.A. and M.M. Smith, *How do genes make teeth to order through development?* J Exp Zoolog B Mol Dev Evol, 2006. **306**(3): p. 177-82.
[115] Le Douarin, N.M., J.M. Brito, and S. Creuzet, *Role of the neural crest in face and brain development.* Brain Res Rev, 2007. **55**(2): p. 237-47.

CHAPTER 8

Consequences of Amelogenin Mutations: Implications in Amelogenesis Imperfecta

J Timothy Wright DDS, MS

Bawden Distinguished Professor and Chair, Department of Pediatric Dentistry, School of Dentistry, The University of North Carolina, Chapel Hill, NC, USA; Fax: 919-966-7992; E-mail: tim_wright@dentistry.unc.edu

Abstract: The amelogenin gene (*AMELX*) was the first extracellular enamel matrix coding gene to be discovered. Mutations in *AMELX* cause a variety of changes in the amelogenin protein that cause abnormal enamel formation. The resulting clinical phenotypes are diverse and are referred to as amelogenesis imperfecta (AI). To date, fourteen allelic *AMELX* mutations have been described that purportedly result in markedly different expression and types of amelogenins. Interestingly, the different protein domains affected by distinct *AMELX* gene mutations result in unique and functionally altered amelogenin proteins that are associated with several rather distinct AI phenotypes. The *AMELX* mutations and associated phenotypes fall generally into three categories. Mutations (e.g. signal peptide mutations) causing a total of loss of amelogenin protein are associated with a predominantly hypoplastic phenotype (though mineralization defects can also occur). Missense mutations affecting the N-terminal region, especially those causing changes in the putative lectin-binding domain and Tyrosine Rich Amelogenin Protein region that contains several critical protease cleavage sites, result in a predominantly hypomineralization / hypomaturation AI phenotype with enamel that is discolored and has retained amelogenin. Mutations causing loss of the amelogenin C terminus result in a phenotype characterized by hypoplasia. The phenotype – genotype correlations indicate there are important functional domains of the amelogenin molecule that are critical for the development of normal enamel structure, composition and thickness and that perturbations in these different domains can result in different clinical phenotypes.

Key Words: Enamel, Amelogenin, Gene, Hereditary, Hypoplasia, Hypomaturation, Hypomineralization

INTRODUCTION

The term amelogenesis imperfecta (AI) is most often used to describe hereditary conditions that affect the dental enamel but that are not associated with other developmental abnormalities such as a syndrome [1]. There are multiple genes known to cause AI and the list continues to grow. Four of the known AI causative genes code for extracellular enamel matrix proteins with two being proteinases (KLK4 and MMP20) and two being proteins that form the extracellular matrix (AMELX and ENAM) [2]. Two recently discovered genes that cause AI (*FAM83H* and *WDR72*) control as yet to be defined cellular functions that are clearly critical for normal amelogenesis [3,4] . This chapter will focus on the consequences of *AMELX* mutations and the resulting clinical phenotypes.

Amelogenin is the predominant extracellular matrix protein in developing enamel and is thought to form an organic scaffold that is essential for controlling and/or sustaining the highly ordered and directional growth of enamel crystallites [5-7]. The amelogenin proteins are coded for by genes on both the X (*AMELX*) and Y (*AMELY*) chromosomes. The function of the *AMELY* amelogenin, if any, remains unclear and deletions that include the *AMELY* gene reportedly do not cause an enamel phenotype [8]. Although the exact functions of the amelogenin proteins have not been fully established, its critical role in enamel development is verified by the association of enamel defects with *AMELX* mutations in humans, and the presence of severe enamel hypoplasia in the amelogenin knock-out mouse [7]. Amelogenin is highly conserved between species, further supporting its importance in enamel formation [9]. Indeed the mutations that cause *AMELX* associated AI occur in highly conserved residues in both mammalian and amniote amelogenin sequences [10]. Human amelogenin has a 16 amino acid signal peptide, and is secreted primarily as a 175 amino acid protein [11]. It is known that there are multiple alternatively spliced amelogenin proteins formed by deleting or adding certain exon products although the function of these proteins remains to be fully defined [12]. As described in detail in previous chapters of this book, amelogenin is a proline rich protein that is hydrophobic and forms multimers that are thought to be important in controlling crystallite growth [13,14]. While the mechanisms by which the amelogenin proteins help orchestrate enamel formation are not fully understood, it is known that complex protein-protein and protein mineral interactions as well as protein processing play important roles [15-17]. The amelogenin proteins form multimers called nanospheres that are approximately 10-20 nm in diameter [18]. During normal enamel formation the amelogenin protein is processed in a controlled fashion thereby generating the regulatory mechanism considered essential for orderly crystallite growth [17]. The acidic amelogenin C-terminus has a high mineral affinity compared with the remaining amelogenin molecule and is rapidly cleaved after secretion of the parent protein from the ameloblasts [19, 20]. During normal enamel development the amelogenin proteins are almost completely removed allowing the enamel crystallites to grow and produce mature enamel that is greater than 95% mineral by weight [21]. All of the known *AMELX* mutations purportedly result in either a protein deficiency or an altered protein with changes in regions that appear to affect critical amelogenin functions (e.g. self assembly, proteinase processing).

AMELX mutations are diverse and include deletions of various sizes, and missense and nonsense mutations [22-25]. These genomic coding errors result in markedly different phenotypes ranging from a deficiency in the amount of enamel (hypoplasia) [13] to defects in enamel mineralization (hypomineralization/hypomaturation) [2]. Some *AMELX*-associated AI types have variable phenotypes [16, 17], while others show a high degree of phenotypic consistency even between families [18]. For example, a markedly consistent phenotype has been observed in males from three families with the same single base C→A substitution in *AMELX* codon 70, causing a Proline to Threonine amino acid change (P70T) [18, 19]. It is felt that mutations causing changes in domains of the amelogenin protein having different and unique functions will likely result in distinct and potentially diverse phenotypes [26]. Identifying different *AMELX* mutations and correlating them with the resulting phenotypes has played an important role in helping define the potential role of amelogenin in enamel formation and its functional domains.

AI NOSOLOGY

The nomenclature for AI has changed little over the past several decades and the classification system proposed and later refined by Carl Witkop Jr. remains the most commonly accepted system in use today [1]. As the molecular etiologies for AI are identified, the utility of a nomenclature that includes molecular information is increasingly recognized and a number of nosological approaches proposed [27]. To date, there is no generally accepted nomenclature that includes the molecular basis of AI. The Online Mendelian Inheritance in Man (OMIM) designation for *AMELX* associated AI is termed hypoplastic/hypomaturation AI (OMIM #301200) [28].

A standard nomenclature system that allows classification of the genomic, cDNA and protein changes for each AI mutation has been proposed and will be followed for defining the *AMELX* mutations reviewed in this chapter (20). This nomenclature is based upon internationally agreed upon guidelines [21, 22] using designated reference sequences. The amelogenin protein numbering begins with the signal peptide and includes exon 4. In humans, the exon 4 product is absent from the majority of secreted amelogenin protein [9]. However, should mutations involving exon 4 be identified, they can be described by this nomenclature.

AMELX GENOTYPES

The *AMELX* gene was discovered and sequenced in the mouse in 1989 [29] and the first human *AMELX* mutation associated with AI was reported in 1991 [22]. Since that discovery, over 14 mutations have been identified in the *AMELX* gene (Table 1).

Table 1: *AMELX* mutations and their associated phenotypes in X-linked amelogenesis imperfecta

Genomic DNA	cDNA	Protein	Male Phenotype	Reference
g.2T>C	c.2T>C	p.M1T	Smooth Hypoplastic (normal mineralization)	Simmer et al. 2004
g.11G>C	c.11G>C	p.W4S	Smooth Hypoplastic (normal mineralization)	Simmer et al. 2004
g.11G>A	c.11G>A	p.W4X	Smooth Hypoplastic (normal mineralization)	Sekiguchi et al. 2001
g.14_22del	c.14_22del	p.I5_A8delinsT	Smooth Hypoplastic (normal mineralization)	Lagerström-Fermer et al. 1995
g.1148_54del	c.55_54del	p.18del	Hypomaturation (some hypoplasia)	Lagerström et al. 1991
g.3455C>T	c.152C>T	p.T51I	Hypomaturation (some hypoplasia)	Lench and Winter 1995
g.3458delC	c.155delC	p.P52fsX53	Hypomaturation (some hypoplasia, variable)	Aldred et al. 1992; Lench et al. 1994
g.3781C>A	c.208C>A	p.P70T	Hypomaturation (some hypoplasia)	Collier et al. 1997; Hart et al. 2000
g.3803A>T	c.230A>T	p.H77L	Hypomaturation	Hart et al. 2001
g.3958delC	c.385delC	p.H129fsX187	Smooth Hypoplastic	Sekiguchi et al. 2001
g.3993delC	c.420delC	p.Y141fsX187	Smooth Hypoplastic	Greene et al. 2000
g.4046delC	c.473delC	p.P158fsX187	Smooth Hypoplastic	Lench and Winter 1995
g.4114delC	c.541delC	p.L181fsX187	Smooth Hypoplastic (some hypomineralization)	Kindelan et al. 2000; Hart et al. 2001
g.4144G>T	c.571G>T	p.E191X	Smooth Hypoplastic	Lench and Winter 1995

These mutations span the gene from the 5' to 3' end and result in a variety of different changes in the translated protein. The known *AMELX* mutations include large deletions, missense, and nonsense mutations that result in a variety of diverse changes in the amelogenin protein. Table 1 lists the different mutations with the genomic and cDNA designations along with the purported protein alteration and resulting phenotype. Direct analysis of the *AMELX* cDNA and enamel protein products is largely precluded in humans with AI mutations as the ameloblasts are not present after the tooth has fully formed and erupted. Therefore, the protein alterations resulting from the different *AMELX* mutations are predicted from the genomic DNA sequence with none being verified at the cDNA or protein level. While mutations spanning much of the *AMELX* coding region have now been identified, mutations have not been described for all exons or regions (Figure 1). There are currently no known *AMELX* mutations in exons 4, 7, 8 or 9.

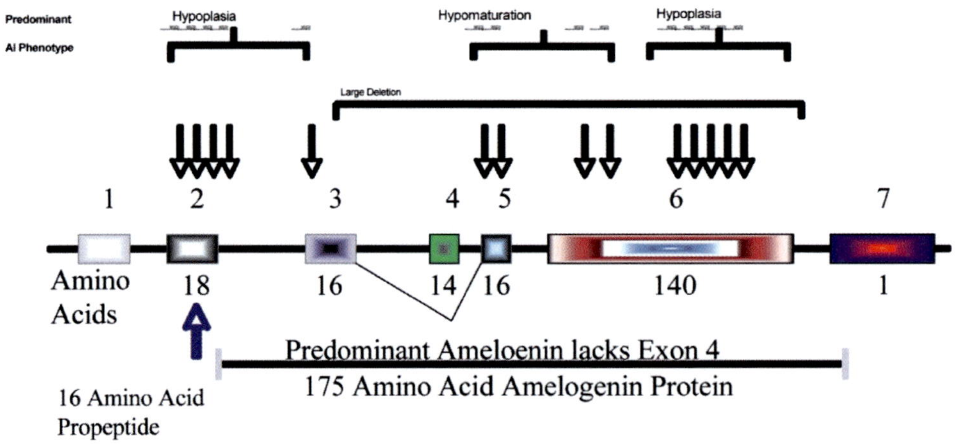

Figure 1: The human *AMELX* gene with the seven exons that code for the signal peptide (blue arrow) and full length secreted amelogenin protein (bottom of figure) is shown with the location of the known human mutations (down arrows ↓). The enamel phenotypes that result from these mutations are illustrated at the top of the figure.

Several mutations lead to a lack of protein production and or secretion, such as large deletions, and several mutations that affect the signal peptide. There are multiple known mutations that alter single amino acids near the middle of the protein and there are multiple single nucleotide deletion mutations that cause a frame shift and introduction of a premature stop codon causing truncation of the C-terminus the amelogenin protein. Interestingly, all of the known exon 6 nucleotide deletions cause frame shift mutations resulting in the introduction of premature stop codons and a protein lacking 18 amino acids at the C-terminus. One point mutation results in truncation of the amelogenin protein's last 14 amino acids. The phenotypes that result from these different *AMELX* mutations vary considerably and can provide insight into critical functional domains of the protein.

While not the focus of this chapter, several recent reports describe *AMELX* genotypes in association with dental caries. There is growing evidence suggesting that *AMELX* genotypes are associated with an increased risk for developing dental caries [30]. These investigations could provide insight as to how enamel composition and structure are related to specific *AMELX* non-AI associated genotypes and how and why these genotypes are associated with an increased risk for developing dental caries.

AMELOGENESIS IMPERFECTA PHENOTYPES

Phenotypes resulting from the different *AMELX* mutations vary considerably in their primary features and severity. The two enamel defects observed with *AMELX* mutations are a deficiency of enamel production that is characterized clinically by thin enamel (hypoplastic) and enamel that has not mineralized to its full potential due to a defect in the maturation process (hypomaturation) [31-33]. The type of enamel defect that develops depends on the *AMELX* mutation's effect on the amelogenin protein. There appears to be a reasonably well-defined relationship between the genotype and phenotype [26] for at least some of the *AMELX* mutations. In addition to phenotypic variation secondary to differences in the amelogenin protein, there is marked variation between males and females with *AMELX* mutations. The male and female *AMELX* AI-associated phenotypes vary because affected males will express only one mutant allele while females will show a mosaic pattern of expression due to X chromosome inactivation (Lyonization) [34, 35]. Indeed, this differential male-female X-linked AI phenotype was one of the early recognized examples of Lyonization [34]. Males show a generalized phenotype where the enamel is characterized by a more uniform reduction in enamel thickness over the entire clinical crown or a generalized hypomaturation defect with discoloration of the enamel. In contrast, females with *AMELX* mutations typically have vertical striations of normal coloured enamel adjacent to opaque or yellow-brown enamel or have enamel of normal thickness adjacent to furrows and grooves of thin enamel, depending on the specific mutation and the effect on the translated protein [34-36]. This differential in phenotype between males and females is extremely helpful when trying to diagnose the specific AI type and narrowing the search for a molecular etiology and candidate gene.

The loss of amelogenin protein due to a variety of *AMELX* mutations results in a hypoplastic phenotype. A number of different mutations are associated with a loss of protein production or protein secretion. A 5 Kb deletion including all genomic DNA from the beginning of exon 3 through part of exon 7 (g.1148_*47del) [22] that would result in no functional amelogenin protein being produced and secreted. This essentially represents a human knockout of the *AMELX* gene with only two amino acids beyond the signal peptide potentially being coded by the mutant gene. The associated phenotype reported in the two Swedish families having this mutation is described as being predominantly a hypomineralization/hypomaturation defect [26]. The enamel was later described as having a mottled white opaque coloration and microradiographic studies indicated the enamel was hypomineralized [37]. There also are reports of variable enamel hypoplasia or generalized thinning of the enamel in these families [32]. Females having a chromosomal deletion that included the entire *AMELX* gene resulted in a lyonized thin hypoplastic phenotype that alternated between normal enamel thickness to thin enamel that lacked a normal prismatic structure as reported in *AMELX* associated AI [38]. Mice lacking amelogenin expression due to either chromosomal deletions involving *Amelx* or having the *Amelx* gene knocked out also have a generalized thin enamel phenotype [7, 39].

Two human *AMELX* mutations would result in alterations of the 16 amino acid signal peptide. The first *AMELX* signal peptide mutation described was a nine base pair deletion and was reported to cause a total lack of amelogenin protein secretion [40]. Another signal peptide mutation has been reported where a single base substitution (g.11G>A) causes the introduction of a premature stop codon [41]. This mutation also is thought to result in a complete loss of amelogenin secretion. Both of these mutations result in a severe reduction in enamel thickness and a clinical phenotype of generalized thin hypoplastic AI. The little enamel that is present is thought to be hard and well-mineralised.

Four *AMELX* mutations involving part of the N-terminus of the amelogenin protein have been described. The first of these was a frameshift mutation described first by Aldred et al. [42] and later by Lench et al., [43] that resulted from a single nucleotide substitution in exon 5 and the introduction of a premature stop codon. This *AMELX* mutation is predicted to result in a secreted amelogenin protein that is only 36 amino acids in length (p.P52fsX53). Both families described with this mutation show primarily a hypomineralization/hypomaturation phenotype but also varying degrees of hypoplasia. There was marked phenotypic variability in the severity between same gender individuals even within the same family [43,44]. Mutations causing a general deficiency of amelogenin production or secretion appear to most often result in a generalized thin enamel phenotype that presumably occurs by a haploinsufficiency type mechanism. These mutations indicate that having the correct amount of amelogenin present is critical for developing a normal enamel thickness. Interestingly, other enamel matrix proteins also are known to be critical for developing a normal enamel thickness (e.g. enamelin) [45].

Three *AMELX* mutations affecting the N-terminal region of the amelogenin protein involve single nucleotide substitutions that cause single amino acid changes. One of these mutations occurs in exon 5 (g.3455C>T) and produces a Threonine to Isoleucine change at amino acid 51 (p.T51I) [44]. The phenotype resulting from this one amino acid change is described as hypomineralization/hypomaturation with brown discoloration of the enamel. Similarly, two other mutations (P70T and H77L) that occur in exon 6 produce an enamel phenotype classified as hypomaturation with brown discoloured enamel (Figure 2) [46, 47]. Based on analysis of the enamel proteins from males with the P70T mutation there is a slight increase in the amount of enamel protein that has an amelogenin-like amino acid composition indicating amelogenin retention [36]. Immunolocalization studies also support the presence of retained amelogenin in the enamel affected by the P70T mutation supporting the contention that this mutation leads to a hypomaturation type defect [36]. The enamel prism structure in the P70T is ranges from relatively normal with prism size areas of porosity to having no discernable prism structure and a random appearing crystallite orientation [36]. The clinical phenotype resulting from the P70T *AMELX* mutation is highly consistent between individuals and families. The author has evaluated 4 families with this mutation and all had the same phenotype. Interestingly, the primary dentition appears opaque white and not brown and the cervical region of the permanent teeth are white opaque while the more coronal portions of the clinical crown appear yellow-brown in colour.

Several studies have sought to explain the mechanism as to how these mutations (T51I ,P70T and H77L) lead to a hypomaturation defect. The term hypomaturation implies that the critical maturation stage of enamel formation, that is essential for final removal of the enamel matrix proteins and crystal growth, is perturbed. So how do these different changes in single amino acids of the amelogenin protein alter amelogenin function or processing during the maturation process. All three of these amino acid changes occur in or just outside a highly conserved region of the amelogenin protein known as the Tyrosine Rich Amelogenin Peptide (amino acid 31-74) [5]. Investigators suggest this region could be critical for cell - protein or protein – protein interactions due to binding cytokeratins or N-acetyl-D-glucosamine [48, 49]. It also has been shown that the T51I and P70T amelogenins do not interact with other amelogenins in a normal fashion as evaluated by the Yeast Two Hybrid Assay and that they do not undergo normal assembly into appropriate sized nanospheres [50]. Others have suggested that the highly conserved proline that is altered in the P70T mutation occurs at a highly conserved proteinase cleavage site for MMP20. Kinetic studies show that this mutation markedly alters the kinetics and greatly reduces MMP20's ability to cleave amelogenin at this location [51, 52]. All three mutations that occur in this region (i.e. T51I, P70T and H77L) result in a hypomaturation enamel phenotype where there is a decreased mineralization of the enamel and an increase in protein retention that includes amelogenin [36]. Therefore, it appears likely that mechanisms such as altered amelogenin assembly and processing by MMP20 lead to the phenotypes observed clinically. Kinetic studies have not been performed on the T51L or H77L amelogenin proteins to determine if they show diminished processing by MMP20 similar to the P70T protein.

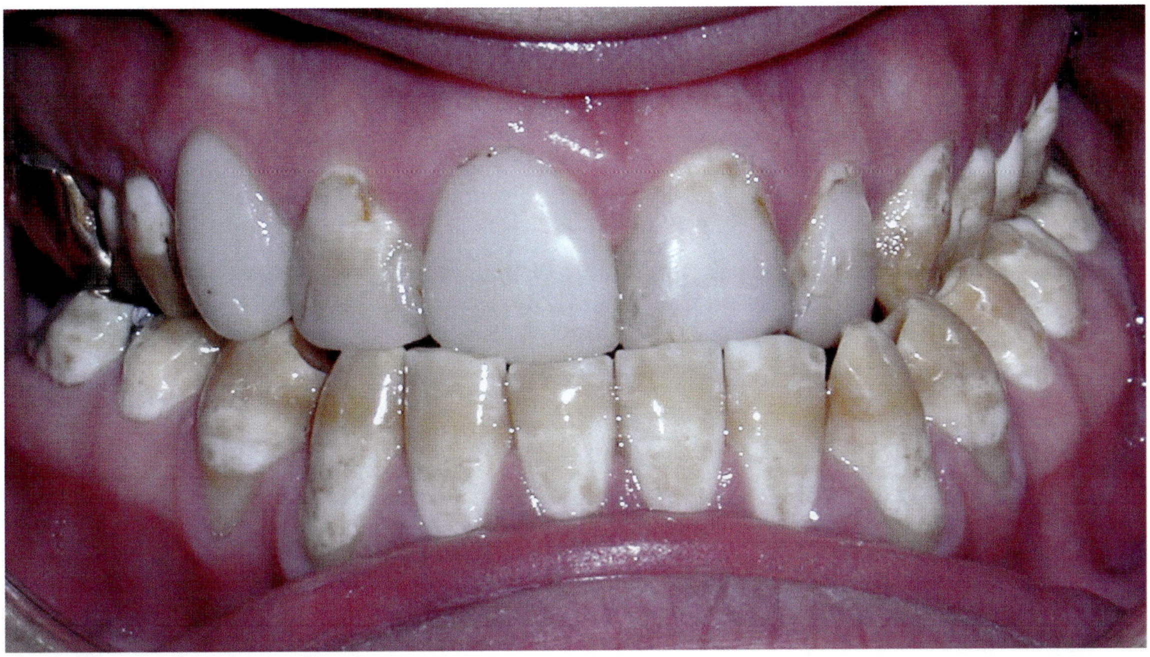

Figure 2: This male with a P70T AMELX mutation has an opaque white colour to the cervical areas of his clinical crowns that becomes yellow-brown in the more coronal areas.

There are five different *AMELX* mutations that introduce a premature stop codon and truncate the C-terminus of the amelogenin protein. Four of these mutations are single nucleotide deletions at various locations in exon 6. All four introduce a premature stop codon at amino acid position 187 [23, 25, 41, 53]. The amelogenin proteins produced by these four mutations are similar in that all lack the C-terminal 18 amino acids. However, they all differ in the extent and type of amino acid changes occurring between the point of the deletion and the stop codon. Despite these differences, these mutations are associated with a generalized thinning of the enamel and hypoplastic phenotype (Figure 3). The severity of the enamel thinning, while not well-quantified, appears to be very severe in the two cases where there are significant portions of the protein altered prior to truncation. The mutation described by Sekiguchi et al. [41] causes alteration of 59 amino acids prior to truncation, while the mutation reported by Greene et al. [53] alters 48 amino acids before terminating. Both of these mutations are predicted to result in the addition of nine cysteine and multiple serine residues in the altered amelogenin sequence in a region that normally has no cysteine and only one serine residue.

Alteration of only 7 amino acids prior to truncation at position 187 is seen with the (p.L181fsX187) mutation. This alteration causes relatively severe enamel thinning so the enamel may be only 10 – 20% of normal thickness [25, 35]. One *AMELX* mutation introduces a single nucleotide change (c.571G>T) and a premature stop codon late in exon 6 (p.E191X), causing truncation of the protein at position 191. This results in a secreted amelogenin protein 14 amino acids shorter than the wild type. This mutation also is associated with a generalized enamel thinning and is classified as a smooth hypoplastic phenotype [44].

The role of the amelogenin C-terminus has long been thought to be critical in enamel formation yet its specific role in this process is not fully understood [54-56]. Many investigations show that the amelogenin C-terminus is critical for the development and progression of amelogenin higher order assemblage and that it may be important in protein mineral interaction [57, 58]. It also has been shown that the proline residues in the C-terminus, which is processed from the protein shortly after it is secreted from the ameloblast, are critical for normal MMP20 cleavage of the C-terminus [20, 59]. The exact mechanism leading to a marked deficiency of enamel formation when the amelogenin carboxy terminus is not produced is not fully understood. However, the generalized hypoplastic phenotype suggests that the ameloblasts likely cease normal function prematurely. This could result from abnormal cell-matrix/mineral interactions that cause the cells to prematurely cease their secretory phase resulting in a thin enamel phenotype.

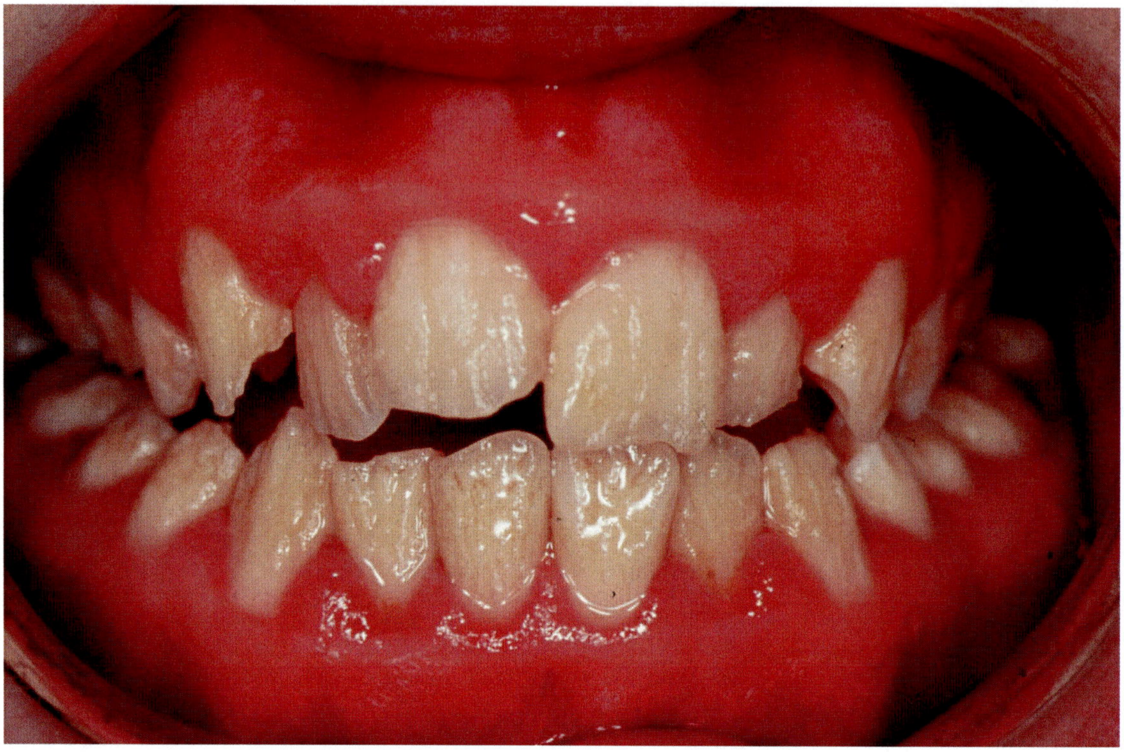

Figure 3: This female dentition is affected by a P158fsX187 *AMELX* mutation and is characterized by a hypoplastic phenotype that shows the classic ridge and furrowing of the enamel that results from lyonization in females. The ridges result from ameloblasts expressing the normal AMELX allele while the furrows are formed by ameloblasts expressing the P158fsX187 *AMELX* allele that causes loss of the C terminus due to introduction of a premature stop codon.

IMPLICATION OF *AMELX* MUTATIONS AND AI

Evaluation of the phenotype and genotype relationship in X-linked amelogenesis imperfecta suggests there is clustering of phenotypes depending on the location and type of *AMELX* mutation and its effect on the amelogenin protein. The demarcation between phenotypes is not always exact with some overlap occurring between hypoplastic, hypomaturation and hypomineralization-type defects. The consistency of these phenotypes does lend itself to assisting with the diagnosis of the X-linked AI conditions and narrowing the search for identifying specific *AMELX* mutations. This is especially true when one encounters X-linked hypomaturation AI phenotypes.

The mechanisms whereby different *AMELX* mutations lead to specific phenotypes is not fully understood, however, our understanding of the connection between the genotype, protein and resulting phenotype is growing. Mutations that result in a loss of functional amelogenin are believed to cause thin enamel due to a haploinsufficiency mechanism. This would be true for the large deletion mutations and the *AMELX* signal peptide mutations. This indicates that a complete absence of amelogenin is not compatible with the formation of a normal enamel thickness. This conclusion is supported by the amelogenin knockout mouse phenotype that is characterized by having only a very thin layer of enamel [7]. Phenotypes in the amelogenin knockout mouse and in humans with the amelogenin signal peptide mutations are remarkably similar. One would predict that the 5Kb deletion mutation that essentially knocks out the human AMELX gene would have the same phenotype as the signal peptide mutations and the knockout mouse model. However, the phenotype described for males in these families is primarily hypomineralized/hypomature enamel with varying degrees of hypoplasia. The presence of hypoplasia in these cases supports the contention that amelogenin is essential for developing a normal enamel thickness. The explanation for the phenotypic variation between the signal peptide mutations and the 5Kb knockout families remains an enigma and more detailed characterization of the phenotypes is required to resolve this issue.

The amelogenin knock-out mouse may provide insight as to why a loss of amelogenin leads to a generalized thin enamel phenotype. Light microscopy studies show that the secretory ameloblasts prematurely loose their tall columnar morphology and take on a cuboidal phenotype in the *AmelX* KO mouse [7]. This suggests that there are as yet poorly understood critical interactions between the extracellular matrix and the ameloblasts that are critical for normal enamel development.

AMELX mutations causing alterations in the N-terminus of the mature amelogenin protein are all associated with a hypomineralization/hypomaturation AI phenotype where the enamel is yellow to brown in coloration and shows varying biochemical disturbances. For the N-terminal defects, the enamel is best characterized for the P70T mutation where the enamel has a slight reduction in mineral content and a slight increase in proline-rich amelogenin-like protein supporting the classification of these defects as being hypomaturation [36]. The H77L mutation lies two amino acids C-terminal to the putative binding site but is also adjacent to a proteolytic cleavage site. Whether this mutation alters amelogenin processing by MMP20 remains unknown. The T51I mutation is located 12 amino acids N-terminal to the putative binding site but appears to result in a similar phenotype as the more C-terminally located mutations in this region. Studies using transgenic mice that express the P70T protein and have a phenotype despite having a normal complement of amelogenin expression suggests a dominant-negative type mechanism occurs [60]. Apparently, having these mutant proteins present does not allow the temporally critical processes of amelogenesis to proceed as necessary thereby resulting in retention of amelogenin protein and an altered enamel ultrastructure [36, 60].

Loss of the C-terminus of the amelogenin protein results in a smooth hypoplastic phenotype not unlike that seen when the total protein is lost. The mechanism leading to this common phenotype is however, apparently quite different. The hypoplastic phenotype seen in all four mutations causing a loss of the 18 C-terminal amino acids, and in the one case causing loss of the C-terminal 14 amino acids also is apparently caused by a dominant-negative type of mechanism. While the specific role of the C-terminus in determining enamel thickness is unknown, the consistent hypoplastic phenotype in all cases lacking this region of the amelogenin protein clearly indicates that it is a critical domain for normal enamel formation. The acidic C-terminal domain has been shown to be important in the amelogenin self-assembly process to form nanospheres and the amelogenin affinity for mineral [40]. It is highly feasible that alteration of any of these processes could sufficiently alter the normal developmental cascades so that enamel formation would prematurely terminate resulting in enamel hypoplasia. Alteration of the C-terminal region from amino acids 157-173 in a transgenic mouse without disturbing the final seven C-terminal amino acids results increased enamel porosity and prism dysmorphology but does not apparently result in thin enamel [61]. The importance of the amelogenin carboxy terminus and its potential role during interactions with membrane-bound proteins such as CD63 and LAMP1 has been reported [62]. The putative binding domain would be partially deleted in all of the amelogenin C-terminal truncation mutations. This could alter the proposed endocytotic activity required for effective removal of the amelogenin protein or other abnormal matrix-cell interactions [62].

Evaluation of the known *AMELX* mutations and the clustering and conservation of phenotypes helps define the important functions of different regions of the amelogenin protein. Two main phenotypes result from the different *AMELX* mutations that span the gene including a deficient amount of enamel or hypoplasia and an abnormal structure and composition of enamel that is called hypomaturation. The phenotype that occurs is dependent on the type and location of the *AMELX* mutation and their affects on the translated amelogenin protein. As our understanding of the amelogenin protein and its activities during enamel formation grows, so does our understanding of the specific mechanisms leading to the markedly different phenotypes that result from changes in the amelogenin protein. Alterations in the human *AMELX* gene and characterization of the resulting enamel phenotypes, continues to provide insight into the critical role of amelogenin during normal enamel formation.

ACKNOWLEDGMENTS

Supported by NIDCR Grant 12879

REFERENCES

[1] Witkop CJJ. Amelogenesis imperfecta, dentinogenesis imperfecta and dentin dysplasia revisited, problems in classification. J Oral Pathol 1989; 17: 547-553.

[2] Wright JT, Daly B, Simmons D, *et al.* Human enamel phenotype associated with amelogenesis imperfecta and a kallikrein-4 (g.2142G>A) proteinase mutation. Eur J Oral Sci 2006; 114 Suppl 1: 13-7; discussion 39-41, 379.

[3] Kim JW, Lee SK, Lee ZH, *et al.* FAM83H mutations in families with autosomal-dominant hypocalcified amelogenesis imperfecta. Am J Hum Genet 2008; 82(2): 489-94.

[4] El-Sayed W, Parry DA, Shore RC, *et al.* Mutations in the Beta Propeller WDR72 Cause Autosomal-Recessive Hypomaturation Amelogenesis Imperfecta. Am J Hum Genet 2009.

[5] Fincham AG, Belcourt AB. Amelogenin biochemistry: current concepts. In: Butler WT, editor. The Chemistry and Biology of Mineralized Tissues. Birmingham: Ebsco Media, Inc.; 1985. p. 240-247.

[6] Robinson C, Shore RC, Kirkham J, *et al.* Extracellular processing of enamel matrix proteins and the control of crystal growth. J Biol Buccale 1990; 18(4): 355-361.

[7] Gibson CW, Yuan ZA, Hall B, *et al.* Amelogenin-deficient mice display an amelogenesis imperfecta phenotype. J Biol Chem 2001; 276: 31871-31875.

[8] Lattanzi W, Di Giacomo MC, Lenato GM, *et al.* A large interstitial deletion encompassing the amelogenin gene on the short arm of the Y chromosome. Hum Genet 2005; 116(5): 395-401.

[9] Delgado S, Girondot M, Sire JY. Molecular evolution of amelogenin in mammals. J Mol Evol 2005; 60(1): 12-30.

[10] Delgado S, Ishiyama M, Sire JY. Validation of amelogenesis imperfecta inferred from amelogenin evolution. J Dent Res 2007; 86(4): 326-30.

[11] Salido E, Yen P, Koprivnikar K, *et al* The human enamel protein gene amelogenin is expressed from both the X and the Y chromosomes. Am J Hum Genet 1992; 50: 303-316.

[12] Simmer JP, Hu C-C, Lau EC, *et al* Alternative splicing of the mouse amelogenin primary RNA transcript. Calcif Tissue Int 1994; 55: 302-310.

[13] Fincham AG, Moradian-Oldak J, Simmer JP, *et al.* Self-assembly of a recombinant amelogenin protein generates supramolecular structures. J Struct Biol 1994; 112: 103-109.

[14] Lakshminarayanan R, Fan D, Du C, *et al.* The role of secondary structure in the entropically driven amelogenin self-assembly. Biophys J 2007; 93(10): 3664-74.

[15] Zhu D, Paine ML, Luo W, *et al.* Altering biomineralization by protein design. J Biol Chem 2006; 281(30): 21173-82.

[16] Robinson C, Connell S, Brookes SJ, *et al.* Surface chemistry of enamel apatite during maturation in relation to pH: implications for protein removal and crystal growth. Arch Oral Biol 2005; 50(2): 267-70.

[17] Lu Y, Papagerakis P, Yamakoshi Y, *et al.* Functions of KLK4 and MMP-20 in dental enamel formation. Biol Chem 2008; 389(6): 695-700.

[18] Fincham AG, Moradian-Oldak J, Diekwisch TGH, *et al.* Ultrastructural evidence for "Nanospheres" as components of secretory-stage enamel matrix and a possible functional role for amelogenin in initial enamel biomineralization. J Struct Biol 1995; 115: 50-59.

[19] Shaw WJ, Campbell AA, Paine ML, *et al.* The COOH terminus of the amelogenin, LRAP, is oriented next to the hydroxyapatite surface. J Biol Chem 2004; 279(39): 40263-6.

[20] Zhu L, Tanimoto K, Le T, *et al.* Functional roles of prolines at amelogenin C terminal during tooth enamel formation. Cells Tissues Organs 2009; 189(1-4): 203-6.

[21] Robinson C, Briggs H, Atkinson P, *et al* Chemical changes during formation and maturation of human deciduous enamel. Archs oral Biol 1981; 26: 1027-1033.

[22] Lagerstrom M, Dahl N, Nakahori Y, *et al.* A deletion in the amelogenin gene (AMG) causes X-linked amelogenesis imperfecta (AIH1). Genomics 1991; 10(4): 971-975.

[23] Kindelan S, Brook A, Gangemi L, *et al.* Detection of a novel mutation in X-linked amelogenesis imperfecta. J Dent Res 2000; 79: 1978-1982.

[24] Kim J-W, Simmer JP, Hu YY, *et al.* Amelogenin p.MIT and p.W4S mutations underlying hypoplastic X-linked amelogenesis imperfecta. J Dent Res 2004; 83: 378-383.

[25] Hart PS, Aldred MA, Crawford PJM, *et al.* Two amelogenin gene mutations cause different amelogenesis imperfecta phenotypes. Archs Oral Biol 2002; 47: 255-260.

[26] Wright JT, Hart PS, Aldred MJ, *et al.* Relationship of phenotype and genotype in X-linked amelogenesis imperfecta. Connect Tissue Res 2003; 44 (suppl.): 72-78.

[27] Aldred MJ, Savarirayan R, Crawford PJM. Amelogenesis imperfecta: a classification and catalogue for the 21st century. Oral Disease 2003; 9: 19-23.

[28] OMIM. Online Mendelian Inheritance in Man, World Wide Web URL. In: McKusick-Nathans Institute of Genetic Medicine, editor. http: //www.ncbi.nlm.nih.gov/omim/ ed. (Baltimore, MD, Bethesda, MD: Johns Hopkins University and National Center for Biotechnology Information, National Library of Medicine; 2009.

[29] Snead ML, Lau EC, Fincham AG, *et al.* Of mice and men: anatomy of the amelogenin gene. Conn Tiss Res 1989; 22: 101-109.

[30] Deeley K, Letra A, Rose EK, *et al.* Possible association of amelogenin to high caries experience in a Guatemalan-Mayan population. Caries Res 2008; 42(1): 8-13.

[31] Witkop CJ, Sauk JJ. Heritable Defects of Enamel. In: Stewart R, Prescott G, editors. Oral Facial Genetics. St. Louis: C.V. Mosby Company; 1976. p. 151-226.

[32] Backman B. Amelogenesis imperfecta-clinical manifestations in 51 families in a northern Swedish country. Scandanavian Journal Dental Research 1988; 96: 505-516.

[33] Sundell S, G K. Hereditary amelogenesis imperfecta: epidemiology and clinical classification in a Swedish child population. Swed Dent J 1985; 9: 157-169.

[34] Witkop CJJ. Partial expression of sex-linked amelogenesis imperfecta in females compatible with the Lyon hypothesis. Oral Surgery, Oral Medicine, Oral Pathology 1967; 23: 174-182.

[35] Wright JT, Aldred MJ, Crawford PJM, *et al.* Enamel ultrastructure and protein content in X-linked amelogenesis imperfecta. Oral Surg Oral Med Oral Pathol 1993; 76: 192-200.

[36] Ravassipour DB, Hart S, Hart TC, *et al.* Unique enamel phenotype associated with amelogenin gene (AMELX) codon 41 point mutation. J Dent Res 2000; 79: 1476-1481.

[37] Lagerstrom-Fermer M, Landegren U. Understanding enamel formation from mutations causing X-linked amelogensis imperfecta. Con Tis Res 1995; 32: 241-246.

[38] Hobson GM, Gibson CW, Aragon M, *et al.* A large X-chromosomal deletion is associated with microphthalmia with linear skin defects (MLS) and amelogenesis imperfecta (XAI). Am J Med Genet A 2009; 149A(8): 1698-705.

[39] Prakash SK, Gibson CW, Wright JT, *et al.* Tooth enamel defects in mice with a deletion at the Arhgap 6/Amel X locus. Calcif Tissue Int 2005; 77(1): 23-9.

[40] Lagerstrom-Fermer M, Nilsson M, Backman B, *et al.* Amelogenin signal peptide mutation: correlation between mutations in the amelogenin gene (AMGX) and manifestations of X-linked amelogenesis imperfecta. Genomics 1995; 26: 159-162.

[41] Sekiguchi H, Alaluusua S, Minaguchi K, *et al.* A new mutation in the amelogenin gene causes X-linked amelogenesis imperfecta. J Dent Res 2001; 80(SI): 617 (Abstract 0722).

[42] Aldred MJ, Crawford PJM, Roberts E, *et al.* Identification of a nonsense mutation in the amelogenin gene (AMELX) in a family with X-linked amelogenesis imperfecta (AIH1). Hum Genet 1992; 90: 413-416.

[43] Lench NJ, Brook AH, Winter GB. SSCP detection of a nonsense mutation in exon 5 of the amelogenin gene (AMGX) causing X-linked amelogenesis imperfecta. Human Mol Genet 1994; 3: 827-828.

[44] Lench NJ, Winter GB. Characterisation of molecular defects in X-linked amelogenesis imperfecta (AIH1). Human Mut 1995; 5: 251-259.

[45] Rajpar MH, Harley K, Laing C, *et al.* Mutation of the gene encoding the enamel-specific protein, enamelin, causes autosomal-dominant amelogenesis imperfecta. Human Mol Genet 2001; 10: 1673-1677.

[46] Collier PM, Sauk JJ, Rosenbloom J, *et al.* An amelogenin gene defect associated with human x-linked amelogenesis imperfecta. Archs Oral Biol 1997; 42: 235-242.

[47] Hart PS, Hart TC, Gibson C, *et al.* Mutational analysis of X-linked amelogenesis imperfecta in multiple families. Archs Oral Biol 2000; 45: 79-86.

[48] Ravindranath RMH, Moraidan-Oldak J, Fincham AG. Tyrosyl motif in amelogenins binds N-acetyl-D-glucosamine. J Biol Chem 1999; 274: 2464-2471.

[49] Ravindranath RMH, Tam W-Y, Nguyen P, *et al.* The enamel protein amelogenin binds to the N-acetyl-D-flucosamine-mimicking peptide motif of cytokeratins. J Biol Chem 2000; 275: 39654-39661.

[50] Paine ML, Lei YP, Dickerson K, *et al.* Altered amelogenin self-assembly based on mutations observed in human X-linked amelogenesis imperfecta (AIH1). J Biol Chem 2002; 277(19): 17112-6.

[51] Li W, Gibson C, Abrams W, *et al.* Reduced hydrolysis of amelogenin may result in X-linked amelogenesis imperfecta. Matrix Biol 2001; 19: 7555-760.

[52] Tanimoto K, Le T, Zhu L, *et al.* Reduced amelogenin-MMP20 interactions in amelogenesis imperfecta. J Dent Res 2008; 87(5): 451-5.

[53] Greene SR, Yuan ZA, Wright JT, *et al.* A gene deletion resulting in amelogenin with nine cysteine residues leads to amelogenesis imperfecta. Archs Oral Biol 2002; 47: 211-217.

[54] Aoba T, Kawano K, Moreno EC. Molecular conformation of porcine amelogenins and its significance in protein-mineral interaction: 1H-NMR photo-CIDNP study. J Biol Buccale 1990; 18(3): 189-94.

[55] Aoba T, Shimoda S, Shimokawa H, *et al.* Common epitopes of mammalian amelogenins at the C-terminus and possible functional roles of the corresponding domain in enamel mineralization. Calcif Tissue Int 1992; 51(1): 85-91.

[56] Fowler CE, Beniash E, Yamakoshi Y, *et al.* Co-operative mineralization and protein self-assembly in amelogenesis: silica mineralization and assembly of recombinant amelogenins in vitro. Eur J Oral Sci 2006; 114 Suppl 1: 297-303; discussion 327-9, 382.

[57] Moradian-Oldak J, Paine ML, Lei YP, *et al.* Self-assembly properties of recombinant engineered amelogenin proteins analyzed by dynamic light scattering and atomic force microscopy. J Struct Biol 2000; 131(1): 27-37.

[58] Moradian-Oldak J, Bouropoulos N, Wang L, *et al.* Analysis of self-assembly and apatite binding properties of amelogenin proteins lacking the hydrophilic C-terminal. Matrix Biol 2002; 21(2): 197-205.

[59] Brookes SJ, Robinson C, Kirkham J, *et al.* Biochemistry and molecular biology of amelogenin proteins of developing dental enamel. Archs Oral Biol 1995; 40: 1-14.

[60] Gibson CW, Yuan ZA, Li Y, *et al.* Transgenic mice that express normal and mutated amelogenins. J Dent Res 2007; 86(4): 331-5.

[61] Paine M, Shu D-H, Luo W, *et al.* Enamel biomineralization defects result from alterations to amelogenin self-assembly. J Struct Biol 2000; 132: 191-200.

[62] Zou Y, Wang H, Shapiro JL, *et al.* Determination of protein regions responsible for interactions of amelogenin with CD63 and LAMP1. Biochem J 2007; 408(3): 347-54.

CHAPTER 9

Degradation of Enamel Matrix Proteins

John D. Bartlett*, Coralee E Tye, Tabitha A. Abrazinski, Jerry Antone, Grace F. Lopez and Ramaswamy Sharma

Department of Cytokine Biology, The Forsyth Institute, 140 The Fenway, Boston, MA 02115; E-mail addresses: CET: ctye@forsyth.org; TAA: tabrazinski@forsyth.org; JA: jantone@forsyth.org; GFL: glopez@forsyth.org; RS: rsharma@forsyth.org

*Corresponding author: JD Bartlertt; Tel: 617-893-8388; Fax: 617-892-8303; Email: jbartlett@forsyth.org

Abstract: MMP20 (matrix metalloproteinase-20; enamelysin) and KLK4 (Kallikrein-4) are the two major, and perhaps only, proteinases present in developing dental enamel. MMP20 cleaves enamel resident proteins during the early developmental stages when the enamel grows in thickness and KLK4 cleaves enamel proteins prior to their absorption by the ameloblasts that sit atop full thickness enamel. KLK4 is expressed when the enamel starts to harden into its final mature form. Mutations in humans that eliminate the function of either MMP20 or KLK4 cause non-syndromic enamel malformations termed *amelogenesis imperfecta*. Homozygous deletion of either of these proteinases from the mouse genome will also result in severely malformed dental enamel. With the exception of malformed enamel, no other phenotype is yet known to occur when either of these proteinases are rendered functionless in humans or mice. Therefore, both MMP20 and KLK4 are essential for enamel formation. This chapter will provide historical insights into the discovery of these proteinases and will provide insights into the mechanistic function of how these proteinases act to direct enamel development.

Key Words: Enamelysin (MMP20), Kallikrein-4 (KLK4), Proteolysis, Enamel, Formation, Maturation, Amelogenesis Imperfecta,

HISTORICAL PERSPECTIVE

Overview

Dental enamel is unique because it is the only epithelially derived calcified tissue in vertebrates and it is the hardest substance in the body. The enamel organ encloses the developing tooth and is required for enamel formation. The ameloblast cells of the enamel organ are adjacent to, and are responsible for, dental enamel development. The ameloblasts pass through a defined set of developmental stages as the dental enamel starts as a soft protein-rich substance and matures into a hard virtually protein-free mineral. These stages include the pre-secretory, secretory, transition, and maturation stages of development. During the pre-secretory stage ameloblasts proliferate. As they progress into the secretory stage, ameloblasts stop dividing and enlarge into tall columnar secretory ameloblasts that align more or less vertically to the adjacent enamel and are responsible for secreting enamel matrix proteins. The transition stage occurs when the ameloblasts transition from tall to shortened cells. This occurs when the enamel has reached its full thickness and when protein secretion into the enamel matrix is greatly reduced. The transition stage progresses rapidly to the maturation stage. During the maturation stage, the ameloblasts are shorter and assist in the removal of proteins from the matrix as the enamel hardens [1, 2]. Once the enamel is fully mature, ameloblasts regress and become part of the reduced enamel organ that covers and protects the completed enamel surface until the tooth erupts [3].

Early Evidence of Proteinase Action

In the early 1960s, Eastoe demonstrated that developing enamel had a high protein content, whereas mature enamel did not [4, 5]. The enamel matrix proteins were demonstrated as removed during the maturation stage of amelogenesis prior to tooth eruption [6]. Studies on developing porcine enamel showed that the percentage protein by weight dropped from 30% during the secretory stage to 2% during the early maturation stage [7]. In the rat incisor, a similar decline was associated with a significant change in the amino acid composition of total enamel matrix proteins [8]. Thus, a role for proteinases in the degradation and export of enamel proteins was advanced. Lysosomes were observed histologically in ameloblasts [9], proteolytic activity was demonstrated in the enamel organ [10], and it was proposed that lysosomal enzymes may be secreted into the enamel matrix [11]. Proteolytic activity was also demonstrated within the forming enamel of 6-8 day old rats [12]. While theories not involving proteinases have been postulated to explain the abrupt loss of matrix during the early maturation stage [13, 14], the progressive decrease in the average size of enamel matrix proteins was more consistent with the involvement of proteinases [7].

Since that time, several investigations have suggested that as the forming enamel passes through the secretory stage and into the maturation stage of development, the enamel proteinases undergo a change in profile. This change was first identified by Overall and Limeback [15] who used enzyme inhibitors to demonstrate that metalloproteinase(s) were present during early enamel development and that serine proteinase(s) were present during the later stages. Although there was some overlap, this change in enzyme profile was confirmed by several other investigators [16-20]. Therefore, prior to identification of any specific protease within developing dental enamel, an abundance of evidence suggested that at least two classes of enzymes were present. A proteinase of the metalloproteinase class was present early during the secretory stage and a proteinase of the serine class was present late during the maturation stage of enamel development.

The Discovery of MMP20

The proteinases in forming enamel are present in very small quantities. This meant that standard cloning procedures, whereby enough purified protein is isolated to identify protein sequence for reverse translation into a viable cDNA probe, were not viable options. Therefore, MMP20 was first cloned from a porcine enamel organ-specific cDNA library by PCR-based homology cloning. The resulting cDNA fragment was 401 bp in length and was similar, but not highly homologous, to other MMPs present in the database. The 401 bp fragment was then used to clone the full-length porcine *Mmp20* mRNA. Alignment of the conceptually translated *Mmp20* mRNA with the amino acid sequence of the other MMP family members revealed that *Mmp20* was a unique member of the MMP family of peptidases. Original northern blots demonstrated that *Mmp20* was expressed only in the enamel organ of developing teeth, hence *Mmp20* was originally named enamelysin [21]. Subsequently, however, *Mmp20* was also found to be expressed in odontoblast [22] and at extremely low levels (approximately 5000-fold less than in the secretory enamel organ) in the large intestine [23].

Interestingly, because the *Mmp20* mRNA was isolated by PCR-based homology cloning, the cellular localization of the protein in the enamel organ and its secretion into the enamel matrix was not known. Two papers published in 1998 resolved these issues. The first demonstrated that MMP20 was expressed by ameloblasts and was secreted into the forming enamel. This was shown by immunogold analysis and by a unique, overloaded enamel protein zymogram that was subsequently assessed by western blot analysis for the presence of MMP20 [24]. The second paper used *in situ* hybridization to show that both ameloblasts and odontoblasts express *Mmp20* transcripts [25]. Thus, in 1998 MMP20 became the first proteinase to be definitively identified as expressed by the ameloblasts of the enamel organ and secreted into the developing enamel matrix.

The Discovery of KLK4

KLK4 was discovered much the same way as MMP20. KLK4 is expressed at lower levels than MMP20 so standard cloning procedures would have been difficult at best. Even so, in a massive undertaking by the laboratories of Fukae, Tanabe, Yamakoshi, and Uchida, over 2000 unerupted porcine incisor tooth buds were collected over a period of five months and KLK4 was purified from transition and early maturation stage porcine enamel. KLK4 protein sequence was obtained and standard cloning procedures were attempted in the Simmer laboratory. However, separately and unbeknownst to these researchers, the Bartlett laboratory had already cloned the *Klk4* mRNA by PCR-based homology cloning. When all became aware of each other's KLK4 results, a highly productive research collaboration resulted that reported the first discovery of KLK4 [26]. The original name for KLK4 was enamel matrix serine proteinase 1 (EMSP1). Unfortunately, a few others cloned *Klk4* from such tissues as the prostate and did not acknowledge the EMSP1 nomenclature, or in some cases, even the original discovery. This led to a nomenclature committee decision to change the name of EMSP1 to KLK4. Ironically, KLK4 has only moderate homology to the other kallikreins; yet KLK4 is located in the kallikrein gene cluster.

Because KLK4 protein had been isolated from forming enamel, it was initially known that KLK4 was secreted into the enamel matrix. This would later be confirmed by western blots and immunogold analysis. In addition, *in situ* hybridization results demonstrated that the ameloblasts of the enamel organ express *Klk4*. These results also showed that *Klk4* was expressed during the maturation stage, but not the secretory stage of enamel development [27]. Thus, in the year 2000, KLK4 was the second, and to date, the last proteinase to be identified as expressed by ameoblasts and secreted into the enamel matrix. It was now known that MMP20 was expressed during the secretory stage through the transition stage of enamel development and that KLK4 was expressed starting at the transition stage through the maturation stage of enamel development. There is, therefore, little overlap in the expression of these two proteinases.

PROTEINASE FUNCTION IN FORMING ENAMEL

Overview

Dental enamel forms in stages within a well-defined extracellular space lined by ameloblasts, which are specialized enamel-forming cells, that control the composition of the enamel extracellular compartment. During the secretory stage, ameloblasts secrete mostly amelogenin, enamelin and ameloblastin [28-31]. These proteins catalyze the extension of ribbon-like enamel crystallites comprised of the mineral calcium hydroxyapatite. Amelogenin is the predominant secretory product of ameloblasts and assembles into spheres that occupy the spaces between the crystal ribbons, serving to separate and support them [32, 33]. The processing of enamel proteins during the secretory stage influences their distribution within the matrix. Intact (uncleaved) enamel proteins are present only on the surface where the crystallites grow in length. Only cleaved products are found in the deeper enamel where they organize into separate compartments [34, 35]. Ameloblastin cleavage products containing the N-terminal side of the protein are found at all depths within the enamel layer, but concentrate primarily in the sheath space between the enamel rods [29]. Enamelin cleavage products, such as 32-kDa enamelin, are found throughout the entire thickness of developing enamel, but are concentrated within the rod enamel. Amelogenin polyclonal antibodies immunostain the entire enamel matrix, but antibodies specific for the amelogenin C-terminus only immunostain the matrix to a depth of approximately 30 microns. These data demonstrate that intact enamel matrix proteins and their C-terminal cleavage products are only present in the most recently formed enamel near the mineralization front, while their cleavage products are distributed throughout the matrix. This suggests that the full-length enamel proteins perform a different function than their cleavage products. It is thought that the full-length proteins promote crystallite elongation and the cleavage products provide support for the extremely thin elongating crystallites.

During the maturation stage the ameloblasts are shortened and they no longer secrete MMP20, amelogenin, ameloblastin or enamelin into the full-thickness hardening enamel matrix. It is during the maturation stage that the long thin crystallites grow in width and thickness and this is when most enamel mineralization occurs. The enamel matrix protein cleavage products that were generated during the secretory stage to support the thin crystallites, now must be removed so that the crystallites can grow laterally and merge with one another to form a complete enamel rod [36]. Once this process is complete for both the rod and inter-rod enamel, the entire dental enamel layer achieves its final hardened form.

Matrix Metalloproteinase-20 Function

MMP20 is expressed during the secretory stage of enamel development when ameloblasts are actively secreting proteins into the enamel matrix. Full-length proteins are found only at the mineralizing front of the elongating enamel crystallites. Thus, they are thought to be essential for promoting crystallite elongation. However, once these proteins are cleaved by MMP20, the cleaved products are found in the deeper more mature enamel and are thought to provide support for the thin crystallites. This is an ongoing process where the newly secreted proteins are cleaved and replaced by proteins that are continously secreted. This creates what is termed a “laddering effect” [37]. The laddering effect can be observed on SDS-PAGE gels loaded with secretory stage enamel protein. Whole proteins are seen at the top of the gel (highest MW bands) and proteolytic cleavage products can be observed as rungs of a ladder going down the gel (lower MW bands).

MMP20 contains an inhibitory propeptide that must be cleaved off for enzyme activity to occur. No activator of MMP20 has been identified although recombinant MMP20 will activate itself. It is, therefore, possible that MMP20 autocatalytically activates itself *in vivo.* MMP20 was first demonstrated to cleave amelogenin. Important studies have definitively demonstrated that digestion of recombinant amelogenin (rP172; Pro^{2}-Asp^{173}) with recombinant MMP20 yields all of the major porcine amelogenin cleavage products that accumulate in secretory-stage enamel [38]. In addition, native MMP20 and amelogenin (P173) purified from developing pig teeth were used to demonstrate that MMP20 digests amelogenin at the exact sites that yields all of the major amelogenin cleavage products that accumulate within secretory stage enamel [39]: the 23-kDa (Met^{1}-Pro^{162}), 20-kDa (Met^{1}-Ser^{148}), 13-kDa (Leu^{46}-Ser^{148}), 11-kDa (Ala^{63}-Ser^{148}/Leu^{64}-Ser^{148}) extended tyrosine-rich amelogenin peptide (TRAP; Met^{1}-His^{62}/Met^{1}-Ala^{63}), and TRAP (Met^{1}-Trp^{45}). MMP20 was shown to process the leucine-rich amelogenin peptide (LRAP) after Pro^{40} and Pro^{45}, and did not degrade LRAP further. MMP20 processes amelogenins into a group of cleavage products that accumulate and are only slowly degraded further by MMP20. Only the tyrosine and leucine-rich amelogenin peptides accumulate within the enamel matrix and this is because MMP20 has little activity to degrade them [39]. MMP20 was also demonstrated to cleave ameloblastin. N-terminal sequencing of recombinant porcine ameloblastin digestion products showed that MMP20 cleaved ameloblastin after Pro^{2}, Gln^{130}, Gln^{139}, Arg^{170}, and Ala^{222}. This shows that MMP-20 generates the 23-kDa ameloblastin starting at Tyr^{223}, as well as the 17-kDa (Val^{1}-Arg^{170}) and 15-kDa (Val^{1}-Gln^{130}) ameloblastin cleavage products that concentrate in the sheath space during the secretory stage [40]. It was concluded that in developing pig teeth, MMP20 is the only significant proteolytic enzyme in the enamel extracellular space during the secretory stage [39]. The importance of the MMP20 processing function is suggested by the loss of prism structure and failure of the enamel layer to achieve full thickness in the *Mmp20* null mice, while its degradative function is evident by the retention of enamel proteins and the tendency of the enamel to chip off in these mice [41]. Therefore, MMP20 and its proteolytic cleavage products are essential for proper dental enamel development.

Kallikrein-4 Function

KLK4 is expressed during the maturation stage of enamel development when the enamel crystallites grow in width and thickness. KLK4 is thought to degrade enamel matrix proteins to facilitate their removal from the hardening enamel. Deletion of KLK4 from the mouse genome results in normally thick enamel containing the normal decussating enamel rod pattern. However, the null mouse enamel retains enamel proteins and the enamel is rapidly abraded following weaning. Upon closer examination it was discovered that the individual enamel crystallites did grow significantly in width and thickness, but they failed to grow together, interlock, and function as a unit. Instead of forming a cohesive enamel rod, individual crystallites were discerned and they appeared to spill out of the enamel when fractured. Therefore, KLK4 is essential for enamel matrix protein removal so that the enamel crystallites may properly mature and merge to form an enamel rod [36].

KLK4 is secreted into the enamel matrix as an inactive zymogen and little is known about how it becomes activated. MMP20 has been shown to activate KLK4 *in vitro* [42]. However, KLK4 and MMP20 expression overlap only briefly during enamel development [43]. Dipeptidyl peptidase I (DPPI), also known as cathepsin C, is a ubiquitously expressed cysteine aminopeptidase that can activate several serine proteases including KLK4 *in vitro* [44]. If DPPI does in fact activate KLK4 *in vivo,* it is likely not the only KLK4 activator. This is because although DPPI null mouse enamel is softer than normal, the phenotype is nowhere near as severe as is observed in the *Klk4* null mouse enamel [36].

Like MMP20, KLK4 was initially demonstrated to cleave amelogenin. Recombinant porcine KLK4 was shown to cleave 11 sites within a recombinant porcine amelogenin substrate. These sites were located after amino acids L23, K24, Y26, R31, Y37, H48, H62, H67, H92, A108, and Q150, respectively. However, some molecular masses measured in the digestion could not be assigned to a single probable peptide, suggesting that many additional sites on the amelogenin protein were cleaved by KLK4 [42]. In addition, native KLK4 and amelogenin (P173) purified from developing pig teeth were used to show that KLK4 digested amelogenin to such an extent that it appeared as a smear on an SDS-PAGE gel whereas that digested by MMP20 appeared as discrete protein bands [45]. Furthermore, unlike MMP20, KLK4 cleaved TRAP after amino acids N14, F15, K24, Y26, N28, and R31 [39]. KLK4 also degrades the 32 kDa enamelin cleavage product that accumulates in secretory enamel. Enamelin starts as 186 kDa parent protein that can only be found within 1 µm of the enamel surface [28]. MMP20 is thought to create the 32 kDa enamelin cleavage product. It was demonstrated with native porcine proteins that KLK4 cleaves 32 kDa enamelin into nine major cleavage products, six of which were successfully characterized. The identified cleavage sites were after amino acids R180, Y205, H206, M219, and R262 [45]. The finding that MMP20 cleavage products persist in the secretory stage, and are further degraded by KLK4 during the maturation stage, is significant. This is because we now know that degradation of these proteins by KLK4 is necessary for their removal so that the enamel can achieve its final hardened form [36].

CONCLUSIONS

Dental enamel development is a dynamic process that occurs in stages to form the hardest substance of the body. The two major stages of enamel development are the secretory and maturation stages. Each of these stages require proteinases if the enamel is to develop normally. MMP20 activity is essential during the secretory stage. It functions to allow the continuously secreted full-length enamel proteins to promote crystallite elongation while providing enamel protein cleavage products as packing material to support the long thin crystallites as they grow in length. This conclusion is based on the observation that the full-length enamel proteins are only present in the most recently formed enamel while the MMP20 cleavage products are found in the more mature and deeper enamel layers. As the ameloblasts progress through the transition stage and into the maturation stage of enamel development, the enamel layer has reached its full thickness and the enamel crystallites start growing laterally in width and thickness. However, if the MMP20 generated "packing material" protein is not removed, the crystallites can significantly increase in their width and thickness, but not to the point where they can actually merge with one another to form a cohesive enamel rod. KLK4 is expressed during the maturation stage to further degrade the remaining MMP20 cleavage products so that they may be efficiently exported out of the mineralizing enamel. This allows the crystallites to merge and form the characteristic solid enamel rod which is necessary for forming strong healthy dental enamel. In part, because the enamel matrix contains only three known proteins (amelogenin, ameloblastin, enamelin) and two proteinases (MMP20 and KLK4), it is one of the best characterized tissues with regard to the mechanistic function of its proteolytic enzymes.

ACKNOWLEDGMENTS

Support (R01DE016276 to JDB) from National Institute of Dental and Craniofacial Research is gratefully acknowledged.

REFERENCES

[1] Bartlett JD, Simmer JP. Proteinases in developing dental enamel. Crit Rev.Oral Biol.Med. 1999; 10:425-441.
[2] Smith CE. Cellular and chemical events during enamel maturation. Crit Rev.Oral Biol.Med. 1998; 9:128-161.
[3] Kallenbach E. Fine structure of rat incisor enamel organ during late pigmentation and regression stages. J Ultrastruct.Res 1970; 30:38-63.
[4] Eastoe JE. Organic matrix of tooth enamel. Nature 1960; 187:411-2.
[5] Eastoe JE. The amino acid composition of proteins from the oral tissues. II. The Matrix Proteins in Dentine and Enamel from Developing Human Deciduous Teeth. Arch Oral Biol 1963; 52:633-52.
[6] Burgess RC, Maclaren CM. Proteins in developing bovine enamel. In: Tooth Enamel I. Stack MV, W. FR (Editors). Bristol: John Wright & Sons LTD; 1965. pp. 74-82.
[7] Fukae M, Shimizu M. Studies on the proteins of developing bovine enamel. Arch Oral Biol 1974; 19:381-386.
[8] Robinson C, Lowe NR, Weatherell JA. Changes in amino-acid composition of developing rat incisor enamel. Calcif Tissue Res 1977; 23:19-31.
[9] Reith EJ. The Ultrastructure of Ameloblasts during Early Stages of Maturation of Enamel. J Cell Biol 1963; 18:691-6.
[10] Sakamoto S, Sasaki S. Changes in catheptic activity in the enamel organ of the bovine tooth germ during development. Arch Oral Biol 1969; 14:987-90.
[11] Katchburian E, Holt SJ. Role of lysosomes in amelogenesis. Nature 1969; 223:1367-8.
[12] Suga S. Histochemical observation of proteolytic enzyme activity in the developing dental hard tissues of the rat. Arch Oral Biol 1970; 15:555-558.
[13] Eastoe JE. In: Comprehensive biochemistry. Forkin M, Stotz EH (Editors). Amsterdam: Elsevier; 1971. pp. 785-834.
[14] Eastoe JE. Enamel protein chemistry--past, present and future. J Dent Res 1979; 58:753-764.
[15] Overall CM, Limeback H. Identification and characterization of enamel proteinases isolated from developing enamel. Amelogeninolytic serine proteinases are associated with enamel maturation in pig. Biochem.J. 1988; 256:965-972.

[16] DenBesten PK, Heffernan LM. Separation by polyacrylamide gel electrophoresis of multiple proteases in rat and bovine enamel. Arch.Oral Biol. 1989; 34:399-404.
[17] Smith CE, Borenstein S, Fazel A, *et al. In vitro* studies of the proteases which degrade amelogenenins in developing rat incisor enamel. In: Tooth enamel V. RW F (Editor) Yokohama: Florence Publishers; 1989. pp. 286-293.
[18] Smith CE, Issid M, Margolis HC, *et al.* Developmental changes in the pH of enamel fluid and its effects on matrix-resident proteinases. Adv Dent Res 1996; 10:159-169.
[19] Tanabe T, Fukae M, Uchida T, *et al.*. The localization and characterization of proteinases for the initial cleavage of porcine amelogenin. Calcif Tissue Int 1992; 51:213-7.
[20] Tanabe T, Fukae M, Shimizu M. Degradation of enamelins by proteinases found in porcine secretory enamel in vitro. Arch Oral Biol 1994; 39:277-81.
[21] Bartlett JD, Simmer JP, Xue J, *et al.* Molecular cloning and mRNA tissue distribution of a novel matrix metalloproteinase isolated from porcine enamel organ. Gene 1996; 183:123-128.
[22] Bartlett JD, Ryu OH, Xue J, *et al.* Enamelysin mRNA displays a developmentally defined pattern of expression and encodes a protein which degrades amelogenin. Connect.Tissue Res. 1998; 39:101-109.
[23] Turk BE, Lee DH, Yamakoshi Y, *et al.* MMP-20 Is Predominately a Tooth-Specific Enzyme with a Deep Catalytic Pocket that Hydrolyzes Type V Collagen. Biochemistry 2006; 45:3863-3874.
[24] Fukae M, Tanabe T, Uchida T, *et al.* Enamelysin (matrix metalloproteinase-20): localization in the developing tooth and effects of pH and calcium on amelogenin hydrolysis. J.Dent.Res. 1998; 77:1580-1588.
[25] Begue-Kirn C, Krebsbach PH, Bartlett JD, *et al.*. Dentin sialoprotein, dentin phosphoprotein, enamelysin and ameloblastin: tooth-specific molecules that are distinctively expressed during murine dental differentiation. Eur J Oral Sci 1998; 106:963-70.
[26] Simmer JP, Fukae M, Tanabe T, *et al.* Purification, characterization, and cloning of enamel matrix serine proteinase 1. J.Dent.Res. 1998; 77:377-386.
[27] Hu JC, Ryu OH, Chen JJ, *et al.* Localization of EMSP1 expression during tooth formation and cloning of mouse cDNA. J Dent Res 2000; 79:70-76.
[28] Hu CC, Fukae M, Uchida T, *et al.* Cloning and characterization of porcine enamelin mRNAs. J Dent Res 1997; 76:1720-1729.
[29] Hu CC, Fukae M, Uchida T, *et al.* Sheathlin: cloning, cDNA/polypeptide sequences, and immunolocalization of porcine enamel sheath proteins. J Dent Res 1997; 76:648-657.
[30] Krebsbach PH, Lee SK, Matsuki Y, *et al.* Full-length sequence, localization, and chromosomal mapping of ameloblastin. A novel tooth-specific gene. J Biol.Chem. 1996; 271:4431-4435.
[31] Snead ML, Lau EC, Zeichner-David M, *et al.* DNA sequence for cloned cDNA for murine amelogenin reveal the amino acid sequence for enamel-specific protein. Biochem Biophys.Res Commun 1985; 129:812-818.
[32] Fincham AG, Moradian-Oldak J, Simmer JP, *et al.* Self-assembly of a recombinant amelogenin protein generates supramolecular structures. J Struct.Biol 1994; 112:103-109.
[33] Fincham AG, Moradian-Oldak J, Diekwisch TG, *et al.* Evidence for amelogenin "nanospheres" as functional components of secretory-stage enamel matrix. J Struct Biol 1995; 115:50-9.
[34] Uchida T, Tanabe T, Fukae M, *et al.* Immunochemical and immunohistochemical studies, using antisera against porcine 25 kDa amelogenin, 89 kDa enamelin and the 13-17 kDa nonamelogenins, on immature enamel of the pig and rat. Histochemistry 1991; 96:129-38.
[35] Fukae M, Tanabe T, Uchida T, *et al.* Enamelins in the newly formed bovine enamel. Calcif Tissue Int 1993; 53:257-61.
[36] Simmer JP, Hu Y, Lertlam R, *et al.* Hypomaturation Enamel Defects in Klk4 Knockout/LacZ Knockin Mice. J Biol.Chem 2009; 284:19110-19121.
[37] Smith CE, Pompura JR, Borenstein S, *et al.* Degradation and loss of matrix proteins from developing enamel. Anat.Rec. 1989; 224:292-316.
[38] Ryu OH, Fincham AG, Hu CC, *et al.* Characterization of recombinant pig enamelysin activity and cleavage of recombinant pig and mouse amelogenins. J Dent Res 1999; 78:743-750.
[39] Nagano T, Kakegawa A, Yamakoshi Y, *et al.* Mmp-20 and Klk4 cleavage site preferences for amelogenin sequences. J Dent Res 2009; 88:823-8.
[40] Iwata T, Yamakoshi Y, Hu JC, *et al.* Processing of ameloblastin by MMP-20. J Dent Res 2007; 86:153-157.
[41] Caterina JJ, Skobe Z, Shi J, *et al.* Enamelysin (matrix metalloproteinase 20)-deficient mice display an amelogenesis imperfecta phenotype. J Biol Chem. 2002; 277:49598-49604.

[42] Ryu O, Hu JC, Yamakoshi Y, *et al.* Porcine kallikrein-4 activation, glycosylation, activity, and expression in prokaryotic and eukaryotic hosts. Eur J Oral Sci 2002; 110:358-365.
[43] Hu JC, Sun X, Zhang C, *et al.* Enamelysin and kallikrein-4 mRNA expression in developing mouse molars. Eur J Oral Sci 2002; 110:307-315.
[44] Tye CE, Pham CT, Simmer JP, Bartlett JD. DPPI may activate KLK4 during enamel formation. J Dent Res 2009; 88:323-327.
[45] Yamakoshi Y, Hu JC, Fukae M, *et al.* How do enamelysin and kallikrein 4 process the 32-kDa enamelin? Eur J Oral Sci 2006; 114 Suppl 1:45-51.

CHAPTER 10

Intrinsic Disorder in Amelogenin

Janet Moradian-Oldak[1] and Rajamani Lakshminarayanan[2]

Center for Craniofacial Molecular Biology, University of Southern California, 2250 Alcazar Street, CSA103, HSC, Los Angeles, CA 90033, USA; Email: joldak@usc.edu. [2]Singapore Eye Research Institute, 7 Hospital Drive Block C, 02-02, Singapore 169611; Email: lakshminus@gmail.com.

Abstract. In addition to its critical structural function during enamel biomineralization amelogenin protein also exhibits distinct signaling activities in a variety of in vitro and in vivo experimental systems. We present computational and biophysical data to demonstrate that amelogenin belongs to the class of Intrinsically Disordered Proteins (IDPs). IDPs lack a well-defined 3D structure under native conditions and are typically flexible, extended, and have little secondary structure in vitro in the absence of partners. This chapter considers details of the conformation, secondary structure, and degree of disorder in amelogenin. We propose that the occurrence of "conformational plasticity" in amelogenin explains its multi-functionality, contributes to its strong tendency to self-assemble, and its potential to specifically interact with different targets.

Key Words: Amelogenin, Intrinsic Disordered Proteins, Biomineralization, Enamel.

INTRODUCTION

The particular functional role of amelogenin protein in controlling calcium phosphate formation during enamel biomineralization has been well recognized [1-5] (see also Chapter 11, this volume). Recent advances in the molecular and structural biology of enamel gene products indicate that control mechanisms are highly dependent on complex protein-protein and protein-mineral co-assembly [6, 7]. Amelogenin self-assembly, which varies depending on the environment, is a critical parameter of the above control processes [8-10].

Using bioinformatic strategies as well as NMR and circular dichroism (CD) spectroscopy in solution, we recently determined that recombinant porcine amelogenin belongs to the class of intrinsically disordered proteins (IDPs), and is extended in its monomeric form [11]. Our finding was also supported by the observation that amelogenin contains a significant amount of polypro type II (PPII) structure and undergoes a conformational transition upon self-assembly [12, 13]. The PPII helix is believed to be the dominant conformation for many proline-rich regions of proteins and it is the major conformation of proteins in denatured states [14]. Intrinsically disordered proteins are typically flexible, extended, and have little secondary structure in vitro in the absence of partners [15]. The advantages of disorder in a protein are that 1) it can bind to differently shaped targets by structural accommodation at the binding interfaces, 2) different disordered sequences can fold to bind a common binding site, and 3) large interaction surfaces can be created by the unstructured molecule as it surrounds its partner or target. We propose that the wide range of inter-converting conformations in amelogenin facilitates protein-protein and protein-mineral interactions [11].

The functional role of intrinsically disordered proteins in the fields of transcriptional regulation, translation, and cellular signal transduction has recently been well recognized. While a series of proteins associated with mineralized tissues have been characterized as IDPs knowledge on their secondary structure and molecular mechanisms of their function are still limited [16]. In general, the functional attributes of IDPs include self-assembly into organized structures or binding to multiple targets with concomitant structural alterations. The amino acid compositions of IDPs are less complex than most proteins and are dominated by disorder-promoting residues such as E, K, R, G, Q, S, P, and A. We notice that some of these compositional and functional attributes mentioned above are also seen in amelogenin, which self-assembles into nanospheres, nanochains, and microribbons [4, 17-21]. In addition, amelogenin binds to apatite crystals through the hydrophilic C-terminal domain, and regions close to the C-terminus (B-domain) have been identified as critical for self-assembly [22-25] as well as for amelogenin's interaction with

Michel Goldberg (ED)

cell components such as LAMP1 and CD63 [26-28]. Small isoforms as well as full-length amelogenin possess signaling activities through specific cell receptors (Chapters 7, 12- 14, this volume).

In this chapter we will first briefly review IDPs and proceed to discuss the various computational and experimental approaches that have been used to define amelogenin as a member of the IDP family. An analysis of disordered regions in alternative splicing of amelogenin will then be presented. We will then provide an overview of strategies used to assess the secondary structure of amelogenin under various conditions and describe situations where amelogenin folding is induced. Given the increasing amount of evidence supporting the existence of intrinsic disorder in a number of proteins and our recent experimental evidence on amelogenin protein, we propose that IDP characteristics may explain the multifunctionality reported for amelogenin and a series of extracellular matrix proteins involved in many biomineralizing systems [27, 29-34].

INTRINSICALLY DISORDERED PROTEINS (IDPs)

Proteins, or significant regions of proteins, that lack a well-defined 3D structure under native conditions are referred to as intrinsically disordered proteins/regions (IDPs/IDRs) [35]. They have also been called rheomorphic, intrinsically unstructured (IUP) or natively unfolded proteins (NUP) [15, 16, 36-42]. Eukaryotic proteomes encompass a high abundance of proteins with long disordered regions (more than 30 amino acid residues) that are frequently associated with regulatory processes. A growing amount of evidence demonstrates that disordered regions play an important role in numerous functions. As many as 30 different functions have been linked to IDPs or ID regions and include protein-protein association, protein-DNA/RNA binding, and phosphorylation [37]. Unlike folded proteins, IDPs exist as an ensemble of inter-converting conformations without a fixed tertiary structure. Binding occurs with a higher-energy, weakly-populated conformation and shifts the equilibrium in favor of the selected conformation [43]. This phenomenon is known as coupled folding and binding. Such disorder-to-order transitions are accompanied by a large decrease in conformational entropy leading to a combination of high specificity and low affinity [44]. This is an important feature that is crucial for cell signaling and regulation and calls into question the traditional principle that well-defined structure is required for function [45-47]. The absence of a stable conformation has numerous advantages including the following: (i) The extended structure provides increased area of interface compared to a folded protein with the same number of residues [48], (ii) there is high specificity to the binding partners with low affinity, (iii) the flexibility allows binding diversity, that is binding to a number of different targets [49], (iv) the extended structure allows ready access of side chains to modifying enzymes as well as to enzymes that recognize the modifications, and (v) the disordered structure facilitates rapid degradation by proteases enabling a facile pathway for down-regulation.

IDPs can be readily identified by examining amino acid composition. A survey of IDPs/IDRs indicates that they are characterized by a low abundance of order-promoting amino acid residues (C, W, F, Y, V, L, and I) and an enrichment in disorder-promoting residues (E, K, R, D, Q, S, P, and T) [50-53]. The depletion of order-promoting residues reduces the non-covalent interactions between amino acids, thus creating a disordered structure. The differences in composition can be readily visualized by comparing the compositional profiles of a set of IDP sequences with those of a set of ordered proteins. The biased amino acid composition has allowed the development of several algorithms to predict IDPs/IDRs based on the premise that absence of a rigid structure is encoded in specific features of the amino acid sequence [54]. Analyzing the amino acid sequences of various IDPs, Uversky et al. proposed that IDPs contain low mean hydrophobicity and high mean net charge and disordered regions do not overlap ordered regions in folded proteins when the two parameters are plotted [55]. The boundary between the folded and intrinsically disordered groups was described by Uversky et al by the empirical equation 1 [55]:

$$\langle H\rangle_b = \langle R\rangle + 1.151/2.785 \ldots \quad (1)$$

where $\langle H\rangle_b$ is the "boundary mean hydrophobicity" value and the mean net charge $\langle R\rangle$ is defined as the net charge on the protein at pH 7.0 divided by the total number of residues. The extended nature of IDPs confers peculiar biochemical properties such as aberrant electrophoretic mobility in SDS-PAGE; high apparent molecular mass; unusual hydrodynamic dimensions and acid and heat resistance; non-cooperative heat and denaturant-induced transitions; hypersensitivity to proteolysis; and "turnout" response to environmental changes such as pH and metal ions or other ligands, osmolytes, and crowding agents [56, 57].

The absence of regular 3D structure in IDPs defeats the use of X-ray crystallography to determine structure. Thus, several other biophysical methods are used to infer the structural details in IDPs/IDRs. These include circular dichroism, intrinsic tryptophan fluorescence, electron spin resonance, Raman optical activity, Fourier-transformed infrared, and nuclear magnetic resonance spectroscopy (for secondary and tertiary structures); and dynamic light scattering, analytical ultracentrifugation, size exclusion chromatography, and small angle X-ray scattering (for hydrodynamic measurements) [57, 58].

INTRINSIC DISORDER IN AMELOGENIN

Bioinformatic Strategies

The bulk of amelogenin is enriched in Pro (P) and Gln (Q), amino acid residues known to promote disorder in protein structure. Other disorder-promoting residues such as Glu (E), Arg (R) and Lys (K) are all concentrated in the hydrophilic C-terminus. We have analyzed amino acid sequences of vertebrate amelogenins from 12 representative species. Mammalian amelogenin sequences are highly conserved, and interestingly, all 12 vertebrate amelogenins contain 50-60% disorder- promoting residues [13].

FoldIndex, PONDR, and IUPred.

We have used bioinformatic tools to reveal the degree of disorder in full-length porcine amelogenin. Bioinformatic analysis using three different predictors of intrinsic disorder; FoldIndex (Figure 1A), PONDR (Figure 1B), and IUPred (Figure 1C), indicated that the central region as well as the 12 amino acid residues at the C-terminus are disordered with a score higher than 0.9 (see the shaded area in Figure 1D). Analysis of amelogenin sequence using the Cumulative Distribution Function (CDF) curve (green line) in PONDR (Fig 1B1) revealed that amelogenin protein is below the boundary (black line) indicating a high proportion of high scores for disorder. Only a segment at the N-terminus (amino acids 6-42) and a segment close to the C-terminus (amino acids 150-160) were predicted to fold and have some level of secondary structure. Interestingly, the regions that separate ordered and disordered segments are close to proteolytic cleavage sites.

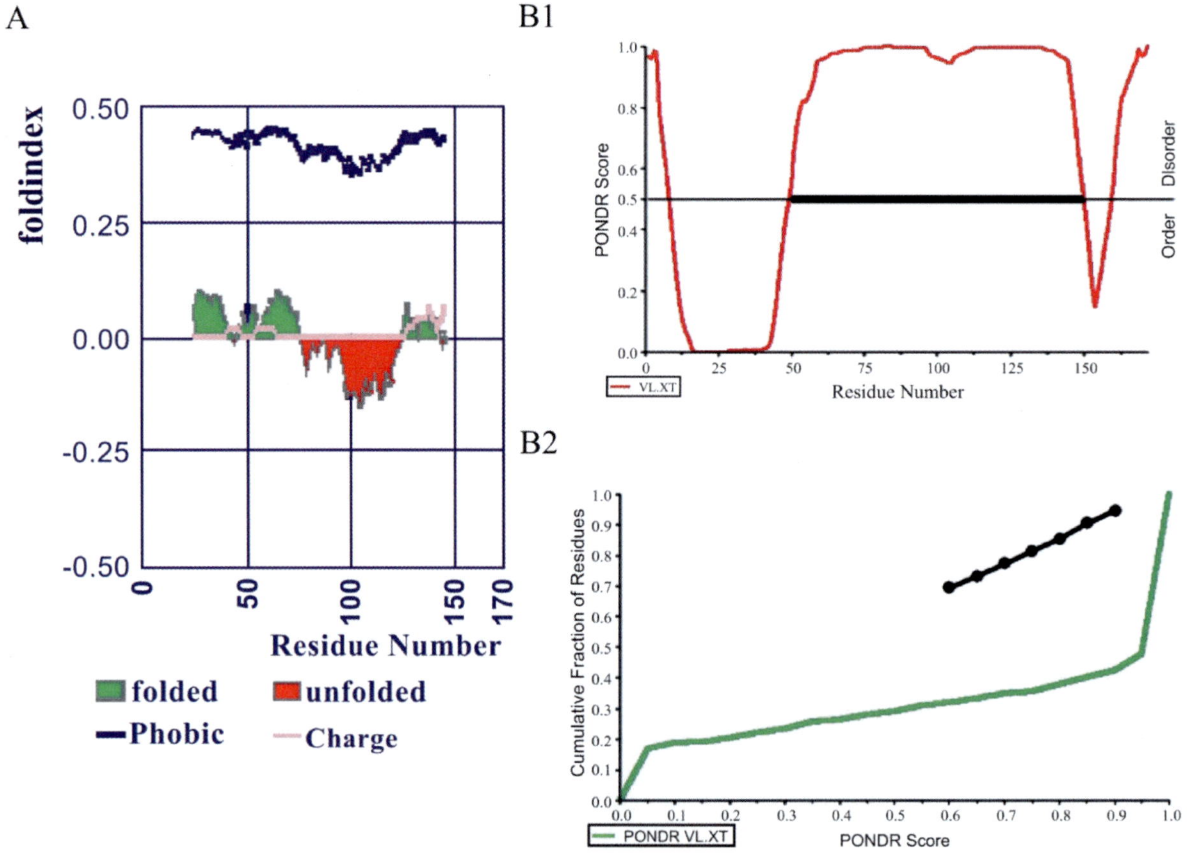

C

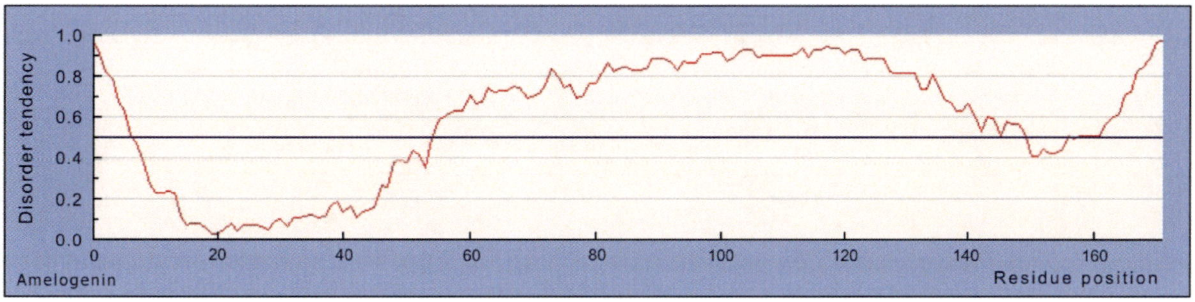

D

[1] PLPPHPGHPGYINFSYEVLTPLKWYQNMIRHPYTSYGYEPMGG**WL**HHQIIPVVSQQTPQS
[61] H**ALQ**PHHHIPMVPAQQPGIPQQPMMPLPGQHSMTPTQHHQPNLPLPAQQPFQPQPVQPQP
[121] HQPLQPQSPMHPIQPLLPQPPLPPMF**SM**QSLLPDLPLEAWPATDKTKREEVD

Figure 1: Bioinformatics analysis of recombinant porcine amelogenin rP172. (A) FoldIndex prediction. (B) PONDR prediction: **B1:** Cumulative Distribution Function (CDF) (PONDR® VL-XT) curve (green line) of amelogenin protein is bellow the boundary (black line) separating ordered proteins (above) from disordered (below) and predicts that amelogenin is fully disordered. **C:** IUPred prediction using the short-range disorder calculation (average taken over 25 amino acids). Sequences falling above the line are predicted to be disordered and those below the line to be more structured. Shaded areas in D represent regions predicted to be disordered by all the predictors (A-C), whereas underlined areas are predicted to fold and have some level of secondary structure. Bold residues in the sequence in D indicate the most common proteolytic cleavage sites during the early stages of enamel formation. The text in blue highlights the sequence of LRAP (Numbering refers to the recombinant rP172.)

CH-Plot Analysis

We used the CH-plot analysis as another approach to investigate whether amelogenin proteins are intrinsically disordered [55]. To gain insight into the folding tendency of amelogenin, we calculated the mean hydrophobicity (<H>) and mean net charge of amelogenins (CH-plot) (see equation 1). Figure 2 shows the CH-plot for the four amelogenins from human, bovine, mouse and porcine. All the amelogenins have low mean hydrophobicity and low mean net charge and lie close to the boundary line indicating that they may have a partially collapsed structure but higher propensity to form a secondary structure when compared to other IDPs.

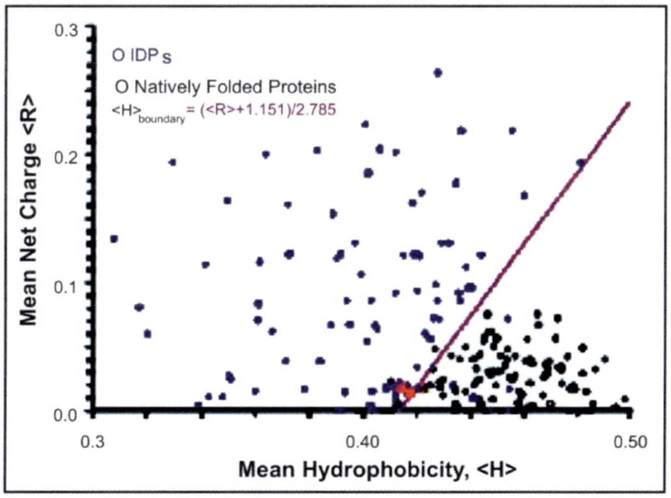

Figure 2: Computational analysis (CH-plot) of of bovine (square), human (circle), mouse (triangle), and porcine (star) amelogenins. The mean net charge (<R>) vs mean hydrophobicity (<H>) plot for IDPs (blue circles), folded proteins (black circles), and the boundary (magenta line, $<H>_{boundary} = (<R> + 1.151) / 2.785$) that demarcates the two class of proteins. The four amelogenins have low mean hydrophobicity and low mean net charge suggesting they may have a higher propensity to form a secondary structure when compared to other IDPs.

Estimation of Polyrpoline Type II (PPII) Content

Spectroscopic studies and *in silico* analyses on model peptides have confirmed that IDPs have ordered or structured regions in their sequence with substantial contribution from polyproline type II structure [59].

Table 1: Comparison of %PPII Content in rP172 Amelogenin, Amyloid Polypeptides, and Calcitonin as Estimated by Three Different Propensity Scales (redrawn from reference [13] with permission, Willey-Liss) . [a] ref [13] at 5 °C, [b] Ref [66], [c] Ref [64].

Proteins/peptides	Experimentally Determined PPII content	Predicted PPII content by		
		Stapley-Creamer	Kallenbach	Schweitzer-Stenner
rP172	[a] 42.6%	39.2%	49%	59%
Aβ(1-40)	[b] 45%	50%	50%	42.5%
Aβ(1-28)	[b] 54% [c](65%)	64.3%	41%	48.2%
Salmon Calcitonin	[c]43%	37.5%	37.5%	43.8%

PPII is a left-handed helical structure with dihedral angles $\phi = -75°$ and $\psi = +145°$, three residues per turn with PPII helices translating 3.1 Å per residue [60]. This results in an extended structure with each turn of a PPII helix spaning around 9 Å. The central region of amelogenin contains several PXXP/PXP repeats the key structural motifs in PPII structure, where X represents amino acids that have high PPII helix forming propensity (Fig's 1D and 3A). Based on the PPII propensity scale for individual amino acid residues (31), we suggested that PPII is the dominant structure in this region [12, 13]. In order to determine to what extent the PPII structure dominates in the ensemble of conformations of amelogenins, we compared different methods reported previously for the estimation of PPII content.

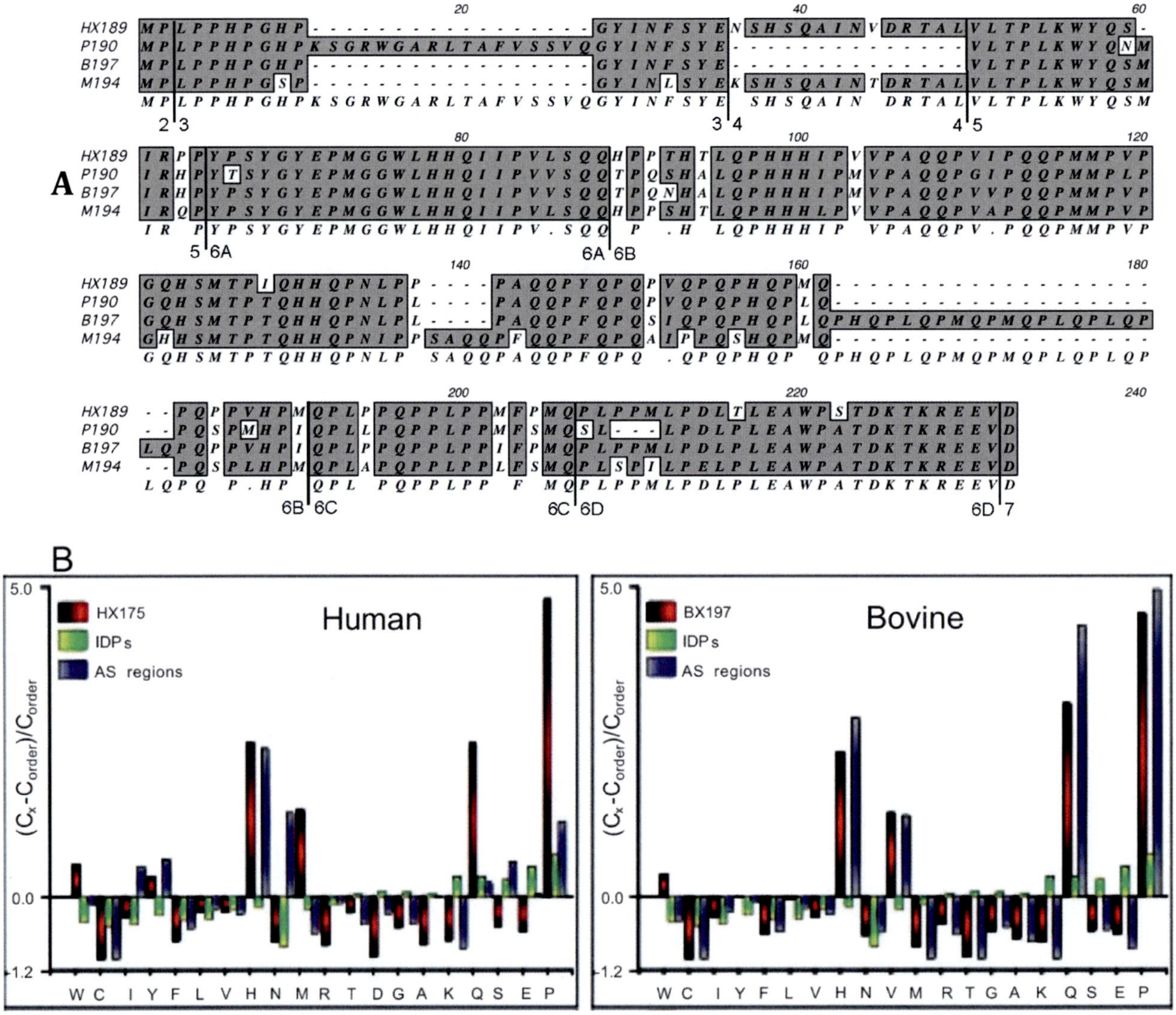

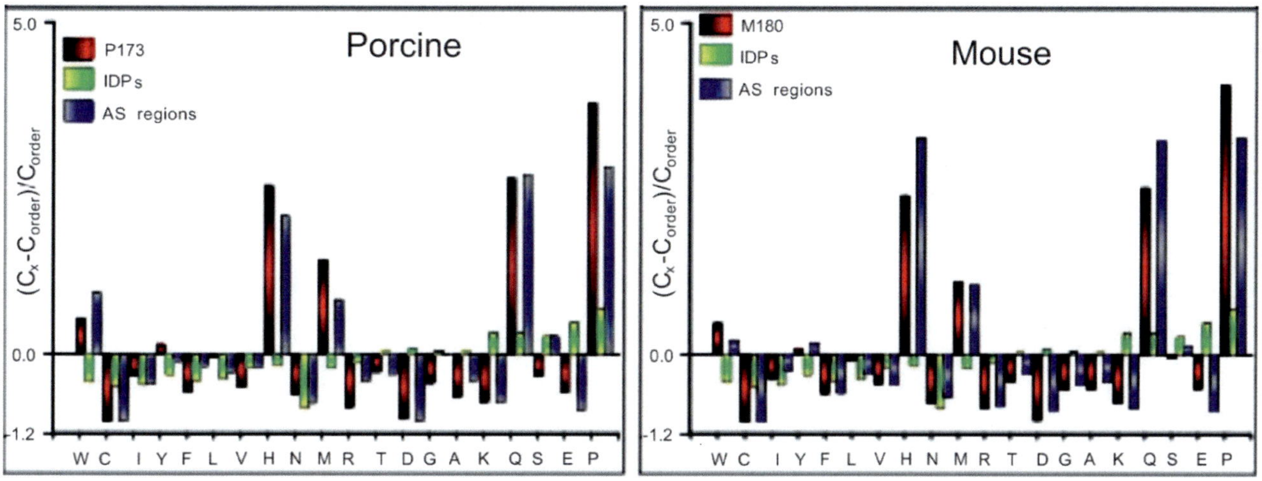

Figure 3: (A) The aligned amino acid sequences of the full-length mouse (M194), Human (HX189), pig (P190) and cow (B197) amelogenins starting with the sequence without the signal peptide. The exon boundaries, and cryptic exon 6 splice boundaries are shown bellow each sequence. Note that exons 8 and 9 are not included. (**B**) Amino acid compositional profiling of the most common full-length amelogenin sequences from cow (BX197), human (HX175), mouse (M180) and pig (P173) and their relation to alternative splice regions. Amino acids are arranged along the X-axis in order of increasing flexibility according to Vihinen's scale [71]. Negative or positive fractional difference indicates depletion or enrichment of the corresponding amino acid in the proteins. The plot shows the fractional difference in amino acid composition of the four amelogenins compared to a set of IDPs relative to a set of ordered proteins (from SwissProt database). Bars represent relative distribution of amino acid residues in IDPs (green), AS regions of amelogenin (blue) and the most abundant forms of amelogenin (BX197, HX175, M180 and P173) (red).

We first used the position sensitive preference for amino acid residues in a polyproline helix described by Stapley and Creamer [61]. We took the average of values provided in Table 3 of this reference for the individual residues and estimated the PPII propensity for the whole sequence of rP172 [13]. Stapley and Creamer analyzed about 274 high-resolution crystal structures and estimated the preference for each amino acid in a PPII helix. We applied this scale to obtain a profile of regions that are dominated by high PPII helix propensity in rP172. We found that the short N-terminal region and the major central regions have average PPII helix propensities above the mean PPII propensity of the whole sequence. Based on the Stapley and Creamer method we have estimated a maximum PPII content of 43.6% and a minimum of 34.8%. The average value (39.2%) is in excellent agreement with the experimentally observed values at low temperatures (see 3.2.1) . We have also estimated the %PPII content in rP172 using the propensity scales reported by Chen *et al.*[62], and Eker *et al.* [63].

Table 1 compares the estimated %PPII content for rP172 and other peptides with the experimentally determined values. A reasonable agreement between the three scales has been observed for short peptides. However, the Schweitzer-Stenner scale predicted a higher PPII content for rP172 [64]. Such a high value was observed only in the presence of 4M guanidine hydrochloride (see section 3.2.1), and there may be disagreement for rP172 because the scales were developed by different experimental procedures. Moreover, based on the method reported by Park et al [65], the PPII conformation as determined experimentally is less dominant in rP172 at physiological temperature (22.3%) but more abundant at low temperature (35.8% at 10º C) (see 3.2.1).

Analysis of Alternative Splicing in Amelogenin

Alternative splicing (AS) is a key event in eukaryotes that increases the coding capacity of the human genome, effectively increasing diversity of functional proteins and signaling network complexity. AS is prevalent in eukaryotes compared to prokaryotes, suggesting its seminal role in the development of multicellular life. Analysis of the AS regions in proteins with known structure has revealed that the spliced regions contain significant amounts of disorder-promoting residues [67]. The amelogenin gene structure is highly conserved in diverse vertebrates. However, alternative splicing of the pre-messenger RNA (mRNA) generates numerous RNA transcripts which are translated to various spliced products, adding further complexity to the biochemical analysis of the organic enamel matrix. Although the coding regions of the human, porcine, bovine and murine amelogenin genes are highly conserved and all contain 7 exons (Fig 3A), the pattern of alternative splicing is unique for each species [27, 68]. The reasons for alternative splicing of the amelogenin gene are not clear.

We have analyzed the distribution of disorder-promoting residues in the AS regions of amelogenin and show that like many other IDPs the spliced regions contain significant amounts of disorder-promoting residues (Table 2). For simplicity, we compared the sequences of human, bovine, murine, and porcine amelogenin. The canonical full-length human amelogenin from the AMGX gene contains 189 amino acid residues and is less abundant than any of the spliced forms. The most abundant spliced product present is obtained by the deletion of exon 4, leading to HX175. Exon4 encodes a 14 residue peptide that has 50% disorder-promoting residues (Table 2). The next most abundant amelogenin (HX159) is obtained by the removal of exons 3 and 4. The deleted regions encode 30 residues and contain 50% disorder-promoting residues. The canonical full length amelogenin from AMGY is not detectable. The most abundant amelogenin derived from the Y chromosome (HY176) is obtained by deletion of exon4 that has a content of disorder-promoting residues similar to HX175. The less abundant HY145 is obtained by the deletion of exon 3, 4, and 5 which encode a 45 residue peptide comprising 40% disorder-promoting residues. Thus, despite sharing similar gene structure, the X- and Y-copies of human amelogenin are spliced differently and the deleted peptides contain different proportions of disorder-promoting residues. Remarkably, for two AS regions of bovine amelogenin, the estimated disorder-promoting contents are ~64%. For the mouse amelogenin gene eleven different isoforms have been reported that include the deletion of exons 3, 4, 5, and internal deletions of 6A, 6B, and 6C. Recent studies have identified exons 8 and 9 in mouse and rat amelogenins. The 8 spliced regions contain 54 – 67% disorder-promoting residues. Similar results (54%-65%) were obtained for the three AS regions of porcine amelogenin (Table 2).

Table 2: Percentages of disordered amino acid residues in encoded amelogenin exons.

Amelogenin	Deleted Exons	% of disordered residues
Human	4	50%
	3,4	50%
	3,4,5	40%
Bovine	5	66%
	3,5	64%
Mouse	4	57%
	6A	54%
	4,6A	55%
	4,5,6A	55%
	4,6A,6B	66%
	6A,6B,6C	66%
	4,6A,6B,6C	65%
	4,5,6A,6B,6C	53%
Porcine	4	53%
	3,4	58%
	4,6A,6B,6C	66%

We applied the compositional profiler technique introduced by Romero et al. [67] to compare the average amino acid profile of the alternatively spliced regions in amelogenin protein sequences with those of a series of globular proteins as well as those of a series of IDPs. Such profiling shows the distribution of different amino acids in a set of disordered proteins and a set of ordered proteins [69, 70]. The "fractional difference" between a given set and the set of globular proteins can be calculated for each amino acid by equation 2 and is defined as:

$$\text{Fractional Difference}=(C_x\text{-}C_{order})/C_{order} \quad ...(2)$$

where C_x is fraction of an amino acid in a given set, such as a series of IDPs, the average composition at the AS region in amelogenin, or the composition of the particular amino acid in the most abundant amelogenin. C_{order} is the corresponding value in the set of ordered proteins. For example, the fraction of alanine present in a set of "ordered" proteins (from the Swiss-Prot) database is 0.0789, whereas fraction of alanine in porcine amelogenins is 0.0489. The fractional difference is now calculated as, (0.0489-0.0789)/0.0789 = -0.38. A negative value indicates depletion of alanine in amelogenins relative to ordered proteins. In the case of AS regions of amelogenin the composition of a particular amino acid was calculated based on the average of all the alternative spliced products available in the data base.

In Figure 3B we compare the amino acid composition of a set of globular proteins from SwissProt with the sets of IDPs, the amino acids in 18 AS regions in amelogenin (from human, cow, mouse, and pig) and the most abundant form of amelogenins from these species [71]. We also compared the compositional profiling of 18 AS regions in human, bovine, murine, and porcine amelogenin sequences with that of IDPs. The analysis predicts that, with few exceptions, the AS regions have increased abundance in disorder-promoting residues. The figure also contains a similar analysis for the most abundant amelogenin present in each organism. Though the four sequences of amelogenin are depleted in order-promoting amino acid residues (C, I, F, L, and V), and enriched in disorder-promoting residues (P and Q), they do not follow the trend usually observed in the disordered vs ordered protein sets. In comparison to IDPs, P and Q are over-represented in amelogenin. However a relatively high frequency of H and M and to a lesser extent W and Y are also apparent in the primary structure of amelogenin. These analyses indicate that amelogenins is not entirely disordered but have some presence of structure–promoting residues, as has been also demonstrated in our recent NMR studies [11] (see 3.2.6).

Experimental Strategies and Biophysical Methods

Experimentally, the presence of intrinsic disorder in proteins can be verified by a variety of biophysical techniques. In this section, we will discuss the experimental techniques that have unequivocally demonstrated that amelogenin belongs to the class of IDPs. These include CD spectropolarimetry, FTIR, intrinsic tryptophan fluorescence, differential scanning calorimetry, small angle X-ray scattering, and nuclear magnetic resonance spectroscopy.

CD Spectropolarimetry and PPII Conformation

Near and far UV-CD have been used extensively to investigate the presence of tertiary and secondary structures, respectively, in proteins. Circular dichroism of proteins in the far UV ranges (180 – 250 nm) provides information about the nature of secondary structure present. For a protein that contains a regular secondary structure the presence of a negative minimum in the π–π* (208 nm) and n–π* (222 nm) regions and a positive maximum around 195 nm are characteristic of an α-helix structure. The presence of a negative minimum around 217 nm and a positive maximum around 195 nm are characteristic of a β-sheet structure [72]. The far UV-CD of an IDP is typified by the presence of an intense negative ellipticity in the π–π* region (195-205 nm) and negligible ellipticity in the n–π* (220-230 nm) region [73]. Goto et al were the first to demonstrate that native porcine amelogenin and various cleavage products (except the TRAP region) lacked typical signatures of an ordered secondary structure [74]. These authors hypothesized that porcine amelogenin contains three independent units: a β-structured N-terminus, a highly repetitive central domain with an undefined conformation, and a coil-like C-terminus. In a subsequent work, Oobatake et al. concluded that the secondary structure of recombinant mouse amelogenin (rM179) is different from globular protein or proline-rich peptides [75]. We have shown that, in water at pH ~3.8, where amelogenin is monomeric, the recombinant full-length porcine amelogenin displays a strong negative minimum around 202 nm in accordance with the spectra reported for native porcine amelogenin (Figure 4A).

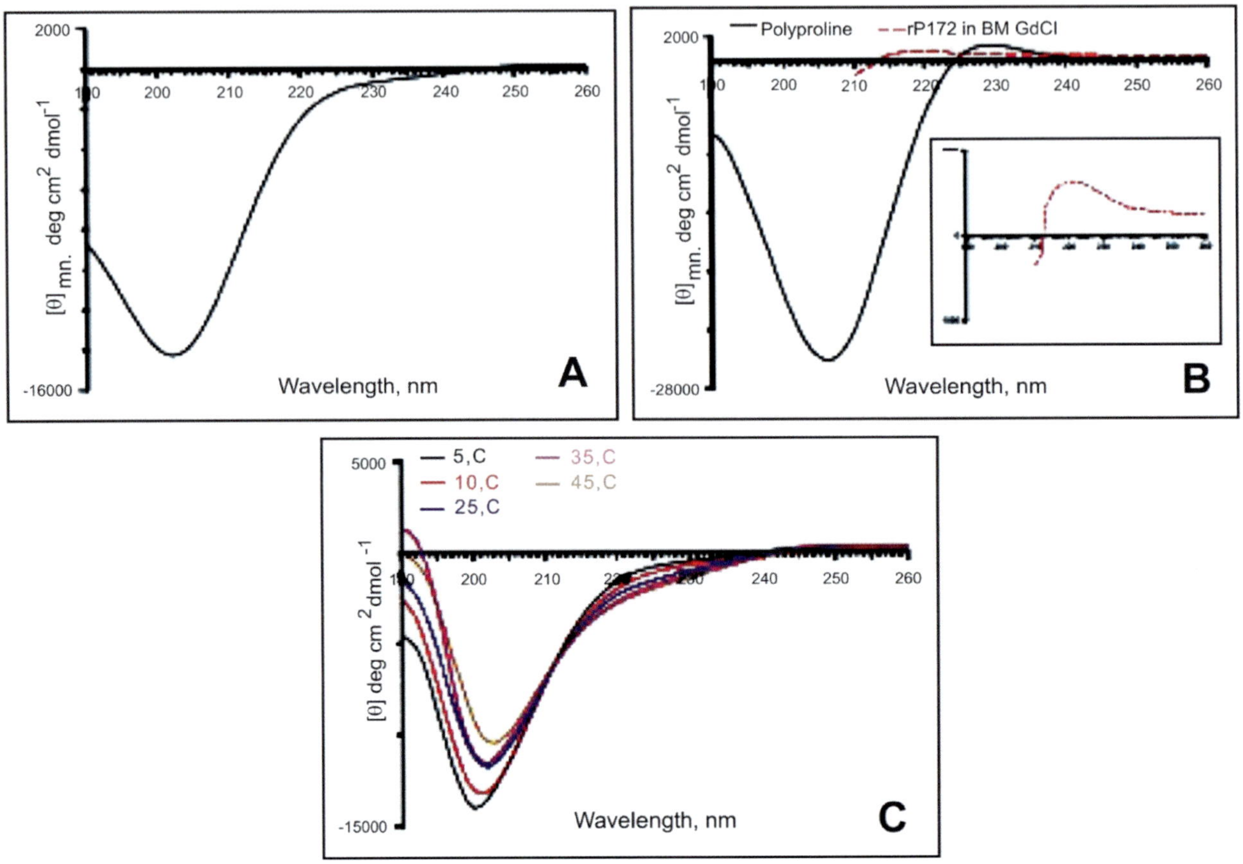

Figure 4: Circular Dichroism of amelogenin. **(A)** CD of rP172 in water. The strong negative ellipticity in the π–π* region (195-205 nm) and a weak shoulder in the n–π* (210-230) region are characteristics of IDPs (spectrum collected at 10 °C). **(B)** CD spectra of polyproline and rP172 in 8M guanidine hydrochloride (GdHCl) at 20 °C. Note the apparent weak positive n–π* transition in polyproline and in denatured rP172. The scale is expanded in the inset to show the weak positive maximum in rP172. (**C**) VT-CD spectra of rP172 in Tris-Hc buffer (pH=7.4) containing 5 mM calcium (redrawn with permission from [13])

Spectroscopic studies and *in silico* analyses on model peptides have confirmed that IDPs are locally ordered with substantial contribution from polyproline type II structure [76-78]. Polyproline, a paradigm for PPII structure, exhibits a weak positive band in the n–π* region (228 nm) and an intense negative minima around 206 nm in the far UV-CD spectra (Figure 4B). Polypeptides containing non-prolyl residues such as polyglutamine, polylysine, polyglycine, polyaspartate, and polyalanine also exhibit CD spectra characteristic of PPII structure [79]. However, the characteristic bands are blue-shifted compared to polyproline, due to differences in transition energies between tertiary, secondary, and primary amides. It has been shown that glutamine, glycine, and alanine flanked by proline residues show a high propensity to form PPII structure. Since PPII is the only secondary structure that has positive ellipticity around 218-228 nm, this band has been used as a marker for the presence of PPII structure [60]. The intensity increase or decrease has been used to estimate the %PPII content in unfolded peptides [59, 60, 65]. Since the low temperature CD spectra of several IDPs resemble PPII structure, it has been suggested that disordered proteins have structured regions with significant population of PPII conformation [80, 81]. The absence of weak positive bands in several IDPs is ascribed to the presence of other local structures or low population of PPII structure at room temperature. In such a scenario, addition of denaturing agents has been shown to promote the formation of an extended PPII structure [82, 83]. In the presence of strong denaturants (8M guanidine hydrochloride), the CD spectra of rP172 (Figure 4B) and the recombinant mouse amelogenins [75] indicated the presence of a weak positive band in the n–π* region, suggesting the presence of PPII structure . In addition, presence of a well-defined iso-elliptic point in the VT-CD spectra is taken as a direct evidence for the existence of an equilibrium between truly unordered and PPII conformations (Fig 4C) (29). Since an isoelliptic point was observed for both native and recombinant porcine amelogenins and for recombinant mouse amelogenin, their secondary structure must contain a significant population of PPII structure [13].

We have performed CD studies of rP172 over a temperature range from 5 °C to 45 °C (Figure 4C). As the temperature was increased, the CD intensity in the 215-230 nm region decreased, whereas the CD intensity at 202 nm increased. The spectra exhibited a well-defined iso-elliptic point around 211 nm indicating a two-state equilibrium between unordered and PPII conformations. Such iso-elliptic points have been observed for several proteins and polypeptides that exhibit unordered-PPII equilibria at low temperature ranges [66]. Using the thermal dependency of ellipticity values, we estimated the PPII content by the method reported by Park et al [65]. Table 3 lists the %PPII content of rP172 at various temperatures based on CD measurements. The PPII content in rP172 varies from 20.2% to 42.6%, depending on the temperature. The estimated PPII content at 37 °C (22.3%) is in good agreement with the estimated values obtained by bioinformatic methods (Table 1).

Table 3: Estimation of PPII content in rP172 based on CD measurements.

Temperature	**%PPII estimated by**		
	Our method[a]	**Kelly et al.[b]**	**Bienkiewicz et al.[c]**
5	42.6	38.4	31.2
10	35.8	35.6	28.6
15	33.4	34.6	27.8
20	30.7	33.5	26.8
25	28.4	32.6	25.9
30	26.8	31.9	24.3
35	23.4	30.5	25.3
37	**22.3**	**30.3**	**24.8**
40	22.0	29.9	23.5
45	20.2	29.2	22.8

[a] Lakshminarayanan et al [13], [b] Kelly *et al.* Ref [60], [c] Equation 1, Bienkiewicz *et al.* Ref [59]

Fourier Transformed Infrared (FTIR) Spectroscopy

FTIR also provides information on the presence of intrinsic disorder in proteins. Evidence is found in the amide I absorption (1700-1600 cm^{-1}) region that originates from >C=O stretching vibration of the amide group, where the frequency of absorption is sensitive to the secondary structure of proteins. FTIR spectra of IDPs exhibit a characteristic maximum around 1645±3 cm^{-1} [84-87]. We have shown that rP172, under weakly acidic conditions, exhibited a maximum around 1642 cm^{-1}, characteristic of proteins that are depleted in ordered conformations (Figure 5).

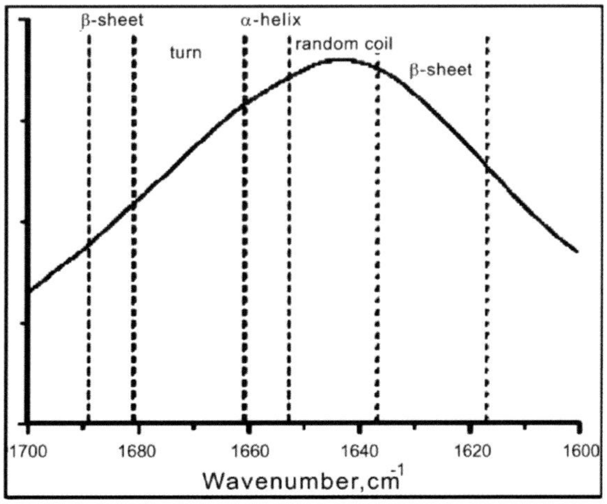

Figure 5: FTIR of amelogenin in water. The absorption maximum for specific secondary structures is highlighted by vertical dotted lines. FTIR of IDPs have a characteristic strong maximum in the random coil region [84-87] .

Intrinsic Tryptophan Fluorescence Spectroscopy

Tryptophan, tyrosine, and phenylalanine are the three chromophoric residues that posses the property of intrinsic fluorescence. Tryptophan has higher quantum yield than tyrosine and phenyl alanine and its wavelength of emission maximum (λ_{max}) depends strongly on the polarity of the environment and ranges from 308-360 nm. Based on the analyses of λ_{max} and spectral band width at the half maximum values of a number of tryptophan-containing proteins, Reshetnyak and Burstein have identified five discrete states for tryptophan in proteins (Figure 6A) [88]. For Class A proteins, the tryptophan fluorophores have highly blue-shifted λ_{max} values (308 nm) and are buried deeply in the protein structure within a non-polar and rigid environment [89]. Class S proteins also have tryptophan fluorophores deeply buried into the protein structure, but the λ_{max} is slightly red-shifted (322.5 ± 4.5 nm) compared to Class A proteins. This results from the fact the tryptophan residues in class S have higher polarity and exist in a more flexible environment than class A proteins. Both these groups of proteins have reduced accessibility to solvent and quenchers. For Class I proteins, the λ_{max} values are further red-shifted to 331 ± 4.8 nm, and the atoms present in the side chain indole rings participate in hydrogen bond formation with surrounding residues or water molecules with a fixed stoichiometry of 2:1. The environment around tryptophan residues for this class has less packing density than the previous two classes. The next two classes, Class II and Class III proteins, correspond to exposed tryptophan residues and several denatured proteins belong to this class. For Class II proteins, the λ_{max} values are around 342.3 ± 3.3 nm and the proteins contain fluorophores surrounded by structured water molecules in the vicinity of indole ring. In contrast, Class III proteins have λ_{max} values around 347 ± 3.1 nm with tryptophan residues fully exposed to highly mobile water molecules. Thus, monitoring intrinsic tryptophan residues provides information on the environment around tryptophan resides and the presence of intrinsic disorder in proteins. Amelogenin contains three tryptophan residues: two in the TRAP region and one in the C-terminus (Fig 3A), and tryptophan fluorescence spectra provide information on the secondary structure around these residues. Figure 6B shows the intrinsic tryptophan fluorescence emission spectra of rP172 in water. The characteristic λ_{max} around 347 nm indicates the exposed nature of these fluorophores and suggests the labile and readily accessible nature of the regions surrounding them. For recombinant mouse amelogenin at pH 4.8, the emission maximum is about 349 nm [75]. Interestingly, both the recombinant porcine and murine amelogenins have λ_{max} values overlapping those of IDPs and denatured proteins (Figure 6A).

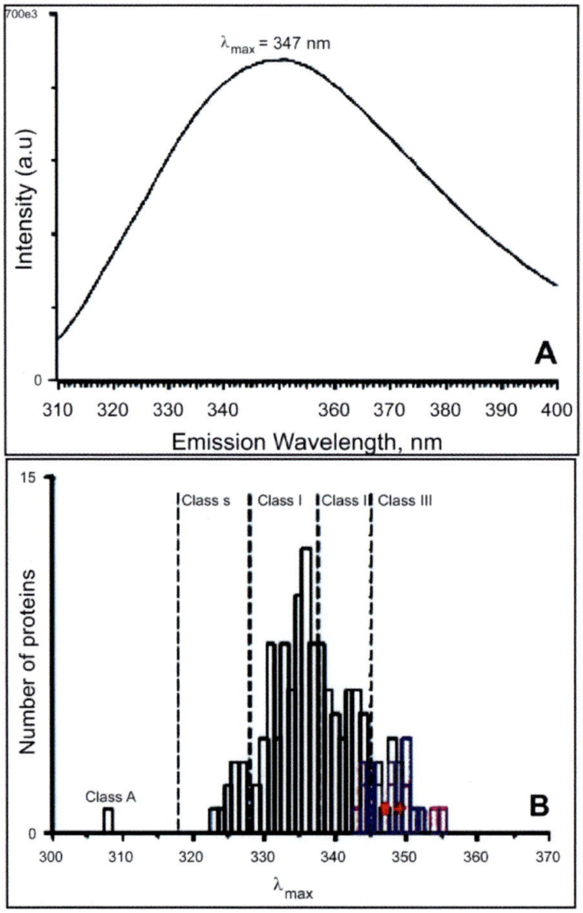

Figure 6: **(A)** Intrinsic tryptophan fluorescence spectra of rP172 in water at an excitation wavelength of 295 nm. **(B)** Classification of proteins based on λ_{max} values in the intrinsic tryptophan fluorescence spectra. The blue and pink bars represent λ_{max} for denatured and intrinsically disordered proteins, respectively. The positions of rP172 (red circle) and mouse amelogenin (red star) are also indicated. The λ_{max} values for the various classes and denatured proteins were taken from [88] whereas λ_{max} values for various IDPs were taken from refs [90-97].

Differential Scanning Calorimetry (DSC)

DSC provides accurate information about the melting behavior and directly measures the enthalpy of denaturation and can be used to distinguish between IDPs and folded proteins. There are two forms of enthalpy of denaturation: the van't Hoff enthalpy (ΔH^{vH}) which is measured from temperature dependence of the equilibrium constant and calorimetric enthalpy ($\Delta H^{cal)}$ which is measured by calculating the area under the DSC thermogram. The direct measurement of ΔH^{cal} and $\Delta H^{van't\ Hoff}$ enthalpies from a single calorimetric trace is possible by this method. The appearance of a well-defined heat absorption peak in the calorimetric trace and $\Delta H^{cal}/\Delta^{Hvant\ Hoff} \approx 1$ are indicative of proteins that contain a single-domain ordered tertiary structure and co-operative melting. Any deviation from this represents the presence of multi-domains in the overall structure [98]. For IDPs, DSC thermograms indicate a broad and weak thermal transition over the entire temperature range [99, 100] . Oobatake *et al.* [75] have shown that for recombinant mouse amelogenin, the DSC trace showed a weak non-cooperative unfolding transition and $\Delta H^{cal}/\Delta H^{vant\ Hoff}$ value of 4.71 indicating the absence of a regular tertiary structure.

Small angle X-ray Scattering (SAXS)

SAXS is one of the most powerful techniques for assessing the shape and size of proteins in solution. Analysis of the scattering curves using Guinier approximation (equation 3) provides information about the radius of gyration (R_g) and hence the size of the particles in solution.

$$I(q) = I(0)\ \exp(-q^2R_g^2/3)\ldots\ (3)$$

Where $I(q)$ is the scattering intensity and $I(0)$ is the scattering intensity at 0°. The slope and intercept obtained from a linear fit of $\ln(I(q))$ vs q^2 at low q values (qR_g) provides information about molecular size (Rg) and association state of the sample. ($I(0)$) depends on whether the protein is aggregated or monomeric (i.e. greater this value means higher aggregation state). The R_g, determined by SAXS for the recombinant mouse amelogenin under acidic conditions (where amelogenin is in monomeric form) has been shown to be identical to that of C-terminus truncated native porcine amelogenin [101, 102]. Figure 7 plots the R_g values for various IDPs against the number of amino acid residues and the reported R_g values for mouse amelogenin. The measured dimension of recombinant amelogenin reasonably agrees with the values for IDPs.

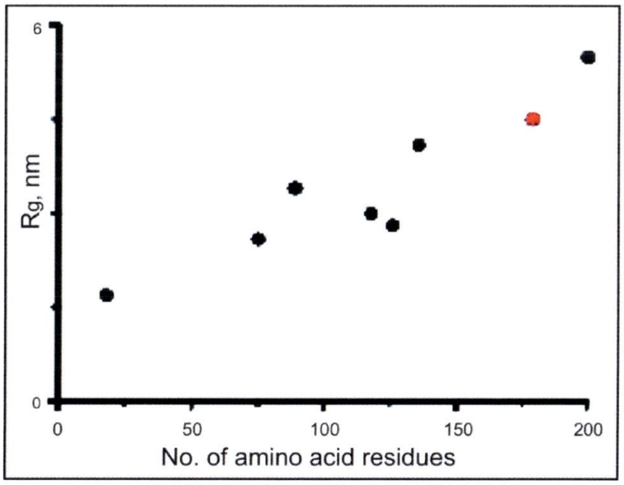

Figure 7: Radius of gyration (R_g) of various IDPs (black circles) derived from SAXS studies plotted against the number of amino acid residues. The R_g values for various IDPs were taken from [103-113] The value for recombinant mouse amelogenin is shown as a red circle (value taken from ref [101])

Nuclear Magnetic Resonance Spectroscopy

NMR provides atomic resolution and thus residue-specific information about macromolecules in solution [56, 58]. However, due to the absence of stable, unique structures and the presence of conformational averaging resulting in compromises in chemical shift dispersion, resonance broadening, and nOe cancellation, IDPs present a challenge for structural determination by NMR. The increased flexibility and populations of several interconverting conformations in IDPs result in poor chemical shift dispersion of proton resonances. Due to the extended and flexible nature of these proteins, the residues in IDPs experience an identical chemical environment, thus resulting in a strong clustering of the proton resonances [114, 115]. The heteronuclear double quantum correlation (HSQC) of a folded protein displays a broad distribution of amide protons. However, for IDPs the chemical shift values are clustered to ~1 ppm. The H-^{15}N HSQC spectra of recombinant porcine amelogenin (rP172) in water (pH= 3.8) at 10 °C and recombinant mouse amelogenin (M180) in 2% deuterated acidic acid solution (pH 3.0) at 25 °C both show clustering of the amide proton chemical shifts (δ), similar to IDPs [11, 116].

Delak et al have utilized a suite of triple resonance NMR experiments that take advantage of the comparatively wide chemical shift dispersions of ^{15}N and ^{13}C spins and analyzed the backbone structure of rP172 [11]. Low temperatures (10° C) were utilized to slow down conformational exchange and prevent unwanted aggregation. Using this approach, the majority of the backbone resonances in U -$^{13}C/^{15}N$ rP172 were resolved and sequentially assigned except for E40, Q126, and H132, which could not be identified. Once the backbone-structure – sensitive data were obtained, Delak et al next determined the extent of deviation of the rP172-specific NMR parameters from protein database random coil values, such that a global picture of rP172 folding could be obtained. It was noted that the majority of secondary shift amplitudes were not particularly intense, indicating that there are no well-defined or stable helical or folded beta sheet secondary structures within rP172 in UDDW.

The Pro $^{13}C\beta$, $^{13}C\gamma$ chemical shifts and the chemical shift difference ($\delta[^{13}C\beta] - \delta[^{13}C\gamma]$) as a reference-independent descriptor of the Xaa-Pro peptide bond conformation have also been analyzed. It was found that while all of the Pro residues were within the canonical chemical shift ranges of both the trans and cis configuration, the majority of Pro residues adopt the trans configuration with the exception of P41, P52, P96, P130, and P154, which resonate within the ^{13}C chemical shift range for the cis configuration [117]. Thus, we conclude that (a) the global structure of rP172 in the monomeric form is largely unfolded, and (b) the majority of Pro residues in rP172 appears to adopt the trans configuration, similar to what is observed within the Pro-rich titin PEVK entropic chain segment [118] a member of the IDP protein class [119]

It is known that unfolded proteins can possess local regions where residual secondary structures reside. Examination of the HSQC spectra for rP172 revealed the presence of duplicated HSQC cross-peaks for residues V54, A63, W161, and T164 suggesting the presence of two rP172 conformations, presumably in slow exchange with one another. The co-existence of global unfolded structure with residual local structure was also confirmed by quantitative NMR data (nOe's, J-couplings). The absence of global folded structure is confirmed by two observations. First, there is a lack of consistent sequential backbone; medium and long-range backbone; and sequential, medium and long-range backbone-side chain nOe's. Second, the ^{3}J coupling constants predominantly fall within the random coil range [120]. However, this dataset also confirms that rP172 does possess short, dispersed sequence regions which exhibit partially ordered secondary structure traits (Fig 8). These have been tentatively assigned and are summarized as follows: (a) a short helical region at L23 - Q27, which correlates with conformational shift deviations in that region, (b) extended beta strand structure in sequence regions P2 – P22, L46 – H62, and G90 – Q101 (which correlates with the low Pro content in these three sequence segments and the large deviation in ΔJ values (ref)), and (c) turn or loop regions assigned to the Y37 – W45 segment. Interestingly, this sequence segment, -YGYEPMGGW-, contains turn- or loop-forming amino acids Y, G, and M [121] .

A comparison of the best protonated/deprotonated models of rP172 with the general secondary structure features found in our NMR dataset (Figure 8) show good agreement with regard to important secondary structure features. For example, we find that rP172 amelogenin adopts an extended beta conformation within the P2 – P22, L46 – H62, and G90 – Q101 regions. There is also evidence of a turn or loop region near the C-terminal end of the TRAP region (Y37 – W45) and extended helical or PPII-like structure at the A63-H69 and M146-D173 regions. The C-terminal domain appears to be coil-like and more condensed in configuration, which is consistent with previous NMR studies of the amelogenin C-terminal region [122].

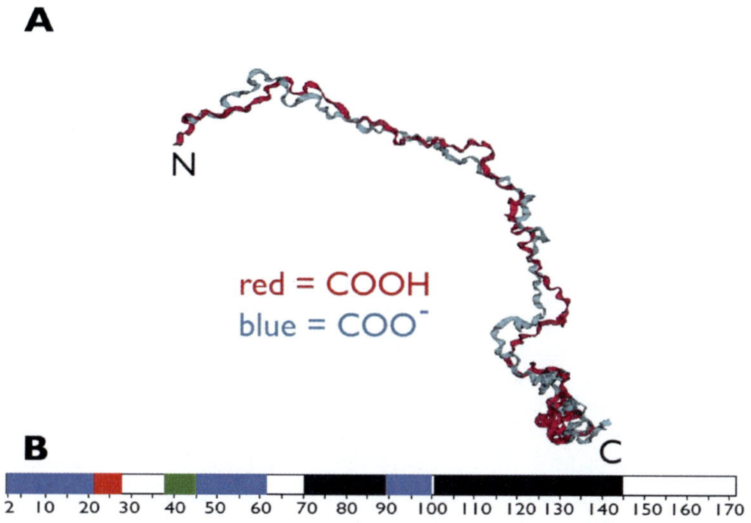

Figure 8: (A) Backbone aligned best structures obtained for the fully protonated (Red) and deprotonated (Blue) forms of recombinant porcine amelogenin (rP172) in monomeric form, showing that the molecule is extended (backbone rmsd = 4.7 Å). (B) Secondary structure assignment based upon nOe and ^3J data in this figure; black = PPII, red = alpha-helix, blue = extended beta strand, green = beta turn or loop, and white = random coil or unstructured. Adapted in part with permission from ref [11] Copyright 2008 American Chemical Society.

Induced Folding in Amelogenin

One important feature of IDPs is that they acquire an ordered conformation (induced folding) upon changing the environmental conditions such as increasing temperature, raising the pH, addition of metal ions, ligands or binding partners, structure promoting solvents (such as trifluoroethanol), osmolytes, crowding agents or lipids [57].

Temperature Effect

A characteristic feature of an IDP is its "turnout" response to temperature [123-125]. Thus, VT-CD spectra of IDPs differ from folded proteins in three different ways: (i) elevated temperature increases partial folding of IDPs, ii) the transition is non-cooperative, and iii) in a number of cases the transition is highly reversible. Monitoring VT-CD spectra, therefore, provides more info about the nature of IDPs. The complete wavelength scan as a function of temperature in the Far UV-CD region for a number of IDPs is characterized by a decrease in the intensity of negative ellipticity in the $\pi-\pi^*$ region whereas the intensity of the shoulder observed around n-π^* region increases, and the spectra exhibit a well-defined iso-elliptic point depending on the value of CD minimum in the $\pi-\pi^*$ region. Full length native porcine amelogenin, recombinant mouse [75] and porcine amelogenins (Figure 4C) all exhibit VT-CD spectra with a well-defined iso-elliptic point around 211-213 nm. The temperature-induced formation of an ordered secondary structure is further confirmed by monitoring the $[\theta]_{222/224}$ as a function of temperature. For IDPs such thermal transition results in a linear increase of $[\theta]_{222/224}$ and heat-induced changes are completely reversible. The full-length native porcine amelogenin, rM179, and rP172 all undergo a linear thermal transition and heat-induced structural change is completely reversible (Figure 9A). This behavior is quite different from folded proteins which undergo a co-operative loss (sigmoidal) in secondary structure, as a function of temperature. The formation of ordered secondary structure in IDPs at elevated temperature is attributed to the increased strength of hydrophobic interactions, a major driving force for folding.

The Effect of Trifluoroethanol (TFE)

IDPs have an increased propensity to form an ordered secondary structure in the presence of trifluoroethanol (TFE), a fluorinated alcohol that promotes α-helical structure by weakening the hydrogen bonding of water molecules to the peptide backbone [125]. The increase in secondary structure is manifested by a decrease in ellipticity at 200 nm and significant increase in the negative ellipticity around 222 nm. The increase in helical content is estimated using the equation 4 [126]:

$$\% \alpha\text{-helix} = {}^{obs}[\theta]_{222} / {}^{max}[\theta]_{222} \quad ...(4)$$

where $^{obs}[\theta]_{222}$ is the observed ellipticity values at 222 nm and $^{max}[\theta]_{222}$ is maximum ellipticity values at 222 for a protein in 100% helical conformation and can be estimated by using the equation 5,

$$^{max}[\theta]_{222} = -40{,}000\ \{1-2.5/N\}\ldots(5)$$

where N is the number of amino acid residues. The amount of TFE required to induce maximum α-helicity depends on the amino acid sequence. For rP172, we have shown that TFE induces significant increase in α-helical content and maximum is reached at 30% TFE (Figure 9B) [12]. Further increase in TFE reduces the α-helical content slightly and remains same at higher concentration of TFE (Figure 9C).

Ionic Strength Effect

For IDPs that posses high mean net charge, the structure is highly extended and unfolded due to the presence of repulsive electrostatic and low attractive hydrophobic interactions [36]. Addition of metal ions, therefore, tends to screen the non-compensated repulsive attraction and induce folding in these proteins. Such metal-ion induced transformations are often accompanied by favorable enthalpy (negative) and unfavorable entropy (negative) changes. However, amelogenin contains very low mean net charge and low hydrophobicity; therefore, it has been hypothesized that it may have weak affinity for the metal ions (36). Le et al have shown that recombinant human amelogenin have weak affinity (K_d = 0.78 mM) to calcium ions and the binding is accompanied by unfavorable enthalpy (+0.462 kcal/mole) and favorable entropy changes (+15.8 cal/deg/mol) [127]. Recently, Buchko et al. have shown that the H-^{15}N HSQC spectra for the recombinant mouse amelogenin is perturbed following the addition of high concentration of Ca^{2+} (165 mM) and Na^{+} (300 mM) ions [116, 128]. These authors have also shown that the backbone dynamics (overall correlation time, τ_c) is increased by the addition of Ca^{2+} and Na^{+} ions or increase in pH of the solution, and attributed these observations to the formation of homodimer. The amide protons of the N-terminus (G8-I51) and the residues close to the C-terminus (L141-T171) have been shown to be involved in the dimerization process at high concentration of Ca^{2+}.

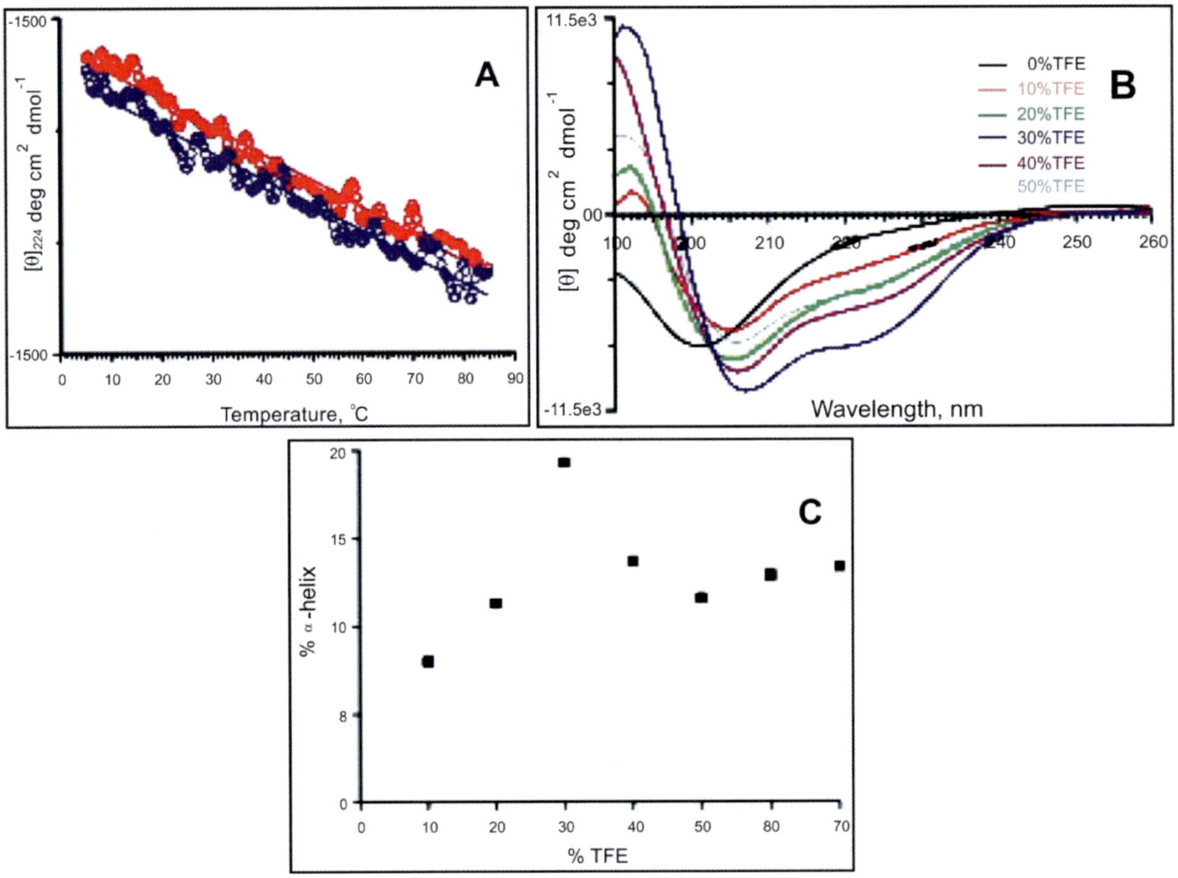

Figure 9: (A), Reversible thermal transition in rP172 based on data in ref. [12]. The red open circles indicate ellipticity values on heating while the blue open circles are for the cooling cycle. The lines indicate linear fit; **B)**, effect of TFE on the conformation of rP172, taken from ref. [13] **C)**, increase in α-helical content with increasing concentration of TFE.

Target-Induced Folding

IDPs undergo conformational change upon interaction with natural binding partners [15, 129]. Although this is well-documented for a number of IDPs, comparable studies are limited for amelogenin due to the low abundance of other enamel matrix proteins and the difficulty in extracting them in homogeneous form. Recent evidence that amelogenin directly interacts with a nonamelogenin protein, the 32 kDa enamelin fragment, is based on a series of biophysical and immunochemical methods. Immunoprecipitation studies revealed that the 32 kDa enamelin and amelogenin eluted together from a Protein A column indicating their direct interaction.

Particle size distribution analysis of amelogenin-enamelin mixtures by dynamic light scattering (DLS) has indicated formation of complexes between the two proteins at acidic pH (5.8). At pH 8.0, moreover, the 32 kDa enamelin displayed a profound influence on the self-assembly of amelogenin. Upon sequential addition of the 32 kDa enamelin at enamelin-rP172 molar ratios of 1:100, 1:50, and 1:10, the particle size of the major population in the rP172-enamelin solution decreased from an initial 17.6 nm to 15.1 nm, 11.8 nm, and finally 4.3 nm, indicating a decrease in average size of amelogenin-containing particles as a function of increasing enamelin concentration. A schematic diagram representing the effect of enamelin at different ratios on particle size distribution is shown in Figure 10. It was assumed that amelogenin nanospheres would be in [130] some form of equilibrium with individual amelogenin molecules [12, 131, 132]. This amelogenin self-assembly equilibrium could be broken and shifted by the presence of proteins, ligands, or a change of pH or temperature. When the 32 kDa enamelin was added to the solution containing assembled amelogenin, the nanosphere size of rP172 in the solution became smaller, indicating a shifting of the amelogenin self-assembly equilibrium towards dissociation in a dose dependent manner. This is a clear indication that co-assembly between enamelin and amelogenin molecules does take place. We speculate that when enamelin binds to amelogenin through its sugar chains, its hydrophilic and acidic nature would stabilize the amelogenin molecules and thus inhibit the hydrophobic interactions among neighboring rP172 molecules. We further suggest that the interactions between amelogenin and enamelin lead to a more stable conformation of the otherwise extended and unfolded amelogenin molecule. Conformational changes of rP172 as a result of its co-assembly with the 32 kDa enamelin were also apparent in the CD experiments. The appearance of an isodichroic point accompanied by slight shifting and intensity decrease of minima in the CD spectra gave a solid indication of the conformational changes of rP172 when enamelin was added. Our results collectively suggest that the 32 kDa enamelin can be a potential binding target for amelogenin *in vivo*.

A single report utilizing in vitro immunochemical studies has indicated that amelogenin also interacts with recombinant ameloblastin (an enamel matrix protein) [133]. However, structural studies resulting from such interactions are lacking. Numerous studies have demonstrated that membrane-bound proteins such as CD-63, Annexin A2, and lysosomal-associated glygoprotein 1 (Lamp1) also interact with amelogenin in a specific manner and such interactions are critical for amelogenin cell-signaling and/or endocytosis [6, 26, 27]. Immunohistochemical studies have also showed that amelogenin interact with cytokeratin 14 and cytokeratin 5 in vivo, but the physiological significance of such findings is not clear . While structural details of amelogenin's interactions with its targets are lacking, it is likely that the flexible structure of this protein facilitates its interactions with different targets, ligands, polypeptides as well as apatite mineral for achievement of internal stabilization of protein configuration.

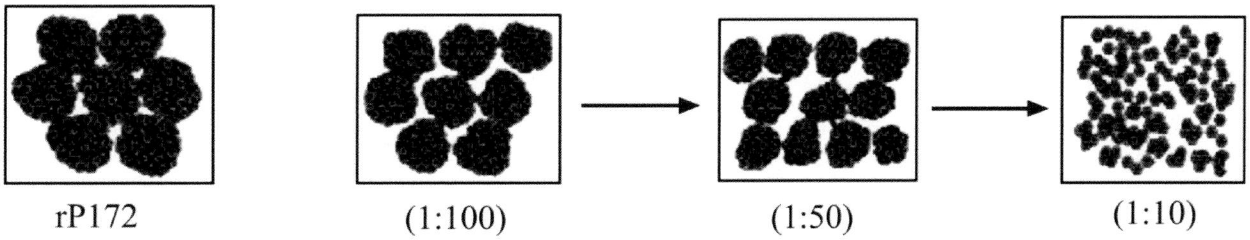

Figure 10: Schematic diagram showing the effect of increasing concentration of enamelin on the size distribution of amelogenin-containing particles based on dynamic light scattering studies. Numbers in parentheses represent the molar ratio of enamelin to rP172. Redrawn with permission from ref [134]

Intrinsic Disorder and Self-Assembly

Thermodynamics of Amelogenin Self-Assembly

An important characteristic of amelogenin is its ability to self-assemble into large structures in response to increasing pH, protein concentration, temperature, and ionic strength [9, 10, 19, 101, 135]. It has been reported that the self-assembly is mainly triggered by pH [135]. However, little was known about the driving force for this self-assembly. Recently, we investigated the thermodynamic driving force for amelogenin self-assembly by isothermal titration calorimetry (ITC) dilution experiments based on the assumption that amelogenin disassembles upon several fold dilution [12, 13]. In this method, stepwise addition of a high concentration of the protein in an appropriate buffer is injected in small aliquots into an adiabatic calorimetric cell loaded with the same buffer. An abrupt dilution of the concentrated protein solution disturbs the equilibrium, triggering the dissociation of the assemblies into monomers or oligomers. Each injection produced exothermic heat of reaction upon dilution (Figure 11A). Both dissociation of the assembled amelogenin and dilution of the monomer contribute to the large heat change observed during the first few injections. As more assembled amelogenin is injected into the cell, the total concentration of amelogenin increases in the cell and the reaction enthalpy decreases (intermediate region); as the total concentration of amelogenin exceeds the critical aggregation concentration (CAC) in the cell, the reaction enthalpy remains constant. Further addition does not dissociate the assembled amelogenin and the heat produced is due solely to the dilution of aggregates [136]. The difference in enthalpy of the two plateaus gives the enthalpy of disassembly (ΔH_{dA}) (Figure 11B). The enthalpy of assembly (ΔH_A), which has the same magnitude but opposite sign as $\Delta H_{dA,}$ is obtained by the method of Heerklotz et al [136]. For amelogenin at 30 °C, a positive ΔH_A value was obtained. For a thermodynamically allowed reaction ($\Delta G = \Delta H\text{-}T\Delta S = \text{-ve}$), this requires a large increase in contribution from ΔS at a given temperature. The positive value of ΔH_A therefore indicates that the self-assembly of amelogenin is entropically driven. Similar positive ΔH_A values have been obtained for casein micelles and co-chaperonin protein 10 [137, 138]. Raising the temperature to 37° C decreases the ΔH_A values suggesting increased hydrophobic interactions. Dissecting the energetics in a salt-free solution, we showed that amelogenin self-assembly is entropically driven due to the hydrophobic effect (i.e., ΔS_{HE}) that occurs as result of removal of excessive water molecules from the monomer/oligomer interfaces [13].

Association of identical subunits in multimeric proteins involves not only the folding of the monomer (intramolecular) but also association between the subunits (intermolecular). The proposed mechanisms of association depend on whether the monomers are folded or unfolded before association [139-142]. Since IDPs provide a greater capture radius for specific binding than a structured protein, Shoemaker et al. proposed that association in IDPs takes place through "fly-casting" in which a weak long range interaction between unfolded peptides followed by folding enhances the speed of assembly [49]. Unlike assembly of folded proteins wherein the process takes place through destabilization leading to unfolding of the globular structure, this mechanism requires a partial refolding of IDPs [139].

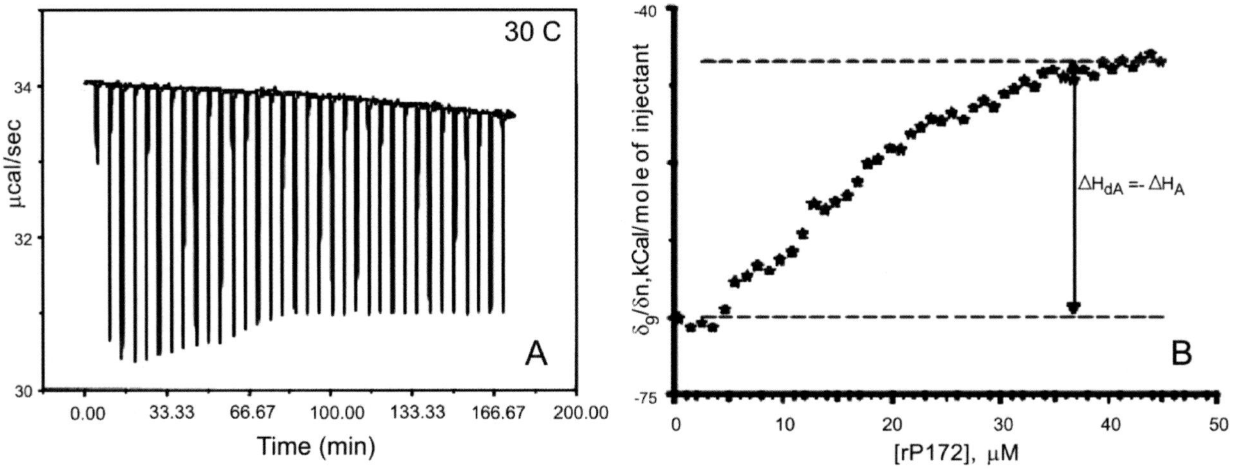

Figure 11: (**A**) ITC raw data for the dissociation of amelogenin (rP172) assemblies at 30 °C. (**B**) Heat of dilution (δq_i), obtained by integration of each peak, per mole of rP172 injected (δn_i) is plotted against the concentration of rP172 in the cell after each injection. The enthalpy of disassembly (ΔH_{dA}) is the difference in reaction enthalpy between the two plateaus. The enthalpy of assembly (ΔH_A) has the same magnitude but opposite sign as that of ΔH_{dA} .

The Putative Pre-Molten Globule-like (PMG) State of Amelogenin

Based on far UV-CD spectra and hydrodynamic properties, Uversky classified IDPs into two non-overlapping subgroups: coil-like and premolten globule (PMG)-like structures [73]. The PMG-like proteins possess considerable amounts of residual secondary structure and are therefore more compact than coil-like proteins but significantly less ordered than native or molten globules. In general, despite the same amino acid composition, the secondary structure and the degree of compactness (hydrodynamic properties) of the four conformational states; native, molten globule, pre-molten globule, and denaturated; are different (Fig 12A). Native structure is the most compact state and possesses proper tertiary and secondary structures. Molten globules (MG) possesses a high content of secondary structure and no tertiary structure. As a result, in the MG state a protein is extended by about 1.5 times compared to native structures and exhibits strong binding to hydrophobic ANS (1-anilino-8-naphthalene sulfonate) dye. The pre-molten globule (PMG) conformation corresponds to the denatured state of a protein. A protein in the PMG state is highly extended (about 3 times more extended than a native state) with little secondary and no tertiary structures. Protein in a PMG state shows weak binding to ANS dye. Protein in the denatured states is highly extended and behaves like a linear polymer chain. A protein in this state has high flexibility, no secondary or tertiary structures, and large hydrodynamic dimensions (7 times larger than the native state).

Since, amelogenin contains a significant amount of order-promoting residues and the NMR structure indicates that the protein is not fully extended and exhibits some local secondary structures, it is reasonable to assume that it may belong to the PMG-like subclass. This can be verified by the "double wavelength" plot introduced by Uversky [73]. In this plot, the CD ellipticity value at 222 nm is plotted against the ellipticity values at 200 nm, which allows classification of IDPs into coil-like or PMG-like structures (Fig.12B). The figure indicates a transition from coil-like structure at low temperatures to a PMG-like structure above 20 °C, suggesting that it possesses a small amount of an ordered secondary structure and is more compact than intrinsic coil-like proteins. Since the PMG-like state is associated with assembly of several disease- and non-disease-related proteins [97, 143, 144], it is tempting to suggest that amelogenin possesses an adaptable structure (PMG-like) which may play an important role in the self-assembly. The driving force for amelogenin self-assembly is, therefore, the presence of extended structure with exposed hydrophobic domains. As the protein self-assembles, interaction between other polypeptide chains is mediated by hydrophobic interactions leading to removal of ordered water molecules from the hydrophobic interface. As a result, considerable breaking of the hydrogen bonding occurs and hence a positive (endothermic) reaction enthalpy, a mechanism characteristic of assembly of protomers that have more than 7 subunits [145-147].

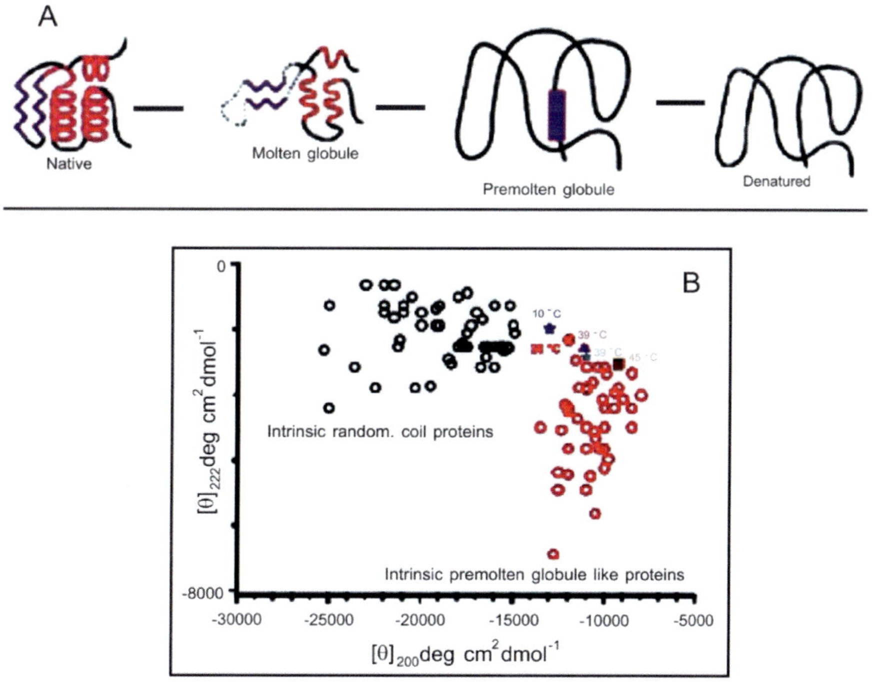

Figure 12: (A) The protein quartet model of protein folding/functioning adopted with permission from [148] **(B)** Double wavelength plot that divides IDPs into two subgroups: intrinsic coil-like and intrinsic premolten-globule (PMG)-like states. The temperature-induced transition from an extended coil-like state at low temperatures to partially compact PMG-like state at higher temperature is shown for rP172.

SUMMARY AND FUTURE PERSPECTIVE

This chapter considers details of the conformation, secondary structure, and degree of disorder in amelogenin. Using computational and biophysical techniques we identify unfolded regions in amelogenin supporting the notion that it is a member of the class of IDP's. Detailed comparative analyses indicate that amelogenins is not entirely disordered but have some presence of structure–promoting residues, as has been also demonstrated in our recent NMR studies. We propose that the occurrence of "conformational plasticity" in amelogenin explains its strong tendency to self-assemble under certain conditions, its potential to specifically interact with different targets including organic macromolecules and mineral. Such interactions allow amelogenin to fulfill different functions.

Amelogenin monomers that are only stable at acidic pH do not fold into a 3D compact structure but are extended and exhibit only local residual secondary structures, including PPII secondary structure (Fig 8) [11, 102, 149]. PPII structure has been linked to protein-protein interaction processes and to the stabilization of sequences against conformational transformation [149]. Thus, the presence of PPII structure within the amelogenin protein may serve dual roles in terms of promoting molecular recognition (i.e. signaling function) and stabilizing unfolded regions against transformation changes until appropriate conditions are realized. Isothermal titration calorimetry studies have revealed that amelogenin self-assembly is entropically driven, and is promoted by hydrophobic interactions. As in many IDP's the disorder-to-order transition that occurs during amelogenin self-assembly would decrease conformational entropy and make highly specific interactions between amelogenin molecules possible. Presumably interaction of amelogenin with other molecular entities, cell surface, or mineral surface would be partially driven by the need to achieve internal structural stabilization within the individual amelogenin molecules.

In general, we find that the assembly behavior of amelogenin is similar to other intrinsically disordered proteins such as prions and amyloid peptides that are also enriched in proline and other hydrophobic amino acids [150]. Amelogenin molecules have a strong tendency to self-associate upon pH increase and eventually assemble into homogeneous particles at pH=8. Increasing protein concentration or slow evaporation of the surrounding solution can lead to the formation of fibrillar structures, or micro-ribbons. We postulate that the extended, unfolded configuration of amelogenin is important for its self-assembly because it offers conformational freedom to allow interactions and multiple contacts to occur between amelogenins during self-assembly. The conformational exchange detected by NMR, which shows more than one protein structural state co-existing in solution, is another good indication for amelogenin conformational flexibility that not only allows self-association, but also interactions with other enamel matrix proteins, or the mineral phase.

Amelogenin is cleaved by specific proteases during enamel formation (Chapter 8, this volume). The location of residual structure and the boundaries between residual structural elements and disordered regions within rP172 amelogenin may also have an important impact with regard to the cleavage sites of proteases. Notably, the common conserved cleavage sites within porcine amelogenin, W45/H46, S148/M149, W161/A162, and H62/H63 [151, 152] are positioned at the boundaries of regions that have secondary structure (Fig's 1D and Figure 8). Due to the unfolded nature of the rP172 amelogenin protein, these cleavage sites that are located at the starting points of residual secondary structure would not be obscured by any residual folding, and would be fully accessible for protease recognition.

We note that amelogenin alternative splicing occurs at regions that are enriched in disorder-promoting amino acid residues. In addition, analysis of the distribution of disorder-promoting residues in the AS regions of amelogenin showed that the spliced regions contain significant amounts of disorder-promoting residues. Omission of these regions would not have a catastrophic effect on the structure of the remaining amelogenin protein. Alternative splicing in amelogenin may contribute to functional diversity of the protein. This is evident by the signaling function of the alternatively spliced leucine rich amelogenin polypeptide (LRAP) that is endcoded from exons 2,3, and 6D.

In summary, a number of chapters in this book highlight the multifunctionality of amelogenin protein. Amelogenin protein is closely associated with the mineralization of vertebrate enamel through a series of protein-protein, protein-mineral, and protein-cell interactions. Such interactions control the processes of protein secretion, macromolecular self-assembly, crystal nucleation and growth, and protein degradation and removal. This proline-rich protein also exhibits signaling activity as determined in numerous cell culture systems. Amelogenin interactions with cell surface proteins such as Lamp1, CD63, Anxa2 can lead to control of cell differentiation. Both the full-length amelogenin and the alternatively spliced isoform, LRAP, promote cell differentiation through the Wnt signaling pathway, although the direct target through which amelogenin triggers this pathway has not yet been identified [153]. We speculate that intrinsic disorder in amelogenin sequence is a key to its multi-functionality and its self-assembly properties.

Future experimental strategies will be necessary to investigate the function of unfolded regions in amelogenin as well as to study a series of multifunctional extracellular matrix proteins involved in other biomineralizing systems such as bone [27, 29, 33, 154-157]. A number of proteins associated with mineralized tissue containing calcium phosphate have been characterized as intrinsically disordered [158, 159]. These proteins are statherin, casein, phosphophoryn (known as dentin phosphoprotein; DPP), bone sialoprotein (BSP) and osteopontin (OPN). Combination of bioinformatics and biophysical strategies will be a promising approach to explore the function of IDP's in biomineralization.

ACKNOWLEDGMENTS

The authors acknowledge funding from the National Institute of Health NIH-NIDCR DE013414, DE-020099 and DE-15644 to JMO. We thank Dr. Carol Wuenschell for assistance in proof reading and editing the manuscript.

LIST OF ABBREVIATION

CD = Circular Dichroism

DLS = Dynamic Light Scattering

DSC = Differential Scanning Calorimetry

FTIR = Fourier Transform Infrared

HSQC = Heteronuclear Single Quantum Coherence

IDP = Intrinsically Disordered Protein

ITC = Isothermal Titration Calorimetry

Lamp1 = Lysosomal-associated glygoprotein 1

LRAP = Leucine Rich Amelogenin Polypeptide

NMR = Nuclear Magnetic Resonance

NUP = Naturally Unfolded Protein

PMG = Premolten Globule -like

PPII = Polyproline Type II

rP172 = Recombinant Porcine Amelogenin (full-length)

SAXS = Small Angle X-ray Scattering

TFE = Trifluoroethanol

UDDW = Unbuffered Deionized Distilled Water

VT-CD = Variable Temperature Circular Dichroism

REFERENCES

[1] Moradian-Oldak J. Amelogenins: assembly, processing and control of crystal morphology. Matrix Biol 2001 Sep;20(5-6):293-305.

[2] Wang L, Guan X, Yin H, *et al.*. Mimicking the Self-Organized Microstructure of Tooth Enamel. J Phys Chem C Nanomater Interfaces 2008 Mar 22;112(15):5892-9.

[3] Moradian-Oldak J, Paine ML. Mammalian Enamel Formation. In: Astrid Sigel, Sigel H, Sigel RKO, Eds. Metal Ions In Life Sciences: Chichester: John Wiley & Sons, Ltd; 2008. p. 507-46.

[4] Beniash E, Simmer JP, Margolis HC. The effect of recombinant mouse amelogenins on the formation and organization of hydroxyapatite crystals in vitro. J Struct Biol 2005 Feb;149(2):182-90.

[5] Iijima M, Moradian-Oldak J. Control of octacalcium phosphate and apatite crystal growth by amelogenin matrices. J Mater Chem 2004;14(14):2189-99.

[6] Bartlett JD, Ganss B, Goldberg M, *et al.* 3. Protein-protein interactions of the developing enamel matrix. Curr Top Dev Biol 2006;74:57-115.

[7] Fowler CE, Beniash E, Yamakoshi Y, *et al.* Co-operative mineralization and protein self-assembly in amelogenesis: silica mineralization and assembly of recombinant amelogenins in vitro. Eur J Oral Sci 2006 May;114 Suppl 1:297-303; discussion 27-9, 82.

[8] Fincham A, Moradian-Oldak J, Simmer J. The structural biology of the developing dental enamel matrix. J Struct Biol 1999 Jun;126(3):270-99.

[9] Moradian-Oldak J, Goldberg M. Amelogenin supra-molecular assembly in vitro compared with the architecture of the forming enamel matrix. Cells Tissues Organs 2005;181(3-4):202-18.

[10] Margolis HC, Beniash E, Fowler CE. Role of macromolecular assembly of enamel matrix proteins in enamel formation. J Dent Res 2006 Sep;85(9):775-93.

[11] Delak K, Harcup C, Lakshminarayanan R, *et al.* The Tooth Enamel Protein, Porcine Amelogenin, Is an Intrinsically Disordered Protein with an Extended Molecular Configuration in the Monomeric Form (dagger). Biochemistry 2009 Mar;48(10):2272-81.

[12] Lakshminarayanan R, Fan D, Du C, *et al.* The role of secondary structure in the entropically driven amelogenin self-assembly. Biophys J 2007 Nov 15;93(10):3664-74.

[13] Lakshminarayanan R, Yoon I, Hegde BG, *et al.* Analysis of secondary structure and self-assembly of amelogenin by variable temperature circular dichroism and isothermal titration calorimetry. Proteins 2009 Aug 15;76(3):560-9.

[14] Makowska J, Rodziewicz-Motowidlo S, Baginska K, *et al.* Polyproline II conformation is one of many local conformational states and is not an overall conformation of unfolded peptides and proteins. Proc Natl Acad Sci U S A 2006 Feb 7;103(6):1744-9.

[15] Dayson HJ, Wright PE. Intrinsically unstructured proteins and their functions. Nature Reviews 2005;6:197-208.

[16] Dunker AK, Brown CJ, Lawson JD, *et al.*. Intrinsic disorder and protein function. Biochemistry 2002 May 28;41(21):6573-82.

[17] Fan Y, Sun Z, Wang R, *et al.* Enamel inspired nanocomposite fabrication through amelogenin supramolecular assembly. Biomaterials 2007 Jul;28(19):3034-42.

[18] Moradian-Oldak J. The emergence of "nanospheres" as basic structural components adopted by amelogenin. J Dent Res 2007 Jun;86(6):487-90.

[19] Moradian-Oldak J, Du C, Falini G. On the formation of amelogenin microribbons. Eur J Oral Sci 2006 May;114 Suppl 1:289-96; discussion 327-9, 82.

[20] Fincham AG, Moradian-Oldak J, Simmer JP, *et al.* Self-assembly of a recombinant amelogenin protein generates supramolecular structures. J Struct Biol 1994 Mar-Apr;112(2):103-9.

[21] He X, Li W, Habelitz S. The cooperative self-assembly of 25 and 23kDa amelogenins. J Struct Biol 2008 Dec;164(3):314-21.

[22] Paine ML, Snead ML. Protein interactions during assembly of the enamel organic extracellular matrix. J Bone Min Res 1997;12:221-7.

[23] Moradian-Oldak J, Tan J, Fincham AG. Interaction of amelogenin with hydroxyapatite crystals: an adherence effect through amelogenin molecular self-association. Biopolymers 1998 Oct 5;46(4):225-38.

[24] Moradian-Oldak J, Bouropoulos N, Wang L, *et al.* Analysis of self-assembly and apatite binding properties of amelogenin proteins lacking the hydrophilic C-terminal. Matrix Biol 2002;21:197-205.

[25] Shaw WJ, Ferris K. Structure, Orientation, and Dynamics of the C-Terminal Hexapeptide of LRAP Determined Using Solid-State NMR. J Phys Chem B 2008 Nov 18.

[26] Zou Y, Wang H, Shapiro JL, *et al.* Determination of protein regions responsible for interactions of amelogenin with CD63 and LAMP1. Biochem J 2007 Dec 15;408(3):347-54.

[27] Veis A. Amelogenin gene splice products: potential signaling molecules. Cell Mol Life Sci 2003 Jan;60(1):38-55.

[28] Tompkins K, Veis A. Polypeptides translated from alternatively spliced transcripts of the amelogenin gene, devoid of the exon 6a, b, c region, have specific effects on tooth germ development in culture. Connect Tissue Res 2002;43(2-3):224-31.

[29] Fukae M, Kanazashi M, Nagano T, *et al.* Porcine sheath proteins show periodontal ligament regeneration activity. Eur J Oral Sci 2006 May;114 Suppl 1:212-8; discussion 54-6, 381-2.

[30] Gibson CW. The amelogenin "enamel proteins" and cells in the periodontium. Crit Rev Eukaryot Gene Expr 2008;18(4):345-60.

[31] Zeichner-David M. Is there more to enamel matrix proteins than biomineralization? Matrix Biol 2001;20:307-16.

[32] Zeichner-David M, Chen LS, Hsu Z, *et al.* Amelogenin and ameloblastin show growth-factor like activity in periodontal ligament cells. Eur J Oral Sci 2006 May;114 Suppl 1:244-53; discussion 54-6, 381-2.

[33] Sfeir C. The mineralized extracellular "matrix" reloaded: a tissue engineering perspective. J Musculoskelet Neuronal Interact 2006 Oct-Dec;6(4):372-3.

[34] Fisher LW, Fedarko NS. Six genes expressed in bones and teeth encode the current members of the SIBLING family of proteins. Connect Tissue Res 2003;44 Suppl 1:33-40.

[35] Uversky VN, Oldfield CJ, Dunker AK. Intrinsically disordered proteins in human diseases: introducing the D2 concept. Annu Rev Biophys 2008;37:215-46.

[36] Dunker AK, Oldfield CJ, Meng J, *et al.* The unfoldomics decade: an update on intrinsically disordered proteins. BMC Genomics 2008;9 Suppl 2:S1.

[37] Dunker AK, Silman I, Uversky VN, *et al.* Function and structure of inherently disordered proteins. Curr Opin Struct Biol 2008 Dec;18(6):756-64.

[38] Iakoucheva LM, Brown CJ, Lawson JD, *et al.* Intrinsic disorder in cell-signaling and cancer-associated proteins. J Mol Biol 2002 Oct 25;323(3):573-84.

[39] Uversky VN, Dunker AK. Biochemistry. Controlled chaos. Science 2008 Nov 28;322(5906):1340-1.

[40] Holt C, Sawyer L. Caseins as rheomorphic proteins-interpretation of secondary structures of the α-S1-caseins, β-caseins and κ-caseins. J Chem Soc Faraday Trans 1993;89(15):2683-92.

[41] Weinreb PH, Zhen W, Poon AW, *et al.* NACP, a protein implicated in Alzheimer's disease and learning, is natively unfolded. Biochemistry 1996 Oct 29;35(43):13709-15.

[42] Wright PE, Dyson HJ. Intrinsically unstructured proteins: re-assessing the protein structure-function paradigm. J Mol Biol 1999 Oct 22;293(2):321-31.

[43] Boehr DD, Wright PE. Biochemistry. How do proteins interact? Science 2008 Jun 13;320(5882):1429-30.

[44] Spolar RS, Record MT, Jr. Coupling of local folding to site-specific binding of proteins to DNA. Science 1994 Feb 11;263(5148):777-84.

[45] Xie H, Vucetic S, Iakoucheva LM, *et al.* Functional anthology of intrinsic disorder. 1. Biological processes and functions of proteins with long disordered regions. J Proteome Res 2007 May;6(5):1882-98.

[46] Xie H, Vucetic S, Iakoucheva LM, *et al.* Functional anthology of intrinsic disorder. 3. Ligands, post-translational modifications, and diseases associated with intrinsically disordered proteins. J Proteome Res 2007 May;6(5):1917-32.

[47] Vucetic S, Xie H, Iakoucheva LM, *et al.* Functional anthology of intrinsic disorder. 2. Cellular components, domains, technical terms, developmental processes, and coding sequence diversities correlated with long disordered regions. J Proteome Res 2007 May;6(5):1899-916.

[48] Gunasekaran K, Tsai CJ, Kumar S, *et al.* Extended disordered proteins: targeting function with less scaffold. Trends Biochem Sci 2003 Feb;28(2):81-5.

[49] Shoemaker BA, Portman JJ, Wolynes PG. Speeding molecular recognition by using the folding funnel: the fly-casting mechanism. Proc Natl Acad Sci U S A 2000 Aug 1;97(16):8868-73.

[50] Romero P, Obradovic Z, Li X, *et al.* Sequence complexity of disordered protein. Proteins 2001 Jan 1;42(1):38-48.

[51] Dunker AK, Lawson JD, Brown CJ, *et al.* Intrinsically disordered protein. J Mol Graph Model 2001;19(1):26-59.

[52] Uversky VN, Radivojac P, Iakoucheva LM, *et al.* Prediction of intrinsic disorder and its use in functional proteomics. Methods Mol Biol 2007;408:69-92.

[53] Radivojac P, Iakoucheva LM, Oldfield CJ, *et al.* Intrinsic disorder and functional proteomics. Biophys J 2007 Mar 1;92(5):1439-56.

[54] Ferron F, Longhi S, Canard B, *et al.* A practical overview of protein disorder prediction methods. Proteins 2006 Oct 1;65(1):1-14.

[55] Uversky VN, Gillespie JR, Fink AL. Why are "natively unfolded" proteins unstructured under physiologic conditions? Proteins 2000 Nov 15;41(3):415-27.

[56] Receveur-Brechot V, Bourhis JM, Uversky VN, *et al.* Assessing protein disorder and induced folding. Proteins 2006 Jan 1;62(1):24-45.

[57] Uversky VN. Intrinsically Disordered Proteins and Their Environment: Effects of Strong Denaturants, Temperature, pH, Counter Ions, Membranes, Binding Partners, Osmolytes, and Macromolecular Crowding. Protein J 2009 Sep 19.

[58] Eliezer D. Biophysical characterization of intrinsically disordered proteins. Curr Opin Struct Biol 2009 Feb;19(1):23-30.

[59] Bienkiewicz EA, Moon Woody A, Woody RW. Conformation of the RNA polymerase II C-terminal domain: circular dichroism of long and short fragments. J Mol Biol 2000 Mar 17;297(1):119-33.

[60] Kelly MA, Chellgren BW, Rucker AL, *et al.* Host-guest study of left-handed polyproline II helix formation. Biochemistry 2001 Dec 4;40(48):14376-83.

[61] Stapley BJ, Creamer TP. A survey of left-handed polyproline II helices. Protein Sci 1999 Mar;8(3):587-95.

[62] Chen K, Liu Z, Kallenbach NR. The polyproline II conformation in short alanine peptides is noncooperative. Proc Natl Acad Sci U S A 2004 Oct 26;101(43):15352-7.

[63] Eker F, Griebenow K, Cao X, *et al.* Preferred peptide backbone conformations in the unfolded state revealed by the structure analysis of alanine-based (AXA) tripeptides in aqueous solution. Proc Natl Acad Sci U S A 2004 Jul 6;101(27):10054-9.

[64] Schweitzer-Stenner R, Measey T, Hagarman A, *et al.* Salmon calcitonin and amyloid beta: two peptides with amyloidogenic capacity adopt different conformational manifolds in their unfolded states. Biochemistry 2006 Mar 7;45(9):2810-9.

[65] Park SH, Shalongo W, Stellwagen E. The role of PII conformations in the calculation of peptide fractional helix content. Protein Sci 1997 Aug;6(8):1694-700.

[66] Danielsson J, Jarvet J, Damberg P, *et al.* The Alzheimer beta-peptide shows temperature-dependent transitions between left-handed 3-helix, beta-strand and random coil secondary structures. FEBS J 2005 Aug;272(15):3938-49.

[67] Romero PR, Zaidi S, Fang YY, *et al.* Alternative splicing in concert with protein intrinsic disorder enables increased functional diversity in multicellular organisms. Proc Natl Acad Sci U S A 2006 May 30;103(22):8390-5.

[68] Simmer JP. Alternative splicing of amelogenins. Connect Tissue Res 1995;32(1-4):131-6.

[69] Vacic V, Uversky VN, Dunker AK, *et al.* Composition Profiler: a tool for discovery and visualization of amino acid composition differences. BMC Bioinformatics 2007;8:211.

[70] Sickmeier M, Hamilton JA, LeGall T, *et al.* DisProt: the Database of Disordered Proteins. Nucleic Acids Res 2007 Jan;35(Database issue):D786-93.

[71] Vihinen M. Relationship of protein flexibility to thermostability. Protein Eng 1987 Dec;1(6):477-80.

[72] Liu Z, Chen K, Ng A, *et al.* Solvent dependence of PII conformation in model alanine peptides. J Am Chem Soc 2004 Nov 24;126(46):15141-50.

[73] Uversky VN. Natively unfolded proteins: a point where biology waits for physics. Protein Sci 2002 Apr;11(4):739-56.

[74] Goto Y, Kogure E, Takagi T, *et al.* Molecular conformation of porcine amelogenin in solution: three folding units at the N-terminal, central and C-terminal regions. J Biochem 1993;113(113):55-60.

[75] Oobatake M, Yamasaki T, Simmer JP, *et al.* Thermal denaturation of a recombinant mouse amelogenin: circular dichroism and differential scanning calorimetric studies. Proteins 2006 Feb 1;62(2):461-9.

[76] Shi Z, Woody RW, Kallenbach NR. Is polyproline II a major backbone conformation in unfolded proteins? Adv Protein Chem 2002;62:163-240.

[77] Creamer TP, Campbell MN. Determinants of the polyproline II helix from modeling studies. Adv Protein Chem 2002;62:263-82.

[78] Rucker AL, Creamer TP. Polyproline II helical structure in protein unfolded states: lysine peptides revisited. Protein Sci 2002 Apr;11(4):980-5.

[79] Woody RW. Circular dichroism of protein-folding intermediates. Methods Enzymol 2004;380:242-85.

[80] Tiffany ML, Krimm S. Effect of temperature on the circular dichroism spectra of polypeptides in the extended state. Biopolymers 1972;11(11):2309-16.
[81] Drake AF, Siligardi G, Gibbons WA. Reassessment of the electronic circular dichroism criteria for random coil conformations of poly(L-lysine) and the implications for protein folding and denaturation studies. Biophys Chem 1988 Aug;31(1-2):143-6.
[82] Andersson D, Carlsson U, Freskgard PO. Contribution of tryptophan residues to the CD spectrum of the extracellular domain of human tissue factor: application in folding studies and prediction of secondary structure. Eur J Biochem 2001 Feb;268(4):1118-28.
[83] Whittington SJ, Chellgren BW, Hermann VM, *et al.* Urea promotes polyproline II helix formation: implications for protein denatured states. Biochemistry 2005 Apr 26;44(16):6269-75.
[84] Carvalho AF, Costa-Rodrigues J, Correia I, *et al.* The N-terminal half of the peroxisomal cycling receptor Pex5p is a natively unfolded domain. J Mol Biol 2006 Mar 3;356(4):864-75.
[85] Goyal K, Tisi L, Basran A, *et al.* Transition from natively unfolded to folded state induced by desiccation in an anhydrobiotic nematode protein. J Biol Chem 2003 Apr 11;278(15):12977-84.
[86] Haaning S, Radutoiu S, Hoffmann SV, *et al.* An unusual intrinsically disordered protein from the model legume Lotus japonicus stabilizes proteins in vitro. J Biol Chem 2008 Nov 7;283(45):31142-52.
[87] Ulrih NP, Barry CH, Fink AL. Impact of Tyr to Ala mutations on alpha-synuclein fibrillation and structural properties. Biochim Biophys Acta 2008 Oct;1782(10):581-5.
[88] Reshetnyak YK, Koshevnik Y, Burstein EA. Decomposition of protein tryptophan fluorescence spectra into log-normal components. III. Correlation between fluorescence and microenvironment parameters of individual tryptophan residues. Biophys J 2001 Sep;81(3):1735-58.
[89] Shen C, Menon R, Das D, *et al.* The protein fluorescence and structural toolkit: Database and programs for the analysis of protein fluorescence and structural data. Proteins 2008 Jun;71(4):1744-54.
[90] Yiu CP, Beavil RL, Chan HY. Biophysical characterisation reveals structural disorder in the nucleolar protein, Dribble. Biochem Biophys Res Commun 2006 Apr 28;343(1):311-8.
[91] Zurdo J, Gonzalez C, Sanz JM, *et al.* Structural differences between Saccharomyces cerevisiae ribosomal stalk proteins P1 and P2 support their functional diversity. Biochemistry 2000 Aug 1;39(30):8935-43.
[92] Watt K, Jess TJ, Kelly SM, *et al.* Induced alpha-helix structure in the aryl hydrocarbon receptor transactivation domain modulates protein-protein interactions. Biochemistry 2005 Jan 18;44(2):734-43.
[93] Fladvad M, Zhou K, Moshref A, *et al.* N and C-terminal sub-regions in the c-Myc transactivation region and their joint role in creating versatility in folding and binding. J Mol Biol 2005 Feb 11;346(1):175-89.
[94] Khaymina SS, Kenney JM, Schroeter MM, *et al.* Fesselin is a natively unfolded protein. J Proteome Res 2007 Sep;6(9):3648-54.
[95] Nyarko A, Hare M, Hays TS, *et al.* The intermediate chain of cytoplasmic dynein is partially disordered and gains structure upon binding to light-chain LC8. Biochemistry 2004 Dec 14;43(49):15595-603.
[96] Reid J, Kelly SM, Watt K, *et al.* Conformational analysis of the androgen receptor amino-terminal domain involved in transactivation. Influence of structure-stabilizing solutes and protein-protein interactions. J Biol Chem 2002 May 31;277(22):20079-86.
[97] Campioni S, Mossuto MF, Torrassa S, *et al.* Conformational properties of the aggregation precursor state of HypF-N. J Mol Biol 2008 Jun 6;379(3):554-67.
[98] Privalov PL. Stability of proteins. Proteins which do not present a single cooperative system. Adv Protein Chem 1982;35:1-104.
[99] Hackel M, Konno T, Hinz H. A new alternative method to quantify residual structure in 'unfolded' proteins. Biochim Biophys Acta 2000 Jun 15;1479(1-2):155-65.
[100] Mendoza C, Figueirido F, Tasayco ML. DSC studies of a family of natively disordered fragments from Escherichia coli thioredoxin: surface burial in intrinsic coils. Biochemistry 2003 Mar 25;42(11):3349-58.
[101] Aichmayer B, Margolis HC, Sigel R, *et al.* The onset of amelogenin nanosphere aggregation studied by small-angle X-ray scattering and dynamic light scattering. J Struct Biol 2005 Sep;151(3):239-49.
[102] Matsushima N, Izumi Y, Aoba T. Small-angle X-ray scattering and computer-aided molecular modeling studies of 20 kDa fragment of porcine amelogenin: does amelogenin adopt an elongated bundle structure? J Biochem 1998 Jan;123(1):150-6.
[103] Lee L, Stollar E, Chang J, *et al.* Expression of the Oct-1 transcription factor and characterization of its interactions with the Bob1 coactivator. Biochemistry 2001 Jun 5;40(22):6580-8.
[104] Garcia W, de Araujo AP, Neto Mde O, *et al.* Dissection of a human septin: definition and characterization of distinct domains within human SEPT4. Biochemistry 2006 Nov 21;45(46):13918-31.

[105] Paz A, Zeev-Ben-Mordehai T, Lundqvist M, *et al.* Biophysical characterization of the unstructured cytoplasmic domain of the human neuronal adhesion protein neuroligin 3. Biophys J 2008 Aug;95(4):1928-44.
[106] von Ossowski I, Eaton JT, Czjzek M, *et al.* Protein disorder: conformational distribution of the flexible linker in a chimeric double cellulase. Biophys J 2005 Apr;88(4):2823-32.
[107] Wells M, Tidow H, Rutherford TJ, *et al.* Structure of tumor suppressor p53 and its intrinsically disordered N-terminal transactivation domain. Proc Natl Acad Sci U S A 2008 Apr 15;105(15):5762-7.
[108] Abercrombie BD, Kneale GG, Crane-Robinson C, *et al.* Studies on the conformational properties of the high-mobility-group chromosomal protein HMG 17 and its interaction with DNA. Eur J Biochem 1978 Mar;84(1):173-7.
[109] Schweers O, Schonbrunn-Hanebeck E, Marx A, *et al.* Structural studies of tau protein and Alzheimer paired helical filaments show no evidence for beta-structure. J Biol Chem 1994 Sep 30;269(39):24290-7.
[110] Longhi S, Receveur-Brechot V, Karlin D, *et al.* The C-terminal domain of the measles virus nucleoprotein is intrinsically disordered and folds upon binding to the C-terminal moiety of the phosphoprotein. J Biol Chem 2003 May 16;278(20):18638-48.
[111] Jin KS, Kim DY, Rho Y, *et al.* Solution structures of RseA and its complex with RseB. J Synchrotron Radiat 2008 May;15(Pt 3):219-22.
[112] Permyakov SE, Millett IS, Doniach S, *et al.* Natively unfolded C-terminal domain of caldesmon remains substantially unstructured after the effective binding to calmodulin. Proteins 2003 Dec 1;53(4):855-62.
[113] Uversky VN, Karnoup AS, Khurana R, *et al.* Association of partially-folded intermediates of staphylococcal nuclease induces structure and stability. Protein Sci 1999 Jan;8(1):161-73.
[114] Dyson HJ, Wright PE. Nuclear magnetic resonance methods for elucidation of structure and dynamics in disordered states. Methods Enzymol 2001;339:258-70.
[115] Dyson HJ, Wright PE. Insights into the structure and dynamics of unfolded proteins from nuclear magnetic resonance. Adv Protein Chem 2002;62:311-40.
[116] Buchko GW, Bekhazi J, Cort JR, *et al.* H, C, and N resonance assignments of murine amelogenin, an enamel biomineralization protein. Biomol NMR Assign 2008 Jun;2(1):89-91.
[117] Schubert M, Labudde D, Oschkinat H, *et al.* A software tool for the prediction of Xaa-Pro peptide bond conformations in proteins based on 13C chemical shift statistics. J Biomol NMR 2002 Oct;24(2):149-54.
[118] Wishart DS, Case DA. Use of chemical shifts in macromolecular structure determination. Methods Enzymol 2001;338:3-34.
[119] Tompa P. Intrinsically unstructured proteins. Trends Biochem Sci 2002 Oct;27(10):527-33.
[120] Serrano L. Comparison between the phi distribution of the amino acids in the protein database and NMR data indicates that amino acids have various phi propensities in the random coil conformation. J Mol Biol 1995 Nov 24;254(2):322-33.
[121] Wustman BA, Santos R, Zhang B, *et al.* Identification of a "glycine-loop"-like coiled structure in the 34 AA Pro,Gly,Met repeat domain of the biomineral-associated protein, PM27. Biopolymers 2002 Dec 5;65(5):362-72.
[122] Shaw WJ, Ferris K, Tarasevich B, *et al.* The structure and orientation of the C-terminus of LRAP. Biophys J 2008 Apr 15;94(8):3247-57.
[123] Uversky VN, Li J, Fink AL. Evidence for a partially folded intermediate in alpha-synuclein fibril formation. J Biol Chem 2001 Apr 6;276(14):10737-44.
[124] Uversky VN, Li J, Fink AL. Metal-triggered structural transformations, aggregation, and fibrillation of human alpha-synuclein. A possible molecular NK between Parkinson's disease and heavy metal exposure. J Biol Chem 2001 Nov 23;276(47):44284-96.
[125] Rajan R, Balaram P. A model for the interaction of trifluoroethanol with peptides and proteins. Int J Pept Protein Res 1996 Oct;48(4):328-36.
[126] Scholtz JM, Qian H, York EJ, *et al.* Parameters of helix-coil transition theory for alanine-based peptides of varying chain lengths in water. Biopolymers 1991 Nov;31(13):1463-70.
[127] Le TQ, Gochin M, Featherstone JD, *et al.* Comparative calcium binding of leucine-rich amelogenin peptide and full-length amelogenin. Eur J Oral Sci 2006 May;114 Suppl 1:320-6; discussion 7-9, 82.
[128] Buchko GW, Tarasevich BJ, Bekhazi J, *et al.* A solution NMR investigation into the early events of amelogenin nanosphere self-assembly initiated with sodium chloride or calcium chloride. Biochemistry 2008 Dec 16;47(50):13215-22.
[129] Dyson HJ, Wright PE. Coupling of folding and binding for unstructured proteins. Curr Opin Struct Biol 2002 Feb;12(1):54-60.

[130] Ravindranath RM, Tam WY, Bringas PJ, *et al.* Amelogenin-cytokeratin 14 interaction in ameloblasts during enamel formation. J Biol Chem. 2001 Sep 28;276(39):36586-97. J Biol Chem 2001;276:36586-97.
[131] Fincham AG, Leung W, Tan J, *et al.* Does amelogenin nanosphere assembly proceed through intermediary-sized structures? Connect Tissue Res 1998;38(1-4):237-40; discussion 41-6.
[132] Aoba T. Recent observations on enamel crystal formation during mammalian amelogenesis. Anat Rec 1996;245:208-18.
[133] Ravindranath HH, Chen LS, Zeichner-David M, *et al.* Interaction between the enamel matrix proteins amelogenin and ameloblastin. Biochem Biophys Res Commun 2004 Oct 22;323(3):1075-83.
[134] Fan D, Du C, Sun Z, *et al.* In vitro study on the interaction between the 32 kDa enamelin and amelogenin. J Struct Biol 2009 Apr;166(1):88-94.
[135] Wiedemann-Bidlack FB, Beniash E, Yamakoshi Y, *et al.* pH triggered self-assembly of native and recombinant amelogenins under physiological pH and temperature in vitro. J Struct Biol 2007 Oct;160(1):57-69.
[136] Heerklotz H, Tsamaloukas A, Kita-Tokarczyk K, *et al.* Structural, volumetric, and thermodynamic characterization of a micellar sphere-to-rod transition. J Am Chem Soc 2004 Dec 22;126(50):16544-52.
[137] Portnaya I, Cogan U, Livney YD, *et al.* Micellization of bovine beta-casein studied by isothermal titration microcalorimetry and cryogenic transmission electron microscopy. J Agric Food Chem 2006 Jul 26;54(15):5555-61.
[138] Luke K, Wittung-Stafshede P. Folding and assembly pathways of co-chaperonin proteins 10: Origin of bacterial thermostability. Arch Biochem Biophys 2006 Dec 1;456(1):8-18.
[139] Levy Y, Wolynes PG, Onuchic JN. Protein topology determines binding mechanism. Proc Natl Acad Sci U S A 2004 Jan 13;101(2):511-6.
[140] Shakhnovich EI. Folding by association. Nat Struct Biol 1999 Feb;6(2):99-102.
[141] Jaenicke R, Lilie H. Folding and association of oligomeric and multimeric proteins. Adv Protein Chem 2000;53:329-401.
[142] Jones S, Thornton JM. Principles of protein-protein interactions. Proc Natl Acad Sci U S A 1996 Jan 9;93(1):13-20.
[143] Nocula-Lugowska M, Rymarczyk G, Lisowski M, *et al.* Isoform-specific variation in the intrinsic disorder of the ecdysteroid receptor N-terminal domain. Proteins 2009 Aug 1;76(2):291-308.
[144] Gazi AD, Bastaki M, Charova SN, *et al.* Evidence for a coiled-coil interaction mode of disordered proteins from bacterial type III secretion systems. J Biol Chem 2008 Dec 5;283(49):34062-8.
[145] Bello M, Perez-Hernandez G, Fernandez-Velasco DA, *et al.* Energetics of protein homodimerization: effects of water sequestering on the formation of beta-lactoglobulin dimer. Proteins 2008 Mar;70(4):1475-87.
[146] Barranco-Medina S, Kakorin S, Lazaro JJ, *et al.* Thermodynamics of the dimer-decamer transition of reduced human and plant 2-cys peroxiredoxin. Biochemistry 2008 Jul 8;47(27):7196-204.
[147] Luke K, Apiyo D, Wittung-Stafshede P. Dissecting homo-heptamer thermodynamics by isothermal titration calorimetry: entropy-driven assembly of co-chaperonin protein 10. Biophys J 2005 Nov;89(5):3332-6.
[148] Booth DR, Sunde M, Bellotti V, *et al.* Instability, unfolding and aggregation of human lysozyme variants underlying amyloid fibrillogenesis. Nature 1997 Feb 27;385(6619):787-93.
[149] Darnell G, Orgel JP, Pahl R, *et al.* Flanking polyproline sequences inhibit beta-sheet structure in polyglutamine segments by inducing PPII-like helix structure. J Mol Biol 2007 Nov 30;374(3):688-704.
[150] Sanchez de Groot N, Pallares I, Aviles FX, *et al.* Prediction of "hot spots" of aggregation in disease-linked polypeptides. BMC Struct Biol 2005;5:18.
[151] Ryu OH, Fincham AG, Hu CC, *et al.* Characterization of recombinant pig enamelysin activity and cleavage of recombinant pig and mouse amelogenins. J Dent Res 1999;78:743-50.
[152] Moradian-Oldak J, Jimenez I, Maltby D, *et al.* Controlled proteolysis of amelogenins reveals exposure of both carboxy- and amino-terminal regions. Biopolymers 2001 Jun;58(7):606-16.
[153] Warotayanont R, Frenkel B, Snead ML, *et al.* Leucine-rich amelogenin peptide induces osteogenesis by activation of the Wnt pathway. Biochem Biophys Res Commun 2009 Sep 25;387(3):558-63.
[154] He G, Ramachandran A, Dahl T, *et al.* Phosphorylation of phosphophoryn is crucial for its function as a mediator of biomineralization. J Biol Chem 2005 Sep 30;280(39):33109-14.
[155] Yamakoshi Y, Tanabe T, Oida S, *et al.* Calcium binding of enamel proteins and their derivatives with emphasis on the calcium-binding domain of porcine sheathlin. Arch Oral Biol 2001 Nov;46(11):1005-14.
[156] Kirkham J, Andreev I, Robinson C, *et al.* Evidence for direct amelogenin-target cell interactions using dynamic force spectroscopy. Eur J Oral Sci 2006 May;114 Suppl 1:219-24; discussion 54-6, 381-2.

[157] Fisher LW, Torchia DA, Fohr B, *et al.* Flexible structures of SIBLING proteins, bone sialoprotein, and osteopontin. Biochem Biophys Res Commun 2001 Jan 19;280(2):460-5.

[158] Bellahcene A, Bonjean K, Fohr B, *et al.* Bone sialoprotein mediates human endothelial cell attachment and migration and promotes angiogenesis. Circ Res 2000 Apr 28;86(8):885-91.

[159] Huq NL, Cross KJ, Ung M, *et al.* A review of protein structure and gene organisation for proteins associated with mineralised tissue and calcium phosphate stabilisation encoded on human chromosome 4. Arch Oral Biol 2005 Jul;50(7):599-609.

CHAPTER 11

The Role of Amelogenin in Dental Enamel Formation: A Universal Strategy for Protein-Mediated Biomineralization

Henry C. Margolis[1] and Elia Beniash[2]

[1]The Forsyth Institute Boston, Massachusetts USA and [2]University of Pittsburgh School of Dental Medicine, Pittsburgh, Pennsylvania USA

Running title: The Regulation of Enamel Formation by Amelogenin

Abstract: Significant advances have been made in understanding the role of amelogenin and other matrix proteins in the regulation of enamel formation, although the mechanism for this process is not fully understood. However, it is apparent that there are several guiding principles associated with the formation of mineralized tissues, although the mechanism by which enamel mineral forms differs from other mineralized tissues in several distinct aspects. This review briefly describes some of the similarities and difference between enamel, bone and dentin formation and highlights recent *in vitro* and *in vivo* studies from our laboratories that show that amelogenin regulates enamel mineral formation using a strategy that appears to be universally utilized in the development of mineralized tissues. More specifically, the presented studies show that full-length amelogenin has the capacity to stabilize the formation of amorphous calcium phosphate (ACP) and guide its organization into linear needle-like structures that subsequently fuse and organize into parallel bundles of apatitic crystals *in vitro*. Importantly, these *in vitro* findings are consistent with recent *in vivo* data presented that show that mineral morphology and organization in enamel are established by the organic matrix prior to its crystallization. These new findings should aid in the development of novel approaches for mineralized tissue regeneration and repair.

Key Words: Amelogenin, Enamel Formation, Bone, Dentin Formation, Apatitic Crystals, Regeneration, Repair.

INTRODUCTION

The mechanism by which dental enamel forms is not fully understood, although significant advances made to date have provided important new insights into the roles of amelogenin (as described in this volume) and other extracellular matrix molecules in this biomineralization process. Strictly speaking, biomineralization is the process by which living organisms produce mineral deposits for specific purposes [1]. However, it has become apparent that the unique structures and properties of mineralized tissues, including those of enamel, result from highly orchestrated extracellular events involving matrix molecules that can regulate the nucleation, growth, shape, and organization of forming mineral crystals [2]. Importantly, the vertebrate mineralized tissues, *i.e.,* enamel, dentin, bone and cementum, derive their functional capabilities from their unique structures that are formed under tight cellular and molecular controls. Although there are a number of similarities in how mineralized tissues develop, the process of enamel formation (amelogenesis) exhibits several distinct features not associated with other mineralized tissues that might suggest that enamel mineral forms by a different mechanism. This brief review will address some of the similarities and differences related to the mechanism of enamel formation and those of other mineralized tissues, and highlight recent *in vitro* and *in vivo* findings that collectively indicate that amelogenin regulates enamel mineral formation using a strategy that appears to be universally utilized in the development of mineralized tissues.

COMPOSITION AND PROPERTIES OF VERTEBRATE MINERALIZED TISSUES

As illustrated in Table 1, mature enamel differs from other vertebrate mineralized tissues, such as bone and dentine, with respect to relative proportions of mineral and organic components, with enamel having a mineral content that is greater than 95% by weight [3]. Although the mineral phase of each of these tissues is crystalline, with a composition and crystal structure [4] similar to that of hydroxyapatite, the organization, size, morphology and trace ion composition (*e.g.,* carbonate) of the mineral crystals vary significantly, leading to sharp differences in physical chemical properties (*e.g.* solubility) [*e.g.*, 5 - 7].

Table 1: Composition of Mature Enamel, Dentin and Bone*

	Mineral		Organic		Water	
	Wt%	Vol%	Wt%	Vol%	Wt%	Vol%
Enamel	95	87	1	2	3	11
Dentin	70	47	20	33	10	21
Bone	65	36	24	36	15	28

* based on data compiled by G. Nikiforuk [3].

Trace ion concentration gradients from the enamel surface to the dentino-enamel junction (DEJ) are also found [8] in dental enamel (*e.g.,* involving carbonate (higher at the DEJ) and fluoride (higher at the enamel surface)) that can lead to gradients in enamel solubility or hardness, for example. Differences in the composition (mineral and organic) and structural organization of the mineralized tissues similarly dictate differences in bulk density, porosity and mechanical properties [9]. Of considerable importance, mature enamel is the hardest vertebrate tissue [10] consistent with its functional role. Enamel is also comprised of *extremely* long and narrow needle-like crystals [2, 11]. Importantly, these long apatitic crystals are bundled into parallel arrays, called enamel rods or prisms, which are arranged to form intricate interwoven patterns, resulting in a complex and highly ordered mineralized tissue [2]. As seen in the rat incisor (Figure 1), mature enamel is made up of two distinct sets of orthogonally arranged enamel rods and inter-rod enamel that is similarly comprised of well-aligned and elongated crystals [2]. Human molar enamel may be considered even more complex in structure since the paths of individual enamel rods from the dentino-enamel junction to the enamel surface, particularly at the base of tooth cusps, undergo multiple bends that contribute to the increase in enamel volume at the cusp where the enamel is thickest [12].

GUIDING PRINCIPLES IN THE FORMATION OF VERTEBRATE MINERALIZED TISSUES

It has been suggested that both hydrophobic and hydrophilic molecules are always involved in biomineralization, where hydrophobic molecules provide a skeletal or space-filling structure (like collagen in bone) and the hydrophilic (acidic) molecules (like phosphophoryn in dentin) are associated with the regulation of crystal nucleation and growth [2]. The protein matrix of forming enamel is comprised predominately of amelogenins, making up over 90% of the enamel matrix [13, 14]. In addition, two key non-amelogenin matrix proteins, enamelin and ameloblastin, although present in considerably smaller proportions, have been shown, along with amelogenin, to also play critical roles in enamel formation. Recent studies have shown that the amelogenin-null mouse [15] exhibits a dramatic enamel phenotype and that enamel does not form in the absence of either enamelin or ameloblastin [16 - 19]. Hence, amelogenin (mostly hydrophobic), enamelin (hydrophilic and acidic), and ameloblastin (amphiphilic and acidic) appear to fit the suggested requirement for the involvement of both hydrophobic and hydrophilic molecules in the regulation of biomineralization (*i.e.,* enamel formation). However, although very little is known about how these key enamel matrix proteins function independently or collectively *in vivo* to control mineral formation and tissue organization, it appears that the formation of dental enamel takes place in a fashion that differs in several key aspects when compared to the mineralization mechanism involved in bone and dentin formation.

As we have previously discussed in light of the role of amelogenin self-assembly in enamel formation [20], considerable evidence has been obtained to show that a highly-ordered pre-assembled collagen matrix in dentin and bone serves as a template to guide subsequent mineralization, resulting in mature mineralized tissues that are ~ 40-50% by volume comprised of mineral crystals (Table 1). In these tissues the initial collagenous organic matrix secreted by the cells is free of mineral. This organic matrix undergoes a series of structural and compositional changes after the secretion prior to mineralization, which occur a few microns away from the cells in a narrow area called the mineralization front [21 – 23]. In contrast, during the initial secretory stage of amelogenesis, long thin ribbons of enamel mineral begin to form almost immediately as ameloblasts lay down enamel matrix [24 - 26], suggesting that mineralization does not take place within a pre-formed enamel matrix, as is the case in collagen-based tissues, like dentin and bone. In addition, although the initially formed mineral ribbons are hundreds of microns long, they are only a few unit cells in thickness (~2 - 7 nm [27, 28]), if the initial mineral phase is considered to be either hydroxyapatite (HA) or octacalcium phosphate. Thus, secretory enamel has a high protein content with relatively little mineral [29, 30], with the mineral phase comprising 10-20% by volume, while the remaining tissue volume is occupied by enamel matrix and water. However, as seen in Figure 2, these thin ribbons of mineral are organized into parallel arrays, which in turn form an intricate interwoven pattern that serves as a template for the mature fully mineralized enamel tissue (Figure 1). During the maturation stage of amelogenesis [31], resident proteases bring about the almost complete removal of the enamel matrix, allowing mineral ribbons to grow in width and thickness, resulting in a tissue that is >95% mineral (by weight) with only 1-2% of remaining protein and a small percent of water (Table 1). The transient nature of the organic matrix is not common in biomineralization [2] and distinguishes amelogenesis from other biomineralization systems. Hence, despite similarities in the hydrophobic / hydrophilic make-up of the extracellular bone and enamel matrices, for example, it appears that the formation of dental enamel and the formation of collagen-based mineralized tissues take place via mechanisms that differ in several fundamental aspects that ultimately lead to the formation of calcium phosphate mineralized tissues that have distinct structures, compositions and properties.

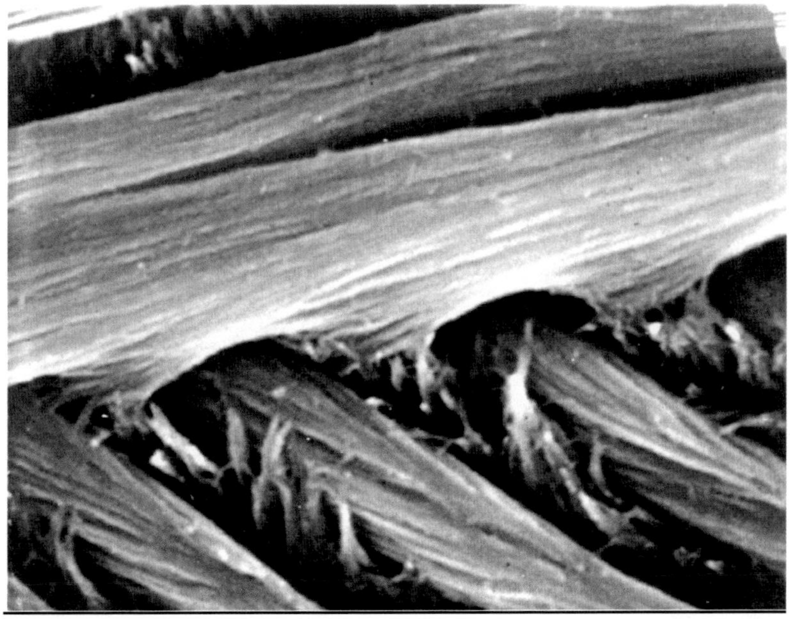

Figure 1: Scanning electron micrograph of mature rat incisor enamel made up of two distinct sets of orthogonally arranged enamel rods and inter-rod enamel that are similarly comprised of well-aligned and elongated crystals (courtesy of Dr. Ziedonis Skobe).

THE ROLE OF AMELOGENIN IN THE FORMATION OF ORDERED ARRAYS OF HYDROXYAPATITE CRYSTALS IN VITRO

Our recent *in vitro* findings [32] support the conclusion that amelogenin-mediated mineralization proceeds through a cooperative mechanism where mineralization and protein assembly occur simultaneously. This finding is consistent with a model developed by others [33] suggesting that the interplay between self-assembly of organic molecules and mineralization, and the subsequent cooperative re-organization of hybrid inorganic-organic nanostructures, can lead to the formation of hierarchical structures. Under experimental conditions designed to simultaneously induce spontaneous mineralization and protein self-assembly, recombinant full-length mouse amelogenin rM179 [32] was found *in vitro* to guide the formation of bundles of parallel-aligned ribbons of HA crystals that are similar in these respects to those seen in developing enamel (Figure 2). In contrast, randomly arranged HA crystals were observed when rM179 was first pre-assembled and then exposed to the same mineralizing conditions [32]. These findings are consistent with a cooperative mechanism for protein-mediated mineralization and add further support to the notion that enamel mineralization does not take place within a pre-formed enamel matrix, as was shown to be the case for collagen-based tissues. In addition, parallel arrays of HA crystals were not observed in *in vitro* experiments [32] when recombinant amelogenin cleavage product rM166 that lacks the hydrophilic C-terminus was used. Instead, in the presence of rM166 randomly arranged HA crystals were observed. These combined studies provide evidence that the full-length amelogenin plays a unique role in regulating the formation of highly-ordered enamel mineral crystals during the secretory stage of amelogenesis through cooperative interactions between enamel matrix molecules (mostly amelogenins) and forming mineral crystals. More specifically, these results demonstrate that the hydrophilic C-terminal domain in amelogenin is essential for the alignment of crystals into parallel arrays. Consistent with these *in vitro* findings, it is of interest to note that the full-length amelogenin was found to be exclusively associated with newly formed enamel mineral [34]. Thus, despite the fact that the parent amelogenin undergoes proteolysis soon after secretion, it appears that the full-length protein plays a critical role in the regulation of HA crystal organization during the very initial stages of mineralization.

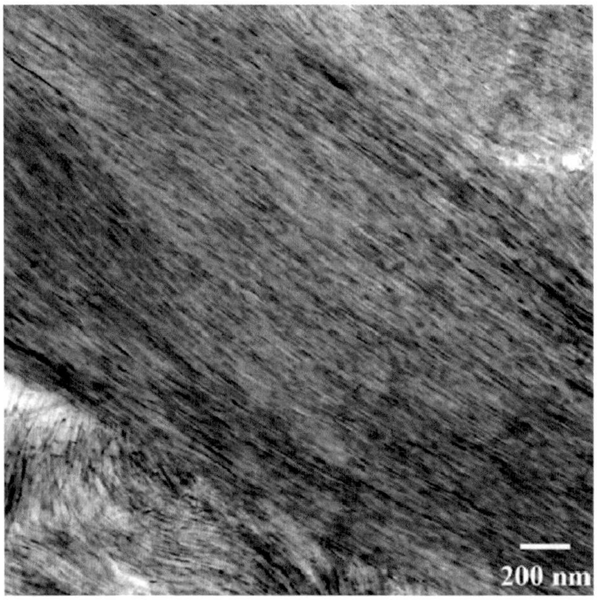

Figure 2: TEM micrograph of secretory murine enamel showing parallel arrays of long and narrow nascent crystals (enamel rods).

As noted in the preceding paragraph, under conditions that support simultaneous protein assembly and mineralization in the presence of the full-length mouse amelogenin (rM179), a mineral product is obtained that is similar to that found in developing enamel. To gain further understanding of this key finding, the effect of porcine amelogenins on the kinetics of mineralization was assessed in greater detail by monitoring changes in solution pH, as an indication of mineralization progress, as well as the nature of mineral products formed over time, using Fourier transform infrared spectroscopy, transmission electron microscopy, and electron diffraction [35]. Notably, in the absence of protein (control), a decrease in solution pH was observed to take place in three distinct steps, corresponding to an initial induction period of ~15 min that was associated with the formation of mono-dispersed spherical particles (32.1±4.3 nm in diameter) of amorphous calcium phosphate (ACP), followed by a rapid and a slower apatitic crystal growth phase. After 45 min, thin plate-like crystals were found to grow from a network of ACP particles. Subsequently (from 1h – 1 day), spherical particles could no longer be seen and were replaced by networks of randomly arranged thin plate-like crystals of HA (determined after 1 day). The results of the control experiments without protein are similar to those reported by others [36]. In the presence of the full-length recombinant porcine amelogenin rP172, a similar change in pH with time was observed, however, following a notably longer ~45-min induction period. During this time period, rP172 was found to stabilize ACP nanoparticles (Figure 3A) and prevent their transformation to plate-like crystals, as was seen in the control. In general, the stabilized ACP particles were also smaller than those seen in the control (8.5±1.1 nm in diameter). Importantly, unlike the control, the observed nanoparticles (presumably ACP) were found to align and form linear needle-like structures at ~45 min (Figure 3B)in the presence of rP172, whereas needle-like crystals were subsequently observed after 1-4 hr (Figure 3C). After 1 day, multiple bundles of well-aligned needle-like crystals of HA were seen (Figure 3D), that were similar to those found in the presence of the full-length mouse amelogenin rM179 [32]. Hence, the experimental results outlined above suggest that in the presence of rP172, ACP nanoparticles appear to align to form linear needle-like structures that subsequently fuse, transform and organize into parallel arrays of apatitic needle-like crystals. In the presence of recombinant porcine amelogenin rP147 that lacks 25 C-terminal amino acids, however, an almost immediate decrease in pH was seen (*i.e.*, no induction period was observed) that corresponded to a rapid (within 15 min) formation and transformation of ACP particles to randomly arranged plate-like HA crystals that were similar to those seen in the control. These findings confirm that, like rM179, full-length amelogenin has the unique capacity to promote the formation of oriented bundles of HA crystals *in vitro*, similar to those found in developing tooth enamel. As described in the following section, results showing that the full-length porcine amelogenin has the capacity to stabilize and guide the formation of linear arrays of initially formed ACP mineral particles have significant biological relevance.

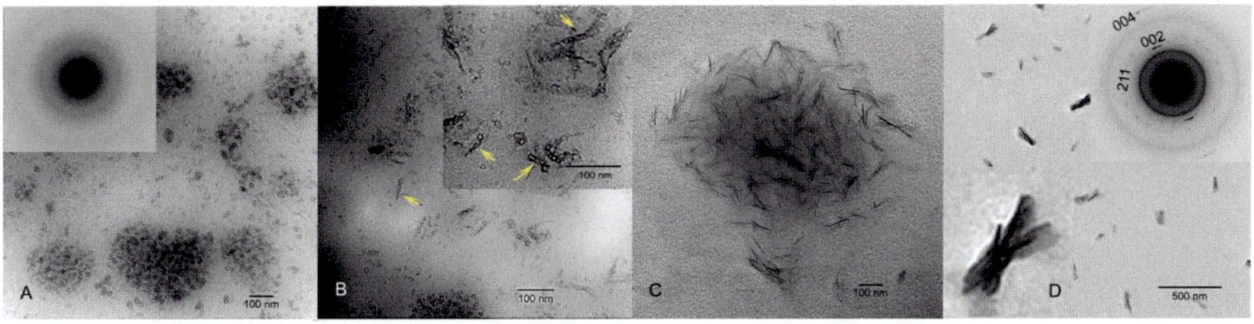

Figure 3: TEM micrographs of calcium phosphate mineral products formed in the presence of recombinant full-length porcine amelogenin rP172 at selected times (15 min, 45 min, 1 - 4 hrs, and 1 day) [35]. At 15 min (A), ACP was initially formed based on the observed (inset) selected area electron diffraction (SAED) pattern. At 45 min (B), ACP particles were observed (inset) to align and form needle-like particles (arrows), whereas needle-like crystals were subsequently observed after 1-4 hrs (C). After 1 day (D), based on SAED and Fourier transform infrared spectroscopy analyses, aligned bundles of needle-like apatitic crystals were formed in the presence of rP172 (insets, showing a higher magnification of a bundle of aligned HA crystals and an arc-like diffraction pattern in the direction of the 002 reflection). In contrast, in the absence of rP172 (control), networks of randomly arranged plate-like crystals of HA were observed at 1 day (data not shown). (Reprinted from [35], with permission from The American Society for Biochemistry and Molecular Biology).

A UNIVERSAL STRATEGY FOR BIOMINERALIZATION IN ENAMEL FORMATION - THE ROLE OF AMELOGENIN IN VIVO

Our findings that have shown that full-length amelogenin has the capacity to stabilize ACP *in vitro* are consistent with earlier electron microscopy studies that suggested that ACP is the first mineral phase formed in secretory enamel [37, 38]. The possible presence of transient mineral phases, including ACP, in vertebrate mineralized tissues has been debated for many years and, in some cases, this issue remains unresolved [39 - 42]. Recent studies, however, have provided strong evidence to support a biomineralization strategy in bone involving transient precursor phases, including ACP [43 - 44].

More importantly, a recent extensive study of early enamel mineralization using four independent physical characterization techniques has conclusively demonstrated that the first enamel mineral formed during the secretory stage is ACP that eventually transforms into apatitic crystals [45]. Specifically it has been shown that the newly formed few micron thick outer layer of secretory enamel in constantly growing murine incisors contains an amorphous mineral phase (Figure 4A) while inner older layers of enamel contain crystalline mineral of an apatitic nature (Figure 4B). Even more intriguing is the fact that the amorphous mineral particles in the outer enamel (Figure 4A) have a ribbon-like shape and organize into interwoven parallel arrays. Hence, in terms of mineral morphology and structural organization this amorphous layer is similar to inner secretory enamel containing crystalline mineral. These observations imply that the mineral morphology and organization in enamel is established by the organic matrix prior to its crystallization.

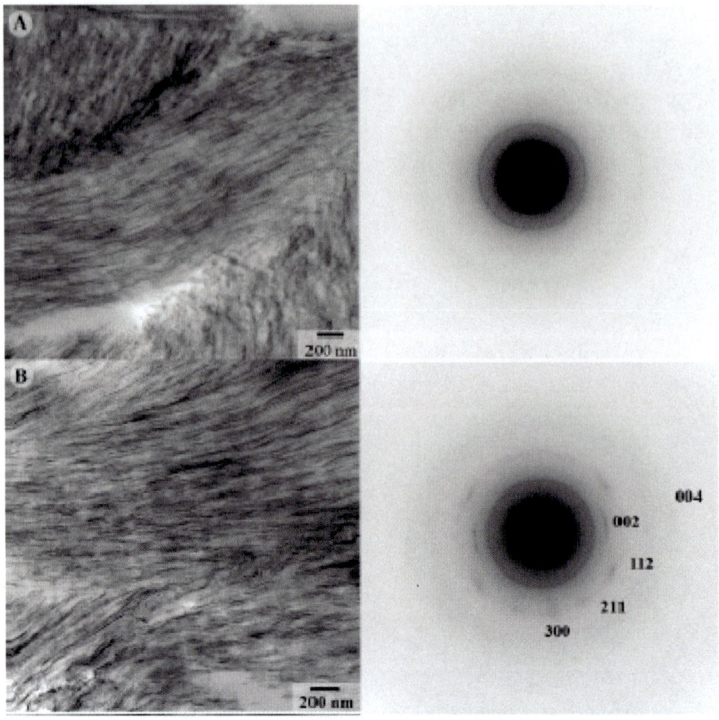

Figure 4: TEM micrographs and corresponding diffraction patterns taken from unstained thin sections through outer enamel layer (A) and inner enamel layer (B). (Reproduced from [45] with permission from Elsevier Limited.)

Based on the *in vivo* findings presented above and the fact that full-length amelogenins *in vitro* have the unique capacity to form higher-order chain-like structures [32, 46 - 49], in contrast to amelogenins that lack the hydrophilic C-terminus, it is reasonable to propose that amelogenin super-assemblies play a role in guiding the formation of linear arrays of amorphous calcium phosphate (ACP) nanoparticles that subsequently fuse and transform into ribbon-like apatitic crystals, as illustrated in Figure 5. This hypothesis is supported by the fact that this sequence of events appears to reflect precisely the mineralization phenomenon observed *in vivo* [45].

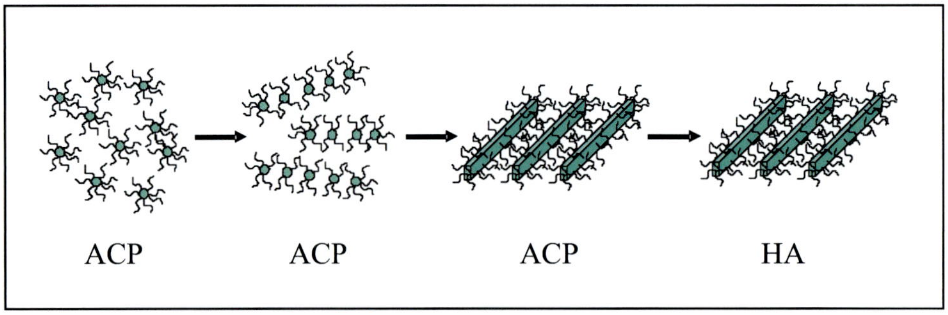

Figure 5: Schematic showing the alignment of amelogenin stabilized ACP nanoparticles into linear arrays that subsequently fuse and form parallel arrays of ACP ribbons, which latter transform into ribbon-like apatitic crystals, based on presented *in vitro* [35] and *in vivo* [45] findings.

In further support of the potential role of amelogenin in the mediation of enamel mineralization *in vivo* via an ACP precursor phase, we have found that the predominant native amelogenin in secretory porcine enamel, P148, dramatically inhibits spontaneous calcium phosphate formation *in vitro* and stabilizes ACP for long periods of time, preventing its transformation to apatitic material [35]. P148 contains a single phosphate group on serine-16 and an additional N-terminal methionine, in comparison to its recombinant analog rP147 that had little to no influence on spontaneous mineralization *in vitro*. Additional studies confirmed that the observed inhibition of calcium phosphate formation and enhanced stabilization of ACP by P148 was due to the presence of the single phosphate group [35]. Studies have now confirmed [unpublished results; personal communication H. Margolis] that the native full-length native porcine amelogenin P173 (also phosphorylated at serine-16) similarly stabilizes ACP for long periods of time (> 1 day), under the same experimental conditions. These *in vitro* results suggest that both the native full-length (P173) and the major proteolytic degradation product (P148), which lacks 25 C-terminal amino acids, may have functional, although distinct, roles in the regulation of nascent enamel mineral crystal formation during secretory amelogenesis. The employment of a biomineralization strategy involving stabilized amorphous mineral precursors has a number of distinct advantages, including greater spatial control of initial mineralization events, as described above for rP172 [35] and seen in developing enamel [45], and in the prevention of precipitation in other areas [50]. As previously discussed [35], P148 may play an important functional role in regulating mineralization during enamel formation through its inhibition of crystal nucleation and the stabilization of ACP, preventing unwanted crystal formation throughout the majority of the extracellular enamel matrix during the secretory stage of amelogenesis, in which the 3D network of nascent mineral particles occupies only 10 - 20% of its total volume [29, 30], as noted earlier. On the other hand, although this has not yet been proven, based on the exclusive localization of full-length amelogenin to newly developing enamel mineral [34] and the importance of the presence C-terminal amino acid domain in the regulation of organized mineral formation *in vitro*, full length phosphorylated amelogenins may play a role in guiding the alignment of ACP nanoparticles during nascent enamel crystal formation. Studies are underway to investigate this possibility.

Our collective finding [35, 45] and proposed mechanism (Figure 5) are also consistent with a model for enamel formation that was proposed [51, 52] based on the examination of developing rat incisor enamel using a freeze fracturing technique [53]. Results obtained suggested that enamel crystals may form through the linear assembly of observed globular structures that contain enamel matrix proteins and amorphous mineral particles, although no evidence for the nature of the mineral phase was provided. It was further proposed that through proteolytic processing of matrix components, mineral deposits would fuse and transform into long apatitic crystals. Support for this mechanism has also been recently obtained [45], based on differential staining patterns of the developing enamel matrix (Figure 6) that suggest that biochemical changes in the enamel matrix may trigger mineral phase transformation.

Transient amorphous mineral phases (*i.e.*, ACP and amorphous calcium carbonate) have been found in a number of other biomineralization systems, including mollusk shells and teeth, echinoderm skeletal elements, sponge spicules [54 - 59] and bone [43, 44, 60], as discussed above. Other biomineralization related molecules, like the highly phosphorylated osteopontin from milk [61] and the N-terminal domain of dentin matrix protein 1 [62], have also been shown to stabilize ACP. These findings, in part, support the suggestion that the transformation of amorphous phases to crystalline materials is an important aspect of biological mineralization [56, 63, 64].

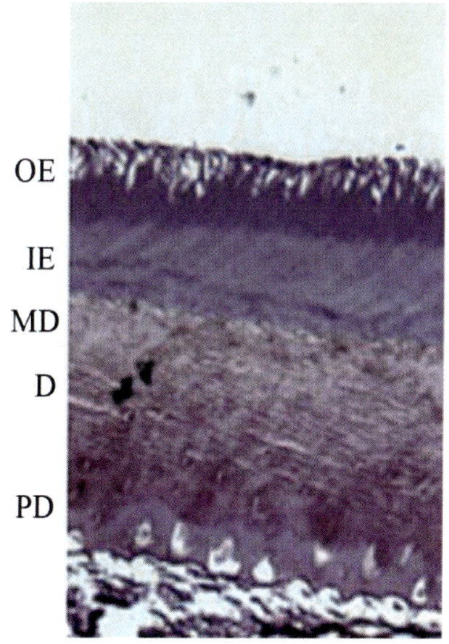

Figure 6: Light micrograph of a semi-thin section of mouse incisor in the region of the cervical loop stained with toluidine blue. OE-outer enamel, IE-inner enamel, MD-mantle dentin, D-dentin.

In light of the results presented here, despite apparent differences in the composition and properties of dental enamel, and unique features associated with enamel matrix mediated mineral formation, it appears that amelogenin can regulate enamel mineral formation using a strategy that is universally utilized in the development of mineralized tissues; *i.e.,* via a transient amorphous phase. Building on such findings, this strategy has been employed in the development of novel bioinspired materials [65, 66]. Accordingly, the findings highlighted in the present paper regarding the role of amelogenin in regulating calcium phosphate mineral formation should aid in the development for new approaches for enamel regeneration and repair

ACKNOWLEDGEMENTS

The authors thank Dr. Ziedonis Skobe for supplying us with the electron micrographs of dental enamel. We also gratefully acknowledge the National Institute of Dental and Craniofacial Research for grant funding (DE-016376 (HM) and DE016703 (EB)) that supported this work.

REFERENCES

[1] Mann S. Inorganic Structures of Life. In: Biomineralization: Principles and Concepts in Bioinorganic Materials Chemistry. Oxford University Press 2001, Oxford, UK, pp 1-4.

[2] Weiner S. Organization of extracellularly mineralized tissues: A comparative study of biological crystal growth. CRC Critical Rev Biochem 1986; 20: 395-408.

[3] Nikiforuk G. Understanding Dental Caries. 1. Etiology and Mechanisms Basic and Clinical Aspects. S. Karger 1985, Basel, Switzerland, pp 13-141.

[4] Elliott JC. Structure and Chemistry of the Apatites and Other Calcium Orthophosphates. Elsevier Science B.V. 1994, Amsterdam, The Netherlands pp 1-389.

[5] Moreno EC, Aoba T. Comparative solubility study of human dental enamel, dentin, and hydroxyapatite. Calcif Tissue Int 1991; 49: 6-13.

[6] Aoba T, Miake Y, Shimoda S, *et al.* Dental apatites in invertebrate species: morphology and chemical properties. In: Mechanisms and phylogeny of mineralization in biological systems, S Suga, H Nakahara (Eds), Springer-Verlag 1991, pp 459-63.

[7] LeGeros RZ. Calcium phosphates in enamel, dentin and bone, In: Calcium Phosphates in Oral Biology and Medicine. HM Meyer (Ed), Karger 1991, Basel, pp. 108-29.

[8] Robinson C, Kirkham J, Brookes, SJ, *et al.* Chemistry of Mature Enamel. In: Dental Enamel Formation to Destruction. Robinson, Kirkham, Shore, Eds. CRC Press 1995, Boca Raton, FL, pp. 167-91.

[9] Birchall JD. The importance of the study of biominerals to materials technology. In: Biomineralization: Chemical and Biochemical Perspectives, S Mann, J Webb, RJP Williams (Eds), VCH Publishers 1989, NY, pp. 491-509.

[10] Cuy JL, Mann AB, Livi KJ, *et al.* Nanoindentation mapping of the mechanical properties of human molar tooth enamel. Arch Oral Biol 2002; 47: 281-91.

[11] Daculsi G, Menanteau J, Kerebel LM, *et al.* Length and shape of enamel crystals. Calcif Tiss Int 1984: 36: 550-5.

[12] Skobe Z, Stern S. The pathway of enamel rods at the base of cusps of human teeth. J Dent Res 1980; 59: 1026-32.

[13] Termine JD, Belcourt AB, Christner PJ, *et al.* Properties of dissociatively extracted fetal tooth matrix proteins. J Biol Chem 1980; 20: 9760-8.

[14] Fincham AG, Moradian-Oldak J, Simmer JP. The structural biology of the developing dental enamel matrix, J Struct Biol 1999; 126: 270-99

[15] Gibson CW, Yuan ZA, Hall B, *et al.* Amelogenin-deficient mice display an amelogenesis imperfecta phenotype. J Biol Chem 2001; 276: 31871-5.

[16] Fukumoto S, Kiba T, Hall B, *et al.* Ameloblastin is a cell adhesion molecule required for maintaining the differentiation state of ameloblasts. J Cell Biol 2004; 167: 973–83.

[17] Wazen R, Moffatt P, Zalzal SF, *et al.* A mouse model expressing a truncated form of ameloblastin exhibits dental and junctional epithelium defects. Matrix Biol 2009; 28: 292–303.

[18] Hu JCC, Hu Y, Smith CE, *et al.* Enamel defects and ameloblast specific expression in Enam knock-out/lacZ knock-in mice. J Biol Chem 2008; 283: 10858–71.

[19] Smith CE, Wazen R, Hu Y, *et al.* Consequences for enamel development and mineralization resulting from loss of function of ameloblastin or enamelin. Eur J Oral Sci 2009; 117: 485-97.

[20] Margolis HC, Beniash E, Fowler CE. Role of macromolecular assembly of enamel matrix proteins in enamel formation. J Dent Res 2006; 85: 775-93.

[21] Beniash E, Traub W, Veis A, *et al.* A transmission electron microscope study using vitrified ice sections of predentin: Structural changes in the dentin collagenous matrix prior to mineralization. J Struct Biol 2000; 132: 212-25.

[22] Septier D, Hall RC, Lloyd D, *et al.* Quantitative immunohistochemical evidence of a functional gradient of chondroitin 4-sulphate dermatan sulphate, developmentally regulated in the predentine of rat incisor. Histochemical Journal 1998; 30: 275-84

[23] Weinstock M, Leblond CP. Radioautographic visualization of the deposition of a phosphoprotein at the mineralization front in the dentin of the rat incisor. J Cell Biol 1973; 56: 838–45.

[24] Nylen MU, Eanes ED, Omnell KA. Crystal growth in rat enamel. J Cell Biol 1963; 18:109-23.

[25] Arsenault AL, Robinson BW. The dentino-enamel junction: a structural and microanalytical study of early mineralization. Calcif Tissue Int 1989; 45: 111-21.

[26] Smith CE. Cellular and chemical events during enamel maturation. Crit Rev Oral Biol Med 1998; 9:128-61.

[27] Daculsi G, Kerebel B. High-resolution electron microscope study of human enamel crystallites: size, shape and growth. J Ultrastr Res 1978; 65: 163-72.

[28] Cuisinier FJG, Steuer P, Senger B, *et al.* Human amelogenesis.1 High Resolution Electron Microscope Study of Ribbon-Like Crystals. Calcif Tissue Int 1992; 51: 259-68.

[29] Robinson C, Kirkham J, Hallsworth AS. Volume distribution and concentration of protein, mineral and water in developing bovine enamel. Arch Oral Biol 1988; 33: 159-62.

[30] Fukae M. Amelogenesis - three dimensional structure of amelogenin micelles and their degradation product by a cascade system. The Proceedings of International Symposium of Oral Science in Tsurumi University School of Dental Medicine, Yokohama 2002, Japan: pp. 73-78.

[31] Robinson C, Kirkham J. The dynamics of amelogenesis as revealed by protein compositional studies. In: The Chemistry and Biology of Mineralized Tissues. Butler WT (Ed), Ebsco Media Inc 1985, Birmingham, Alabama, pp 248-63.

[32] Beniash E, Simmer JP, Margolis HC. Effects of recombinant mouse amelogenins on the formation and organization of hydroxyapatite crystals in vitro. J Struct Biol 2005; 149:182-90.

[33] Colfen H, Mann S. Higher-order organization by mesoscale self-assembly and transformation of hybrid nanostructures. Angew Chem Int Ed 2003; 42: 2350-6.

[34] Uchida T, Tanabe T, Fukae M, *et al.* Immunochemical and immunohistochemical studies, using anti-sera against porcine 25 kDa amelogenin, 89kDa enamelin and the 13-17 Kda nonamelogenins, on immature enamel of the pig and rat. Histochemistry 1991; 96: 129-38.

[35] Kwak SY, Wiedemann-Bidlack FB, Beniash E, *et al.* Role of 20 kDa amelogenin (P148) phosphorylation in calcium phosphate formation in vitro. J Biol Chem 2009; 284:18972–9.

[36] Bar-Yosef Ofir P, Govrin-Lippman R, Garti N, *et al.* The influence of polyelectrolytes on the formation and phase transformation of amorphous calcium phosphate. Cryst Growth Des 2004; 4: 177-83.

[37] Diekwisch TG H. Subunit compartments of secretory stage enamel matrix. Connect Tissue Res 1998; 38: 101 –11.

[38] Bodier-Houllé P, Steuer P, Meyer J M, *et al.* High-resolution electron-microscopic study of the relationship between human enamel and dentin crystals at the dentinoenamel junction. Cell Tissue Res 2000; 301: 389-395.

[39] Termine JD, Posner AS. Infrared analysis of rat bone—age dependency of amorphous and crystalline mineral fractions. Science 1966; 153: 1523–5.

[40] Boskey AL. Amorphous calcium phosphate: the contention of bone. J Dent Res 1997; 76: 1433–6.

[41] Grynpas MD. Transient precursor strategy or very small biological apatite crystals? Bone 2007; 41: 162–4.

[42] Weiner S. Transient precursor strategy in mineral formation of bone. Bone 2006; 39: 431–3.

[43] Crane NJ, Popescu V, Morris MD, *et al.* Raman spectroscopic evidence for octacalcium phosphate and other transient mineral species deposited during intramembranous mineralization. Bone 2006; 39: 434-42.

[44] Mahamid J, Sharir A, Addadi L, *et al.* Amorphous calcium phosphate is a major component of the forming fin bones of zebrafish: Indications for an amorphous precursor phase. Proc Natl Acad Sci USA 2008; 105: 12748-53.

[45] Beniash E, Metzler RA, Lam RS, *et al.* Transient amorphous calcium phosphate in forming enamel. J. Struct Biol 2009; 166: 133–43
[46] Fincham AG, Moradian-Oldak J, Simmer JP, *et al.* Self-assembly of a recombinant amelogenin protein generates supramolecular structures. J. Struct. Biol 1994; 112: 103–9.
[47] Aichmayer B, Margolis HC, Sigel R, *et al.* The onset of amelogenin nanosphere aggregation studied by small-angle x-ray scattering and dynamic light scattering. J Struct Biol 2005; 151:239-49.
[48] Moradian-Oldak J, Du C, Falini G. On the formation of amelogenin microribbons. Eur J Oral Sci 2006; 114: 289–96.
[49] Wiedemann-Bidlack FB, Beniash E, Yamakoshi Y, *et al.* pH triggered self-assembly of native and recombinant amelogenins under physiological pH and temperature in vitro. J Struct Biol 2007; 60: 57-69.
[50] Addadi L, Beniash E, Weiner S. Assembly and mineralization processes in biomineralization: strategies for forming biological composite materials. In: Jones, W., Rao, C.N.R. (Eds.), Supramolecular Organization and Materials Design. Cambridge University Press 2002, Cambridge, pp. 1–34.
[51] Robinson C, Shore RC, Wood SR, *et al.* Subunit structures in hydroxyapatite crystal development in enamel: implications for amelogenesis imperfecta. Connect Tissue Res 2003; 44: 65–71.
[52] Robinson C. Self-oriented assembly of nano-apatite particles: a subunit mechanism for building biological mineral crystals. J Dent Res 2007; 86: 677-9.
[53] Robinson C, Fuchs P, Weatherell JA. The appearance of developing rat incisor enamel using a freeze fracturing technique, J Cryst Growth 1981; 53: 160-5.
[54] Lowenstam H.A, Weiner S. Transformation of amorphous calcium phosphate to crystalline dahllite in the radular teeth of chitons. Science 1985; 227: 51-3.
[55] Lowenstam HA, Weiner S. On Biomineralization: Oxford University Press 1989, New York, NY pp 324.
[56] Beniash, E, Aizenberg J, Addadi L, *et al.* Amorphous calcium carbonate transforms into calcite during sea urchin larval spicule growth. Proc R Soc Lond Ser B-Biol Sci 1997; 264: 461-5.
[57] Wu LN, Genge BR, Dunkleberger DG, *et al.* Physicochemical characterization of the nucleational core of matrix vesicles. J Biol Chem 1997; 272:4404-11.
[58] Levi-Kalisman Y, Raz S, Weiner S, *et al.* X-Ray absorption spectroscopy studies on the structure of a biogenic amorphous calcium carbonate phase. J Chem Soc -Dalton Trans 2000; 21: 3977-82.
[59] Aizenberg J, Lambert G, Weiner S, *et al.* Factors involved in the formation of amorphous and crystalline calcium carbonate: A study of an ascidian skeleton. J Am Chem Soc 2002; 124:32-9.
[60] Kim HM, Himeno T, Kokubo T, *et al.* Process and kinetics of bonelike apatite formation on sintered hydroxyapatite in a simulated body fluid. Biomaterials 2005; 26: 4366-73.
[61] Gericke A, Qin C, Spevak L, *et al.* Importance of phosphorylation for osteopontin regulation of biomineralization. Calcif Tissue Int 2005; 77: 45–54.
[62] Gajjeraman S, Narayanan K, Hao J, *et al.* Matrix macromolecules in hard tissues control the nucleation and hierarchical assembly of hydroxyapatite. J Biol Chem 2007; 282: 1193–204.
[63] Weiner S, Sagi I, Addadi L. Choosing the crystallization path less traveled. Science 2005; 309: 1027-8.
[64] Deshpande AS, Beniash E. Bio-inspired synthesis of mineralized collagen fibrils. Cryst Growth Des 2008; 8: 3084–90.
[65] Aizenberg J, Muller DA, Grazul JL, *et al.* Direct fabrication of large micropatterned single crystals. Science 2003; 299: 1205–8.
[66] Loste E, Meldrum FC. Control of calcium carbonate morphology by transformation of an amorphous precursor in a constrained volume. Chem Commun 2001; 10: 901–2.

CHAPTER 12

Role of Spliced Forms of Amelogenins as Signaling Molecules

Arthur Veis[1]*, Kevin A. Tompkins[2] and Stanca Iacob[3]

[1]Department of Cell and Molecular Biology, Feinberg School of Medicine, Northwestern University, Chicago, IL 60611, USA; [2]Departments of Oral Biology and Implantology, Faculty of Dentistry, Chulalongkorn University, Bangkok, Thailand and [3]Department of Biochemistry,Rush University Medical Center 1735 W. Harrison Street, 5th Fl-CRB, Chicago, IL 60612, USA

Abstract: The amelogenin (AMEL) gene intron-exon structure, order and nucleotide sequence has been well preserved during evolutionary development. The variations of splicing of the nuclear pre-mRNA to produce the mRNA and subsequently translated proteins, depend on the sequence lengths of both the introns and exons, the presence of possible cryptic splice sites in large exons, the intrinsic "strengths" of the splice boundary sequences in interaction with the spliceosome components and the intervention of a variety of tissue and species specific accessory factors. A large number of splice isoforms has indeed been found; 16 alternative protein isoforms have been reported in mouse amelogenin, but the actual splicing patterns do differ in different animals. The major higher mass isoforms are used in building the amelogenin ECM and directing the organization and mineralization of the enamel. The question raised here is the role of the smaller isoforms? Their role appears to be largely as participants in regulatory processes during development of the enamel organ and in odontogenesis. However, it is becoming clear that amelogenin expression is not restricted to the enamel organ. Amelogenin peptides have been found in such diverse organs as brain, eye, cartilage and bone during embryogenesis. The knockout of amelogenin gene is not lethal, and these non-odontogenic tissues do form and appear to function normally, suggesting that the normal *in vivo* effects of the smaller splice isoforms may be subtle, modifying developmental rates, but it is evident that individual small amelogenin protein isoforms, added exogenously in vivo and in culture can markedly alter phenotypic expression in non-odontogenic tissues, as well as induce various forms of tissue repair in teeth. Thus, the study of the AMEL gene small isoforms and their mechanisms of action are fields worthy of extended study.

Key Words: Amelogenin, Splice Isoforms, LAMP1, Nitric Oxide Synthetase, Nitric Oxide, Enamel Formation, Non-Odontogenic Tissues, Tissue Repair.

INTRODUCTION

The amelogenin (AMEL) gene is of very ancient origin, with the primordial gene appearing well before the evolutionary development of enamel-covered vertebrate teeth [1]. Like most eukaryotic genes, the primary amelogenin gene (e.g. huAMEL, 7349 nucleotides, Ref Seq NM_182680) contains both exons and introns and the processing of the primary gene pre-mRNA transcript leads to a variety of splice product mRNAs. These in turn produce a variety of proteins of multiple sizes, differing to some extent from species to species relative to their expression level. In comparing the splicing patterns from an evolutionary perspective and over many species it is striking that the exon sizes and boundary sequences and their expression or deletion have been highly conserved. Amelogenin exon 6 is rather large and contains irregular, or cryptic, splice sites, while exon 4 is small, and is frequently skipped.

The amelogenin proteins form an extracellular structural matrix (enamel matrix) functioning as a template for deposition of the enamel mineral. The mechanism of mineral formation in enamel is still not totally understood, but one way to consider the problem is to ask about the properties of the amelogenin protein domains encoded by the conserved exons, and to examine how the differently spliced isoforms might modify function. For example, all of the primates from human to lemur express exon 4, as do rat, cow and pig, whereas the genes of mouse, dog and horse, and non-mammals such as frogs and lizards or the putative ancestral form do not. Since all the extant species have physiologically serviceable enamel, does the late acquisition of the exon 4 sequence have a structural role? If

***Corresponding Author:** Arthur Veis, Department of Cell and Molecular Biology, Feinberg School of Medicine, Northwestern University, 303 E. Chicago Avenue, Chicago, IL 60611, USA; E-mail: aveis@northwestern.edu not, why did it appear and become conserved in mammals. Do the AMEL splice isoforms possibly have non-structural functions? It appears that this may be the case and the information related to that possibility will be the main focus of this chapter. First, however, we will briefly review the mechanisms of alternative gene splicing and the relationships of that to the specific nucleotide sequences of the amelogenins and the predicted and actual splice isoforms.

Recent studies have suggested that some of the lower mass isoforms may not only have signaling effects during tooth development, but also that cells other than the ameloblasts might transiently express amelogenin isoforms with cell regulatory bioactivities in different tissues. The possible amelogenin bioactivities during development and tissue repair or regeneration will be examined in detail. Finally, the chapter concludes with a discussion of the mechanisms by which the amelogenin splice isoforms might act during cell function.

THE PATTERNS OF ALTERNATIVE GENE SPLICING IN AMELOGENINS

The splicing of a multi-exon pre-mRNA gene transcript requires the recognition of the splice boundaries of the introns to be excised (intron definition) or recognition of the exon boundary sequences (exon definition). In either case the intron to be looped out is cut from the nucleotide sequence at both 5'- and 3'-ends. The 3'-end of the upstream exon is then linked to the 5'-end of a downstream exon [2, 3]. To facilitate this process five small nuclear ribonucleoproteins assemble on the pre-mRNA in a stepwise fashion: 1) U1 snRNP binds to the intron at its 5'GT splice site; 2) factor SF1 [BBP] binds to the intron 3' region at the first A upstream of the polypyrimidine tract just upstream of the 3'AG nucleotide terminus of the intron; 3) factors U2AF 65 and U2AF 35 bind to the polypyrimidine tract and the 3'AG nucleotide terminus of the intron. The bound SF1 then interacts with more factor U2 snRNP and that intron 3' complex interacts with the U1 already at the intron 5'-end site, essentially folding the intervening sequence back on itself, forming a loop bringing the upstream exon in juxtaposition with the 5'-end site of the next exon, effectively changing the polarity of the mRNA at that point. Factor aggregate U4/U5/U6 Tri-snRNP joins the complex, and then effects a rearrangement of the spliceosome complex, during which the U6 displaces and releases the U4. This reorganized complex catalyzes the joining of the exons and releases the bound factors. The strength and efficiency of the entire process is dependent on the length of the intron that must be folded out and removed. Since the complexes are quite bulky, a short intron may be unable to loop and properly position itself *vis-à-vis* the downstream exon, thus a potential intron might be incorporated into the mRNA sequence, perhaps acting as a chain mutation. Conversely, an exon which is too short may be skipped for steric reasons. An intron which is too long may also be difficult to align with the "adjacent" exon and hence skip more than 1 exon during splicing. Exon skipping keeps the nucleotides in proper translation phase, whereas intron skipping may generate an out of phase translation.

Since alternative splicing of pre-mRNA is a very common but essential process carried out in the nuclei of all vertebrate cells it is unlikely that the availabilities of the principal spliceosome components are ever a problem. However, there are numerous non-spliceosome proteins also involved in the regulation of "binding strength" and splicing activity [2]. These protein factors are present in different tissues at different levels and it is difficult to sort out their possible involvement with a specific target gene without specific study. A review of such effects is far beyond the scope of this chapter. Very little has been done with respect to investigating these accessory factors in the case of amelogenin to this point but our surprising finding that mRNA expressing exon 4 [4, 5] was present in rat incisor odontoblast mRNA, subsequently supported by the observation of Oida *et al.* [6] that porcine odontoblasts also expressed a similar amelogenin, suggests that odontoblast factors can not only activate transcription of the amelogenin gene but also can modulate splicing of the amelogenin pre-mRNA differently than in ameloblasts. Recent detailed immunochemical study of the appearance of mouse amelogenin M180 isoform in cranio-facial development during embryogenesis [7] showed that amelogenin is expressed in various mouse tissues such as brain, eye, ganglia, peripheral nerve trunks, cartilage and bone. The M180 mRNA isoform was detected as early as embryonic stage E10.5 in brain and eye, long before tooth formation begins at E11.0. These data strongly suggest amelogenin protein is multifunctional and may have functions other than the structural templating of enamel mineral formation. It is likely that different amelogenin isoforms will have different functions.

Early biochemical studies of enamel proteins extracted from teeth indicated that the amelogenins were heterogeneous mixtures probably due to proteolytic processing [8], but it became evident [9] from high reproducibility of the molecular weight distributions of the isolated protein that the major components had fixed molecular masses in fixed relative amounts. Although proteolytic degradation was firmly established as a basis for some heterogeneity Shimokawa *et al.* [10] demonstrated the presence of multiple amelogenin mRNA transcripts for bovine amelogenin all arising from a single copy gene leading to multiple amelogenin proteins. Over the following few years a series of papers described the mRNA and translated products from bovine [11, 12], mouse [13, 14] and human [15] tooth organs. Two features were very striking. First, in some species, particularly in the human, the amelogenin gene is sex dimorphic, with genes on both X (AMELX) and Y (AMELY) chromosomes, while in other animals such as the mouse, the amelogenin gene is exclusively on the X chromosome. In the species with amelogenin genes on both X and Y chromosomes, the genes do differ in sequence but nevertheless, the principle splice products are quite similar with regard to the size and type of splice products. In all species the primary translated secreted amelogenin proteins arise from exons 2 through 7, terminated by a stop codon within exon 7, and most of the early work reflects the splice patterns from those exons. A series of papers from the DenBesten laboratory elaborated on their initial finding [16] that some amelogenin proteins isolated from immature secretory stage enamel were different from and in some cases larger than the splice products anticipated from exons 1 through 7. These were attributed to novel 3'-region alternatively spliced isoforms including material from usually untranslated sequences downstream from the exon 7 stop codon. It was found that in fact two series of splice isoforms were present [17]. The cDNAs were grouped into those accounting for and including exon 7 (Group 2) and those encoded for splice sites in the novel 3'-end downstream sequences (Group 1). These were finally determined to include the products from two new exons, exons 8 and 9. [18, 19] When these exons were utilized, the exon 7 and its stop codon were skipped and the 5'-end of exon 8 became attached to the 3'-end of exon 6. The new stop codon is included in exon 9 [19].

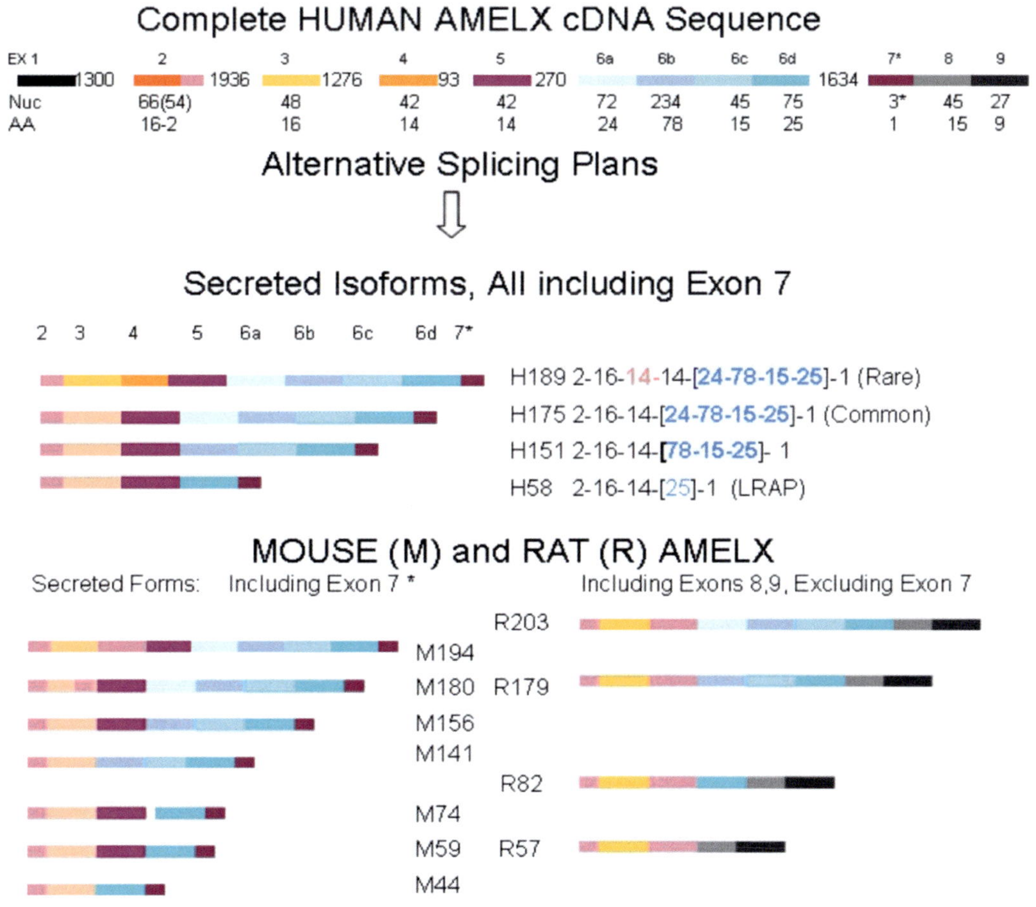

Figure 1: Patterns of splicing and the various splicing isoforms including exons 4, 8 and 9 in human (H), mouse (M) and rat (R) amelogenins.

Figure 1 illustrates the two alternative patterns of splicing now recognized as distinct pathways. The most common path followed is that incorporating exon 7. The human AMELX does not appear to express exons 8 and 9, but this is an active area of investigation. Most of the work examining the expression of the proteins containing exons 8 and 9 has dealt with the well studied rat and mouse systems, which are highly homologous [20].

Figure 2: A.

```
Nucleotide sequences at Splice Boundaries, Human AMELX,
                                Exon boundaries                   Intron Boundaries

Exon 1        2----57   AAaggattc--------cattcaaAG 56
Intron 1     58--1364                                   GTatgtggg--------catttcaGA 1307

Exon 2     1366-1431   AAccatcaa--------gccatgcCT 66
Intron 2   1432-3367                                   GTgagtaaa--------ctgtaaaAG 1936

Exon 3     3368-3415   GTaccacct--------cttttgtAG 48
Intron 3   3416-4691                                   GTaatttt--------cttttgtAG 1276

Exon 4     4692-4733   AActcacat--------actgcatTA 42
Intron 4   4733-4823                                   GTgagtcta--------tctcttaAG   91

Exon 5     4825-4866   GTgcttaac--------aggccacCG 42
Intron 5   4866-5135                                   GTatagtag--------tctcaccAG  270

Exon 6     5137-5562   TAcccttcc--------gaggaagTG  426
     6A    5137-5208      TAcccttcc--------tcccaacAG   72
6B     5209-5450      CAccccccg--------gcccctgCC 242
6C     5451-5495      GCcacagcc--------gcccctgCC  45
     6D    5496-5562      TCccatgct--------gaggaagTG* 67
Intron 6   5563-7195                                   GTgagtata-----ttttttcAG 1633

Exon 7     7196-7349   GAttaa*aag--------taaaaatCA  155
                            END
```

```
B 1. Sequence of Human Exon 7 after stop codon.
7196 gat taa aag atc aga aga tga gag ggg aat gaa tac ttc aga tgc ttt cag gag
     cac tga aag aac aca atg att ttt gct tat aat cac tta ctt agc aaa ttc tgt
     aac taa aaa agt acc att agc aga caa taa aat gca tta aaa atc a 7346

B 2a. Sequences of Rat Exon 7 after FIRST stop codon.
7195 gat taa aag atc aga aga tga agg gat gaa tac ttc aga tgc ttt cag gag tga
     caa gaa cac aat gat ttt tgc tta taa tca ctt tac tta gca aat tct gta act
     aaa aaa gta cca tta gca gac aat aaa atg cat taa aaa tca   7344

B 2b.Sequences of Rat Exons 8 and 9 including stop codon at residue 74
     gca ttt tct cct atg aag tgg tac cag ggc acg gca agg cat ccg*ctt aac atg
     A   F   S   P   M   K   W   Y   Q   G   T   A   R   H   P   L   N   M
     gaa acC aca ACA gaa aaa tga
     E   T   T   T   E   K   STOP
```

Figure 2 examines the nucleotide sequences at the splice boundaries within the human AMELX gene. The principal exon boundaries are direct examples of a normal, strong exon recognition mechanism, modulated primarily by the small sizes of exons 4 and 5 coupled with the short intron sequence between exons 4 and 5. The cryptic splice sites in exon 6 are another matter. Exon 6a (Ex 6a), terminating in AG appears to be relatively easily recognized and it is most frequently cut out (yielding H151, M156, R82). Exons 6b and 6c are weaker in terms of recognition. Exon 6d alone appears in two distinct amelogenin isoforms, where exon 4 is either incorporated or skipped. However, the human protein H58 and corresponding mouse M59 isoform, also known as LRAP (Leucine-Rich Amelogenin Peptide) or [A-4], are prominent constituents of extracts from the enamel organ. The isoform constructed from exons 2-3-4-5-6d-7 (M73, [A+4]) incorporating exon 4, has been identified both as mRNA and protein in extracts from rat enamel and odontoblasts. The expression of the mouse isoforms has been the most thoroughly studied [20], and Table 1 lists the 16 mouse isoforms detected by PCR analysis. Are these many isoforms merely a consequence of the robust splicing mechanism in ameloblasts, or do some provide distinct activities?

Table 1: Mouse Amelogenin Alternative Splice Isoforms. (Adapted from Bartlett et al. (20)

Isoform Acids	Amino	Exons	Mr (D)
1	217	1-6,8-9	24648
2	203	1-3,5-6,8-9	23122
3	194	1-7	21907
4	193	1-5,6b-6d,8-9	21864
5	180	1-3,5-7	20381
6	179	1-3,5,6b-6d,8-9	20338
7	170	1-5,6b-6d-7	19123
8	156	1-3,5,6b-6d-7	17597
9	141	1-3,6b-6d-7	15753
10	96	1-5,6d,8-9	11083
11	82	1-3,5,6d,8-9	9557
12	74	1-3,5,6c-6d-7	8431
13	73	1-5,6d-7	8341
14	59	1-3,5,6d-7	6816
15	57	1-3,5,8-9	6747
16	44	1-3,6d-7	4972

Ex 1 is always expressed but is not present in the translated protein.

- Indicates continuous exons

, Indicates exon splicing

Series in green, excludes exon 7, includes ex 8 and 9

Series in black, includes exon 7, excludes ex 8 and 9

POTENTIAL ACTIVITIES AND SIGNALING FUNCTIONS OF AMELOGENIN ISOFORMS

Early studies of the role of the remnants of inner and outer epithelium cells in Hertwig's epithelial sheath led to the suggestion that ameloblast cell products including amelogenin might have a role in cementum development [21] via an inductive effect. Schonfeld and Slavkin [22] showed that enamel matrix proteins were indeed produced by these cells and were part of the amorphous cementum. The presence of the secreted enamel proteins as having functions outside the enamel organ was not readily accepted, amelogenin was considered to be produced exclusively by the ameloblast [23]. However the concept of heterotypic epithelial-mesenchymal instructive interactions leading to ectopic induction of epithelia by mesenchyme and vice-versa had taken hold. In fact, studies related to this kind of induction by cross-talk between epithelium and mesenchyme dates back further than 100 years. The first observation was noted in rabbit kidneys in which the renal vasculature had been ligated. Bone was seen to form directly below the renal pelvis mucosa [24]. Later work involved the hemisection of the kidney in dog, which revealed that bone was developing in connection with epithelial buds in the mucosa of the renal pelvis [25]. The most important work was that of Huggins *et al.* [26, 27] which demonstrated that the epithelium of the bladder contained osteogenic potential. The epithelial cells of the bladder mucosa were isolated and implanted intramuscularly with resultant bone formation. These results were quite intriguing, considering that, at that time, osteogenesis was routinely associated with cells of mesenchymal, not epithelial, origin.

Following the development of procedures to separate functional epithelium cleanly from the underlying mesenchyme [28], Kollar and Baird [29, 30, 31] showed the direct ability of recombined dental epithelia and dental mesenchyme to re-constitute developmentally functional tooth germs. Later experiments showed that at certain stages in embryonic development dental epithelium could instruct embryonic mesenchyme from other non-dental tissues to differentiate to dental mesenchyme, and vice versa. These experiments clearly confirmed the idea that tissue specific factors at specific stages in development were involved in instructive cross-communication during development but the specific nature of the factors involved was not evident.

The investigation of the osteogenic factors in bone tissue proper advanced the field of organ development with findings that demineralized bone matrix was competent to induce osteogenesis when implanted intramuscularly [32]. When demineralized bone matrix was placed into diffusion chambers and transplanted intramuscularly, bone was observed on the outer surfaces of the chambers indicating that the bone-forming factor was a diffusible non-collagenous molecule, ultimately termed "Bone Morphogenetic Protein" (BMP) [33]. Subsequently, a method for the extraction of BMP from bone matrix was established and tested for bone inductive efficacy by implantaion at non-bone sites [34]. In earlier work Zussman [35] demonstrated that odontoblasts could stimulate ectopic osteogenesis when implanted intramuscularly in rats. Rat incisor tooth pulps were isolated and transplanted to other rats. By 24 days, layers of compact bone surrounded by spongy bone were present. It was shown that the osteogenesis was induced by the odontoblastic cells themselves, not by cells that were recruited to the implant site.

In response to these data, investigations into the osteogenic potential of demineralized dentin matrix were performed. Indeed, when cell-free demineralized dentin was implanted intramuscularly into both rats and rabbits, bone was formed in contact with the dentin matrix [36]. Additional experiments used implanted demineralized enamel and dentin. The enamel implants induced a different type of bone formation. This bone formed on the enamel prism sheaths that remained following the demineralization process [37], and contained regions of cellular and acellular bone, which were highly calcified and resembled fish bones. Dentin matrix implants resulted in woven bone formation. However, in some areas there were also regions of cartilage formation. Remarkably, dentin matrix had a greater osteogenic inducing activity than bone matrix on a comparable weight basis [37].

The search for the osteogenic protein fraction in dentin was undertaken in the authors' laboratory some years later, but, based on these earlier observations noted above, was focused on the questions of osteogenic and chondrogenic activity, not on those of tooth development. This focus determined our initial approach. Rat incisor dentin was isolated and the proteins therein extracted and separated chromatographically [38]. One of these fractions was capable of inducing rat embryonic muscle fibroblasts (EMFs) to undergo a chrondrogenic transformation in an *in vitro* assay measuring the incorporation of ^{35}S into proteoglycans [39, 40]. The molecular masses of the proteins in the active fraction were determined to be in the 6-10 kDa range [41]. This study demonstrated the active fraction was capable of inducing EMFs to produce collagen type II, another sign of chondrogenesis. Refinement of the protein extraction and purification processes from rat dentin resulted in the isolation of an active protein fraction pure enough for amino acid analysis and sequencing. The active fraction had an amino acid content high in glycine, proline, glutamine and alanine residues, and the sequence obtained showed this active protein was not a member of either the BMP or TGFβ families [42].

Bovine dentin was then used to increase the yield of active fraction protein. The extraction method of Urist was followed in order to allow for isolation of any BMPs in the dentin matrix from the so-called Chondrogenic Inducing Agent (CIA). This resulted in the isolation of sufficient amounts of protein for successful amino acid sequencing [4]. The sequencing unequivocally showed that the CIA was actually a low-molecular mass segment of bovine amelogenin. This was an extremely surprising result, because amelogenin function had been ascribed solely to enamel structural formation. However, it could not be determined if it was a proteolytic degradation product of amelogenin present in dentin or a specific splice product isoform.

The origin of the amelogenin peptide identified by Nebgen *et al.* [4] was addressed in a further study. Polymerase chain reaction (PCR) primers were prepared per the protein sequences obtained by Nebgen. A rat incisor odontoblast-pulp cDNA library was probed using these primers and 2 low molecular mass amelogenin clones were isolated [5]. These clones corresponded to rat amelogenins comprising exons 2, 3, 5, 6d, 7 and exons 2, 3, 4, 5, 6d, 7 with molecular masses of 6.7 kDa and 8.1 kDa respectively. These molecular masses fell exactly into the 6-10 kDa range that had been earlier determined [41, 42]. These data established that the amelogenin peptides found by Nebgen *et al.* [4] were neither proteolytic degradation products nor a result of enamel contamination of the extract; they were specific amelogenin protein produced by the odontoblasts. The PCR data also showed that the odontoblast derived mRNAs corresponding to full length R195 and R181 amelogenins were also present, but it appeared that neither was translated into detectable levels of protein. Our focus was on the activity of the low molecular mass amelogenins in signaling, not on amelogenins per se, so we did not explore the question as to why the abundant full length amelogenin mRNAs were not translated into protein. The PCR data also showed that the [A+4] and [A-4] mRNAs were transcribed at nearly the same level in the odontoblasts, whereas the normal rat enamel organ produced much less of the proteins containing the exon 4 product. These observations probably reflect the differential activity of some tissue specific spliceosome activity-regulatory factors between odontoblasts and ameloblasts. This is a subject worthy of further study.

The two small amelogenin splice products differed only by the presence or absence of exon 4 derived protein, a hydrophilic sequence of 14 charged and polar amino acids. The 2 amelogenin clones were thus named [A-4] and [A+4]. The amelogenin isoforms were expressed recombinantly and used in the EMF chrondrogenic assay [39] with differing results. The [A-4] was more effective than the [A+4] at the same concentration, with the maximum effect seen at a concentration of 10 ng/ml or 1.5nM [5]. *In vitro* experiments assayed for chondrogenic/osteogenic marker mRNAs showed the EMFs cultured in the presence of [A+4] up-regulated the expression of Sox9, while [A-4] induced Runx2 expression [5]. Sox9 is an early marker for chondrocyte differentiation, and Runx2 is expressed in hypertrophic chondrocytes as well as being the so-called master switch gene in osteoblast differentiation [43, 44]. Biodegradable poly(lactide)-poly(glycolide) polymer matricies containing [A-4] and [A+4] were implanted intramuscularly into rats. After 28 days the [A-4] implants were diffusely mineralized over much of the implant, while the [A+4] implants had a more focal and punctuate mineralized character as shown by radiographic analysis and Von Kossa staining [5]. Hematoxlyin/Eosin and Goldner's Trichrome staining of the implants revealed the [A+4] implants contained islands of osteoid/woven bone surrounding capillary invasion of the implants to a much greater degree than those containing [A-4]. Both implants were positively stained by the osteogenic markers bone sialoprotein (BSP) and bone acidic glycoprotein-75 (BAG-75). Additional studies indicated that the effects of [A+4] and [A-4] were dependent on the developmental history of the cell types tested or on the milieu into which they were placed [45].

In retrospect, the observation that the amelogenin peptides have the ability to interact with cells of non-oral, non-neural crest origin such as embryonic muscle-derived fibroblasts and induce chondrogenesis and osteogenesis, was not germane to the function of the peptides in tooth development. However, since the amelogenin peptides were shown to be synthesized by odontoblasts, a primary question was the possibility of an autocrine-like effect of the peptides on odontoblast function. Lower first molar tooth germs from postnatal day 1 and 2 mice, were cultured in the Begue-Kirn organ culture system [46] and exposed to either of the amelogenin isoforms under serum-free conditions. Exogenous [A-4] induced the mesenchymal cells of the dental follicle to express cementum attachment protein (CAP), whereas [A+4] induced the expression of dentin matrix protein 2 (DMP2) in the odontoblast layer in the dental papilla [47]. Unfortunately, the serum-free medium did not support the development of the epithelial component of the tooth germ, while 10% fetal bovine serum (FBS) overrode the effects of the amelogenin peptides. Further experiments found that medium with 2% FBS was sufficient to sustain the development of the enamel organ. Early bell-stage embryonic (embryonic day 15, 16) mouse lower first molars were dissected and cultured *in vitro* in the presence of either [A+4] or [A-4] alone or in combination for six days. Distinct developmental effects were observed between [A+4] and [A-4]. Odontoblast differentiation was induced in the presence of [A+4] with enhanced dentin production compared to controls. The expression of a marker of odontoblast differentiation, dentin matrix protein 2 (DMP2), was increased in both differentiating odontoblasts and preameloblasts [48, 49]. The [A-4] treated tooth germs showed an unexpected result. In these tooth organs, while odontoblast development and dentin production was above that in the negative control samples, the development of the preameloblasts was inhibited and their expression of DMP2 was negligible [48, 49]. These data led to the development of a model of amelogenin signaling during the earliest stages of tooth development during which preameloblasts and preodontoblasts face each other separated by a basement membrane. The preodontoblasts begin to mature to secretory odontoblasts before the preameloblasts become secretory ameloblasts. We postulate that as the odontoblasts begin to differentiate, the autocrine secretions of [A+4] may also play a role in the further differentiation of odontoblasts while their [A-4] expression and secretion inhibits the final differentiation of preameloblasts until dentin mineralization results in the cessation of [A-4] signaling [49, 50].

Goldberg and colleagues [51-59] began a series of *in vivo* experiments in which agarose beads soaked in either [A-4] or [A-4] were implanted into rat upper molar pulps following intentional pulp exposures. In this work, [A+4] bead implantation led to the formation of a tubular dentin bridge which physiologically occluded the perforation, but the [A-4] beads induced a general mineralization of the tissue in both the pulp chamber and pulp canal [51, 53]. These results suggest the amelogenin isoforms tested could have important clinical uses in restorative dentistry as a dentin regenerating medicament ([A+4]) or in endodontic therapies as a pulp capping agent ([A+4]) or used to stimulate natural pulp canal obturation following removal of infected pulpal tissue ([A-4]). Similar experiments one week in length indicated both splice products stimulated pulp cell proliferation with [A-4] inducing osteogenic phenotype in some cells more quickly than [A+4] [55]. Amelogenin laden beads implanted into the buccal mucosa in mice had the ability to induce cellular expression of Sox9, RP59 and BSP, markers of chondro-osteodifferentiation for both [A-4] and [A+4] [57]. These studies suggest that different amelogenin splice isoforms could be used differentially in the design of systems for dentin repair and regeneration [59].

A separate line of research based on the hypothesis of amelogenin having a role in root cementum development resulted in a commercially available product composed of a mixture of porcine developing enamel matrix proteins. Enamel Matrix Derivative (EMD) has been utilized clinically for the regeneration of the periodontal attachment apparatus lost as a result of periodontal disease [60]. The effectiveness of EMD has been shown as a solo medicament in the treatment of the bone and attachment loss associated with periodontal disease, in conjunction with other treatment modalities, and with the use of titanium implants [61-66]

The hypothesis for the use of EMD was derived from evidence noted earlier suggesting that enamel associated proteins are involved in the development of acellular cementum. Acellular cementum is a noncellular ground substance through which the collagenous Sharpey's fibers of the periodontal ligament attach to the tooth. Enamel matrix proteins have been detected in the apical extension of the enamel organ inner enamel epithelium (IEE) and external enamel epithelium (EEE) known as Hertwig's epithelial root sheath [22]. More specifically, amelogenin protein was shown to be present in the developing root of human premolars [67]. Experiments showed acellular cementum was formed in root dentin defects in monkeys filled with a crude enamel matrix derived from pigs [68].

The constituent proteins of EMD include various amelogenin isoforms, the majority of which were the 20 kDa amelogenin, and also proteins with protease activity. Other proteins phenotypic for enamel matrix such as enamelin or ameloblastin were absent, as EMD was prepared in a manner to allow for the enrichment of amelogenins at the expense of the other more acidic enamel proteins [69]. EMD is, however, a heterogeneous mix whose elements have not been completely identified, making it difficult to ascribe any EMD induced effect to a particular component [70].

Somerman and colleagues have conducted extensive *in vitro* studies into the effects of full length amelogenin, the spliced form LRAP, and the amelogenin degradation product TRAP (Tyrosine Rich Amelogenin Protein) on cells implicated in cementum formation; cementoblasts and their precursor follicle cells. Full length amelogenin induced BSP expression at low concentrations, while reducing BSP at higher levels, and suppressed mineralized nodule formation by immortalized cementoblasts [71]. Similar experiments using LRAP, [A-4], or TRAP showed induced expression of OPN (osteopontin), with a reduction in OCN (osteocalcin), and mineralized nodule formation by cementoblasts [72]. Amelogenin-null mice had a decrease in BSP expression and an increase in osteoclastic activity resulting in areas of external root resorption [71]. Other *in vitro* experiments revealed amelogenin was capable of reducing the expression of the osteoclast differentiating factor RANKL (Receptor Activator of Nuclear Factor Kappa B Ligand) by osteoblasts, or upregulating the expression of osteoclast inhibiting agent OPG [72, 73, 74]. The *in vivo* application of amelogenin to reimplanted teeth resulted in an observed decrease in root resorption [75]. Full length amelogenin used in the treatment of experimentally induced periodontal disease in a dog model allowed for periodontal regeneration involving cementum, PDL and alveolar bone [76].

Snead and co-workers reported detection of LRAP expression during osteogenic differentiation of mouse embryonic stem (ES) cells. *In vitro* experiments showed LRAP treatment of WT ES cells induced BSP and osterix gene expression, and mineralized nodule formation, while LRAP was capable of improving the impaired osteogenesis observed in amelogenin knockout ES cells [77]. Additional experiments revealed the involvement of canonical Wnt signaling in mediating the observed osteogenic effects of LRAP on ES cells. LRAP stimulation of ES cells resulted in an increase in ß-catenin expression, which could be blocked with the addition of a Wnt inhibitor, sFRP-1 [78]. PCR array analysis demonstrated that LRAP was capable of increasing expression of Wnt agonists while suppressing expression of Wnt antagonists. Another report supported these results, in which *in vitro* experiments using osteoblasts and periodontal ligament cells exposed to full-length recombinant mouse amelogenin revealed amelogenin activated ß-catenin signaling. Further amelogenin reporter transgenic mice showed that amelogenin expression *in vivo* localized around the tooth root, the periodontal ligament and the alveolar bone [79].

To explore the mechanisms of amelogenin signaling, experiments using radiolabeled [A-4] determined that [A-4] bound to mouse fetal myoblast C2C12 cells in a concentration-dependent, saturable fashion. Importantly, some of the bound [A-4] was internalized [80]. Immunohistochemistry on E18 mouse tooth sections revealed specific binding of biotinylated [A-4] on developing odontoblasts, ameloblasts, stratum intermedium cells, and cells of the dental follicle lining the tooth germ. The binding of [A-4] was most intense in polarizing presecretory ameloblasts and odontoblasts and was no longer present at the point of dentin mineralization. Affinity column chromatography identified a 95 kDa protein present at the C2C12 surface which could bind [A-4]. This protein was found to be murine lysosomal-associated membrane protein 1 (LAMP1) [80]. LAMP1 and CD63/LAMP3 were determined to be full length amelogenin binding proteins using the yeast 2 hybrid system [81]. The amelogenin gene is alternatively spliced, with both full-length and M59 amelogenin isoforms sharing exon 6d. Using the yeast 2-hyrbid system, Zou *et al.* [82] identified the exon 6d amino acid region as that which binds to LAMP-1. This shared interaction domain could be an explanation for the similar effects of these two amelogenin isoforms observed by the Somerman laboratory in experiments with cementoblasts and follicle cells. Other reports noted that the uptake of full-length recombinant murine amelogenin by ameloblast-like HAT-7 cells resulted in stabilization of amelogenin mRNA leading to an increased expression, which was reduced when the amelogenin exon 6abc segment was removed from the mRNA transcript, suggesting this segment plays a role in the mRNA stabilization [83, 84]. A further report from this group extended their findings by experimentally using antibody blockade and siRNA knockdown to show LAMP3 antibody was able to block full-length amelogenin internalization, but did not reduce amelogenin-induced mRNA stabilization [85]. Notably, the induced reduction of LAMP1 activity or expression had no affect on amelogenin protein-induced amelogenin mRNA stabilization, suggesting that full length amelogenin and LRAP may transduce their effects by discrete mechanisms [85].

STRUCTURAL DIFFERENCES IN THE AMELOGENIN ISOFORMS

The highly conserved exon-encoded amino acid sequences of the amelogenins of diverse species origin [1] and their placement witin the molecule suggest that the structures of the different encoded regions might be important for the differential function of the various splice products. The signaling activity of any amelogenin isoform will begin with its proper interaction with a cognate receptor, based on its sequence which determines both secondary and tertiary structure. The exact structures of the various amelogenin isoforms remain to be solved by crystallographic methods. Renugopalakrishnan *et al.* [86] applied CD, FTIR and other physical methods to solutions of bovine amelogenin and deduced that the predicted secondary structure of the intact molecule was a mixture of ß-sheet, ß -turn and "unordered" domains. Goto et al. [87], approached this problem from a similar perspective, but isolated the principal proteins of a pig enamel extract, and identified the full length p173, a 20 kDa proteolytic fraction corresponding to residues 1-148, a 13 kDa fraction consisting of residues 46 to148 and a C-terminal fragment residues 149-173. The CD data were interpreted as indicating that the N-terminal portion, which contained the same amino acid sequence as the N-terminal part of [A-4], was probably in a ß-sheet conformation. The predicted structure of the C-terminal 25 amino acids, also shared by [A-4], was suggested to be random coil. This same group later subjected the 20 kDa fragment of porcine amelogenin to small-angle X-ray scattering (SAXS) [88]. Using computer modeling, the SAXS data and the CD data the N-terminal structure of the 20 kDa fragment was represented as a folded ß-strand with a pitch of 0.35 nm.

The inherent high percentage of the proline residues, which favors unfolded or unordered polypeptide conformation, led to the hypothesis that amelogenin belongs to a group of proteins called intrinsically disordered proteins (IDP) [89, 90, 91]. IDPs are proteins without a folded structure under physiological conditions, being enriched in proline residues [92, 93]. An intriguing characteristic of IDPs is that they may have multiple binding partners or functions due to their structurally plastic nature, and can be involved in signaling pathways [94]. The lack of innate global secondary structure could account for amelogenin having its reported roles in both enamel biomineralization and cell signaling. Interestingly, several of the SIBLING proteins involved in biomineralization of dentin and bone, BSP, OPN, DMP-2 and DMP-1, have characteristics of the flexible IDP class [95, 96]. It has been seen that IDPs can fold upon binding to their targets in a stepwise fashion named "fly-casting" based on their flexible nature [94, 97, 98]. Since LAMP1 is not known to have innate signaling ability, one possibility is that it functions by binding and restraining amelogenin in a specific structured form by which the amelogenin could subsequently bind correctly to a receptor which initiates an intracellular signaling cascade. The probability is that the high proline content and hydrophobicity of the large exon 6abc domain contributes to the strong aggregation properties of the amelogenins yielding the nanosphere structure [99, 100] so important in enamel mineral deposition, while the N- and C- terminal domains confer other properties related to their potential of signaling activities in different situations.

THE SIGNALING MECHANISMS OF THE [A-4] (LRAP, M59) ALTERNATIVELY-SPLICED, LEUCINE-RICH ISOFORM OF AMELOGENIN POLYPEPTIDE

The process of tooth development begins at specific sites marked by localized thickening of the oral ectoderm in response to expression of the proliferative growth factor Sonic Hedgehog (SHH), whose focal expression is delineated by expression of Wnt7b in the rest of the oral ectoderm (Wnt7b inhibits SHH expression) [101, 102]. Distal ectodermal expression of BMP-4 induces mesenchymal expression of Msx-1 and Msx-2 while proximal mandibular ectodermal expression induces Dlx-2 expression in the mesenchyme. These homeobox gene products demarcate fields in which single or multi-cusped teeth respectively develop [101]. These signals, and their potential origin, initiating the ectodermal signaling in early tooth development remain elusive. As the oral epithelium invaginates into the underlying mesenchyme to initiate a tooth germ, the two tissue elements are separated by a basement membrane. The epithelial cells lining the basement membrane fold into the tooth shape and become the inner enamel epithelium (IEE) of the enamel organ encasing the dental mesenchyme. The resident IEE cells become the pre-ameloblasts.

Odontogenesis is regulated at all stages by complex reciprocal paracrine and autocrine signaling communications between the IEE and the dental mesenchyme. The pre-ameloblast IEE cells become committed toward maturation to secretory ameloblasts as they respond to signals derived from the pre-odontoblasts, which in turn, enter the process of their terminal differentiation to secretory odontoblasts, possibly as instructed by signals stemming from the pre-ameloblasts. Although initial ameloblast-instructive signaling events are generated by molecules present in the predentin matrix localized at the dentino-enamel junction, the pre-ameloblasts enter the phase of terminal differentiation and start synthesis of their characteristic matrix molecules which are secreted from the developing apical Tome's process into the extracellular space abutting the mantle dentin matrix. Molecules within the predentin extracellular matrix appear to generate signals which regulate further enamel organ development. As developing pre-ameloblasts polarize and begin to secrete their own enamel extracellular matrix, molecules they synthesize and secret into that matrix generate instructive signals that may also regulate pre-odontoblast maturation. The extracellular matrix contains both structural and regulatory elements. Recently, novel signaling properties have been attributed to molecular entities integral to the structural architecture of the extracellular matrix in the connective tissue. These interactions are essential during the developmental period, as matrix-generated signaling might affect cellular fate. In particular, "outside-in" communication events between the extracellular matrix and the pre-amelobalsts are important for establishing cellular homeostasis. Hence, extracellular molecules, produced by the pre-ameloblast and deposited in the surrounding matrix, might in an autocrine fashion regulate terminal cellular differentiation to the mature, secretory phenotype.

During odontogenesis, the enamel organ undergoes several developmental stages. In the proliferation stage, pre-ameloblasts organize into stratified cell layers. Following cessation of cell division, IEE pre-ameloblasts acquire an elongated polarized phenotype and organize into the characteristic single ameloblast cell layer. Concurrently, a reversal of the ameloblasts polarity occurs and the cells acquire the secretory phenotype [103]. Cellular polarity is established through the deposition of the ameloblast extracellular matrix into a space that surrounds the cells Tome's process and abuts the dentin [104]. The secretion of amelogenin and other matrix proteins is directed toward the enamel matrix through the formation of distal junctional complexes in the ameloblasts [105]. Deposition of amelogenin into the extracellular matrix is a dynamic process that involves several developmental stages. The communication between the IEE cells and the preodontoblasts in the dental mesenchyme is limited during odontogenesis by the basement membrane acting as a diffusion barrier separating the layers and the appearance of mineralized dentin covering the predentin and its components. It is during this limited developmental time frame, between the initial breakdown of the basement membrane between preameloblasts and preodontoblasts, cessation of odontoblast cell division followed by secretory odontoblast maturation and predentin formation, and the deposition mineralized dentin which shuts off the paracrine part of the ameloblast-odontoblast regulatory communication [49].

The roles of amelogenin in the formation of the enamel has been widely examined and discussed in detail [106, 107, 108]. Amelogenin proteins are synthesized and secreted into the extracellular matrix during a well-defined period of tooth organ development, and within that time frame their expression and secretion follows both temporal and spatial patterns of regulation. In addition to the full-length structural amelogenin, several alternatively-spliced mRNA isoforms are present, prominently LRAP (109, 110). Full-length amelogenin, as well as LRAP species have been isolated and characterized in the mouse [111], rat [112] and bovine tooth organs [4, 113]. In the rat tooth organ, the expression of structural, full-length amelogenin mRNA commences immediately after birth [114]. In the developing mouse tooth organ, at post-natal day 0.5 (PN0.5) and post-natal day 1.5 (PN1.5), full length amelogenin (M180) mRNA was strongly expressed in the enamel organ, at boundaries between ameloblasts and the *stratum intermedium*, and between ameloblasts and the odontoblasts, respectively [115]. In PN0.5 and PN1.5 mouse ameloblasts and odontoblasts, cellular mRNA expression of the small, spliced isoforms of M59 ([A-4], LRAP) and M73 ([A+4], (LRAP+4)) was found to vary according to the developmental stage of the tooth organ. However, from PN0.5 to PN1.5, the expression of M59 mRNA strongly co-localized with the expression of M180 mRNA [116]. The expression of M59 mRNA demonstrated a temporal and spatial plasticity that varied according to the developmental stage of the ameloblasts. It co-localized strongly with M180 mRNA and this expression pattern suggests that M180 and M59 mRNA expression are both initiated in cells committed toward terminal differentiation.

Morphologically, perinatal pre-ameloblasts demonstrate a stratified cuboidal configuration, although cessation of cell division has already set in. As co-expression of M180 and M59 in ameloblasts was identified at the PN0.5 developmental stage, as well as in cells at the PN1.5 developmental stage, when pre-ameloblasts start to elongate and organize into a simple columnar layer, it might be inferred that M59 might play a regulatory role during the process of terminal differentiation of the ameloblasts. Interestingly, while expression of M180 mRNA persists throughout tooth development up to PN14 [116], the expression of M59 mRNA subsides at PN5, when the ameloblasts have reached their full secretory activity. This might suggest that the small, spliced isoform M59 ([A-4], (LRAP) might play a regulatory role in the acquisition of the mature ameloblast phenotype.

A better understanding of the role of [A-4] (M59, LRAP) in the development of the mouse tooth organ has been acquired from studies with transgenic animals. The enamel organ of mice expressing LRAP under the regulatory control of the amelogenin gene demonstrated an altered enamel rod pattern [117]. Furthermore, studies demonstrated that exogenous M59 (LRAP, [A-4]), administered *in vitro* to mouse molar buds, starting with the embryonic day 16 (E16) developmental stage, reduced ameloblast height, again, supporting the hypothesis that LRAP might be involved in the terminal differentiation process of ameloblasts. If the normal progression of events dictating ameloblast terminal differentiation into mature, secretory cells is altered, ensuing deposition of enamel proteins in the matrix space surrounding the ameloblasts could be impaired [118].

As noted above, during organ development the formation of connective tissues is regulated by growth factors secreted into the extracellular spaces. The growth factors become sequestered in the structural mesh of the matrix and are believed to act according to their concentration gradient. It is probable that mixtures of growth factors, rather than a single growth factor, and their overlapping fields of concentration [101] regulate the overall activity. In the tooth organ, growth factor activity leads to the induction of a series of reciprocal epithelial-mesenchymal communications events between ameloblasts and odontoblasts. These interactions between extracellular matrix molecules and the cells generate intracellular signaling events that might affect cellular fate. As M59 mRNA was found to be strongly expressed in pre-ameloblasts and the M59, [A-4] polypeptide was identified in the extracellular matrix of developing ameloblasts, it might be inferred that the pattern of [A-4] expression mirrors that of M180 mRNA and protein expression, and that the [A-4] modulates M180 gene expression and/or protein synthesis.

Several putative receptors for binding of discrete amelogenin isoforms to the ameloblast plasma membrane have been identified so far. LAMP1, a highly glycosylated trans-membrane protein, is a member of the family of Lysosomal-Associated Membrane Proteins. It is a marker for late endosomes and lysosomes, which are vesicular structures involved in the process of endocytosis. LAMP1 was identified by affinity pull-down and far-Western assays as the binding partner for the M59 ([A-4], LRAP) polypeptide in mouse myoblasts [80]. Conversely, in the yeast 2-hybrid system [81], full-length M180 protein bound to human LAMP3 (CD63) receptors [82]. *In vitro* treatment of intact tooth germs with either recombinant [A-4] (r[A-4]) or recombinant [A+4] (r[A+4]) demonstrated distinct activities in the ameloblasts and odontoblasts, in particular, pre-ameloblasts demonstrated a disorganized orientation within the cell layer, concurrent with a lack of ameloblast polarization [117]. The cell-surface binding partner for r[A-4], identified as LAMP1, was also shown to internalize bound [A-4] into fibroblasts, most probably, through the process of endocytosis [80]. Although LAMP1 demonstrates a predominantly intracytoplasmic localization pattern, alternate traffic of LAMP1 to the plasma membrane has been identified during cytokine exocytosis [119] and LAMP1 might participate in cell-mediated adhesion to the endothelium [120]. Expression of cell-surface receptors, following activation by stimulating ligands, such as growth factors, is partly regulated through the process of endocytosis of receptor-ligand complexes. The ubiquitous signaling molecule nitric oxide was shown to regulate vesicle budding at the plasma membrane and thus, affect receptor trafficking [121]. Receptor intracellular traffic and vesicular localization to distinct intracytoplasmic compartments determine whether receptors enter the pathway of degradation or are re-distributed to the plasma membrane (receptor recycling).

The biological outcome of any signaling activity is determined by the intensity and the duration of the signal, as well as by the developmental stage of the cell. The intracellular signaling cascades activated by distinct amelogenin isoforms have not been fully explored, but as described earlier; immunofluorescence studies showed that M180 amelogenin was present in tooth-related tissues such as periodontal ligament and alveolar bone cells in the mouse. In parallel, β-catenin activity was identified in these cells and attributed to the induction of the Wnt signaling pathway [78]. Additional evidence supporting the signaling properties of amelogenin has come from another set of studies with the enamel matrix preparation EMDOGAIN which showed that the enamel matrix derivative stimulates intrinsic TGFβ1 production [122]. However, the signaling cascades elicited by the alternatively-spliced, small, leucine-rich polypeptides [A-4] and [A+4] in the ameloblasts have not been extensively studied. Clearly, co-expression M180 and M59 ([A-4], LRAP)) in mouse ameloblasts, and their deposition in the enamel matrix, suggest that these two isoforms might engage in reciprocal regulation.

Evidence of the importance of transcriptional regulation of gene expression during development has come from studies addressing the temporal and spatial regulation of the myelinating protein *Plp* [122]. Similar to amelogenin, *Plp* lacks tissue-specific expression; however, a molecular switch occurs early in development, with the predominant *Plp* isoform being expressed in the central nervous system. From the developmental perspective, signaling mechanisms are also tightly regulated. One excellent example comes from the study of the regulation of the enzyme nitric oxide synthase (NOS) and its ubiquitous signaling product nitric oxide (NO), implicitly. The catalytic activity of NOS is dependent on the formation of homodimers. The oxygenase domain performs the oxidation of L-arginine, while the reductase domain facilitates the flow of electrons, which catalyze the reaction. Thus, L-arginine is converted to L-citrulline and NO [123]. The oxidative conversion of L-arginine requires one electron transfer from NADPH to the NOS oxygenase domain. The NOS homodimer also contains a calmodulin-binding unit, which regulates Ca^{2+}-mediated NOS activation. The developmental role of NOS has been examined in a *Drosophila* model of cell division in imaginal disks. As a result of the expression of a truncated isoform of the *Drosophila* NOS4 (DNOS4) protein, which is the product of the *d*NOS locus, a dominant-negative regulation of NOS (DNOS) enzymatic activity ensues, due the formation of heterodimers [124]. This results in the suppression of the antiproliferative activity of DNOS.

In mammalian cells, two isoforms of NOS are expressed constitutively: neuronal NOS (nNOS, NOS1) and endothelial NOS (eNOS, NOS3). The molecule released as a result of the enzymatic activity of eNOS was initially named the endothelium-derived relaxing factor, but later, was identified as NO [125]. Subsequent to its release, NO binds to soluble guanylate cyclase and increases cyclic guanosine-3,5'-monophosphate. NO was shown to regulate vesicle budding at the plasma membrane and thus, affect receptor trafficking [126]. The signaling properties of NO have been examined extensively. It is activated in almost every organ/system and modulates both physiologic and pathologic processes in tissues and cells: vasodilation, angiogenesis, immunity, inflammatory process, anti-tumor activity and cell death. Consequently, eNOS-induced NO release results in vasodilation. The intracellular localization of eNOS has been shown to be regulated by the signaling activity and of receptor tyrosine kinases (RTK) [127]. Specifically, the activation of RTKs induced an intracellular re-distribution of eNOS and upregulated eNOS activity, resulting in increased NO production [128, 129]. The eNOS isoform has been shown to localize mainly to the cytoplasmic surface of the Golgi apparatus, but also to both caveolae and cell junctions, indicating perhaps that distinct activating pathways regulate diverse eNOS enzymatic activities [130]. An interesting model for eNOS regulation was proposed, suggesting that eNOS-interacting proteins, *i.e.* dynamin and NOSTRIN (eNOS TRaffic INducer), mediate the co-internalization of eNOS with RTKs, but determine distinct sorting routes for subsequent delivery of eNOS to the Golgi apparatus and recycling back to the plasma membrane, or the degradation of RTK [129].

Inducible NOS (iNOS, NOS2) regulates many important cellular functions. The inducible form iNOS is activated during inflammatory processes in response to proinflammatory cytokines, *i.e.* interleukin-1 beta (IL-1β) tumor necrosis factor alpha (TNFα). Injury and trauma are other inducing factors. Activated iNOS has been associated with tumor progression and malignant transformation [132]. The iNOS isoform has been shown to inhibit cell proliferation in smooth muscle cells [133]. Through induction of matrix metalloproteinases, iNOS modulates matrix remodeling processes in the connective tissues.

The induction of iNOS activity is regulated mostly at the transcriptional level. The expression of iNOS protein is modulated at the posttranslational level through inhibition of NOS dimerization. [133]. Phosphorylation by *src* and formation of intracellular iNOS-protein complexes further regulate iNOS activity. Activated iNOS was shown to associate with CAP70, a protein expressing PDZ domains, which promoted dimerization and increased iNOS enzymatic activity. Association of iNOS with EBP50 promoted traffic of the complexed proteins to the apical pole of epithelial cells, thus, establishing directional NO release [134]. More so, PDZ domain-containing proteins, such as angiomotin, have been shown to establishing the polarity of endothelial cells through regulation of tight junction formation [135], while in macrophages, association of PDZ domain-containing proteins with iNOS was essential for the process of phagocytosis. It has been shown that in polarized cells, activation of iNOS induces NO production [136].

The authors' recent work, which examined the biological effect of [A-4], demonstrated that in developing mouse ameloblast-like cells (LS8 cells), exogenous recombinant mouse [A-4] (r[A-4]) activated iNOS and eNOS, albeit to different extents [137]. The mRNA expression of the structural, full-length isoform of amelogenin (M180) was partly regulated through the activation of iNOS in response to r[A-4]. As yet, the iNOS-activating effect of [A-4] has not been completely explored. Hence, mechanistic aspects underlying iNOS induction by exogenous r[A-4] in developing ameloblasts remain to be elucidated. One possible mechanism in developing mouse molars might involve binding of [A-4] to the ameloblast cell surface activating traffic of LAMP1-containg vesicles toward the plasma membrane, resulting in the intracellular uptake of [A-4]. Supporting evidence comes from *in vitro* studies demonstrating that r[A-4] can bind the cell surface of intact tooth germs and was shown to be internalized into mouse myofibroblasts [50]. Also, the intracellular distribution of LAMP1 was affected by exogenous r[A-4] in the ameloblast-like LS8 cells [137]. Another possible scenario implicating NO in the regulation of M180 gene expression in the mouse molar might include a requirement for the cytoplasmic re-distribution of iNOS and directional production of NO. Hence, the consequences of ameloblast stimulation by exogenous [A-4] might involve the association of activated iNOS with vesicular components near the apical pole, facilitate NO production and provide directional release of NO. This might represent an instructive signal for the cells, indicating that an apical pole has been established in the elongating ameloblasts, and it faces the space abutting dentin. This hypothesis is supported, in part, by our observations derived from *in vitro* models of mouse molar organ cultures or LS8 monolayer cultures, which show a change in the orientation and morphology of amelobasts undergoing development [50,137].

The regulatory function, exercised by r[A-4] on M180 gene expression, might be inferred from observations implicating NO in the development of cellular polarity. As yet, the iNOS-activating effect of [A-4] has not been completely explored. However, recently, we proposed a mechanism for the regulation of M180 gene expression in developing mouse ameloblasts [137]. Full-length, structural amelogenin gene expression was up-regulated *in vitro*, following exogenous r[A-4]. The modulation in M180 gene expression was partly mediated through the induction of

NOS2 and the production of NO. Whether the r[A-4]-stimulated production of NO regulates intracellular localization of LAMP1, thus enabling the uptake of exogenous r[A-4] into the LS8 ameloblast-like cells, or whether LAMP1 translocation and M180 gene expression are co-regulated by NO remains to be established. Clearly, NO production, resulting from the induction of NOS2 by r[A-4], partly modulates the initiation of M180 gene activation in developing ameloblasts. Ultimately, deposition of amelogenin into the enamel matrix initiates enamel mineral nucleation. The question of how signaling pathways affect the regulation of M180 expression and the integration of these signaling cascades into the signaling network of the ameloblasts still remains to be elucidated.

CONCLUDING REMARKS

The amelogenin gene in all species is very similar, with an essentially common pattern of exons and introns, and with more DNA sequence in the introns than in the exons of the primary gene transcript. Cutting out the introns to obtain the mRNA that will be translated to functional protein involves splicing mechanisms common to all eucaryotes, thus, differences in splicing patterns of the amelogenins in animals may relate to the tissue specific activity of proteins regulating splicing, rather than to differences in the main spliceosome proteins that interact with the exon or intron boundary sequences. Thus, for example, some species or some tissues regularly express exon 4, whereas others delete this exon. In the human, rat and bovine, AMEL exon 4 is not present in the amelogenin mRNA of the IEE, yet in the odontoblasts of those animals, exon 4 mRNA can be detected during early developmental stages. The small isoform, M59 (LRAP, [A-4]) was detected early on and many studies have suggested that it has important roles in tooth development. As indicated in our studies and the extensive works of Hammerstrom on EMDOGAIN, the LRAP-enriched amelogenin derivative, has a number of biological activities, and, as shown by Goldberg and colleagues, the individual peptides, in the form of recombinant M59, r[A-4] and M73, r[A+4], have different functions in dentin repair in *in vivo* implants. The recent findings, noted above, that amelogenin protein can be found in systems as diverse as brain tissue and bone tissue indicate that the information instructive for the transcription of genomic AMEL DNA, its conversion to AMEL mRNA and ultimately translation to one or more of the AMEL isoforms, can be activated in non-tooth tissues.

In addition to the very beautiful work on the role of the full-length amelogenin in structuring the enamel mineral, it is clear that comparable in depth studies of the factors controlling expression of AMEL genes in non-dental tissues need to be explored, while the mechanisms by which the individual small isoforms interact with cells in either paracrine or autocrine fashion is also a fertile field for further study, with relevance for tooth development, as well as broader aspects of tooth repair and wound healing in general.

ACKNOWLEDGEMENT

All of the work of the authors reported in this chapter has been supported by NIH - NIDCR Grants DE-01374 & DE-08525 to AV.

REFERENCES

[1] Sire J-Y, Delgado S, Girondot M. The amelogenin story: origin and evolution. Eur J Oral Sci 2006; 114 (Suppl 1):64-77.
[2] Black DL, Mechanisms of alternative pre-messenger RNA splicing. Annu Rev Biochem 2003; 72:291-336.
[3] Berget SM. Exon recognition in vertebrate splicing. J Biol Chem. 1995; 270:2411-14.
[4] Nebgen DR, Inoue H, Sabsay B, *et al.* Identification of the chondrogenic inducing activity from bovine dentin (bCIA) as a low molecular mass amelogenin polypeptide. J Dent Res 1999; 78:1484-94.
[5] Veis A., Tompkins K, Alvares K, *et al.* Specific amelogenin gene splice products have signaling effects on cells in culture and in implants in vivo. J Biol Chem 2000; 275: 41263-72.
[6] Oida S, Nagano T, Yamakoshi Y, *et al.* Amelogenin gene expression in porcine odontoblasts. J Dent Res 2002; 81:103-8.
[7] Gruenbaum-Cohen Y, Tucker AS, Haze A, *et al.* Amelogenin in cranio-facial development: The tooth as a model to study the role of amelogenin during embryogenesis. J Exp Zool (Mol Dev Evol) 2009; 312B:445-57.
[8] Shimizu T, Tanabe T, Fukae M. Proteolytic enzyme in porcine immature enamel. J Dent Res 1979; 8:782-9.

[9] Termine JD, Belcourt AB, Christner PJ, *et al.* Properties of Dissociatively Extracted Fetal Tooth matrix Proteins **I.** Principal molecular species in developing bovine enamel J. Biol. Chem. 1980; 255: 9760-8.

[10] Shimokawa H, Sobel ME, Sasaki M, *et al.* Heterogeneity of amelogenin mRNA in bovine tooth germ. J Biol Chem 1987; 262:4042-7.

[11] Gibson C, Golub E, Herolr R, *et al.* Structure and expression of the bovine amelogenin gene. Biochemistry 1991; 30:1075-9.

[12] Gibson CW, Golub E, Ding W, *et al.* Identification of the leucine-rich amelogenin peptide (LRAP) as the translation product of an alternatively spliced transcript. Biochem Biophys Res Commun 1991; 174:1306-12.

[13] Lay BC, Simmer JP, Bringas P, *et al.* Alternative splicing of the mouse amelogenin primary RNA transcript contributes to amelogenin heterogeieity. Biochem Biophys Res Commun 1992; 188:1253-60.

[14] Simmer JP, Hu CC, Lau BC, *et al.* Alternative splicing of the mouse amelogenin primary RNA transcript. Calcif Tissue Int 1994; 55: 302-10.

[15] Salido BC, Yen PH, Koprivnikar K, *et al.* The human enamel protein gene amelogenin is expressed from both the X and Y chromosomes. Am J Hum Genet 1992; 50:303-16.

[16] DenBesten PK, Li RS. Characterization of amelogenin from secretory- and maturation stage rat incisor enamel. Arch Oral Biol 1992; 37:1097-100.

[17] Li R, Li W, and DenBesten PK. Alternative Splicing of amelogenin mRNA from rat incisor ameloblasts. J. Dent Res 1995; 74:1880-5.

[18] Li W, Mathews C, Gao C, *et al.* Identification of two additional exons at the 3' end of the amelogenin gene.; Arch Oral Biol 1998; 43: 497-504.

[19] Papagerakis P, Ibarra JM, Inozentseva N, *et al.* Mouse amelogenin exons 8 and 9: sequence analysis and protein distribution. J Dent Res 2005; 84(7):613-617.

[20] Bartlett JD, Ball RL, Tye CE, *et al.* Origin, Splicing, and expression of rodent amelogenin Exon 8. J. Dent Res 2006; 85: 894-9.

[21] Grant D.and Bernick S. Morphodifferentiation and Structure of Hertwig's Root sheath in the cat. J Dent Res 1971; 50(6):1580-8.

[22] Schonfeld SE, Slavkin HC. Demonstration of enamel matrix proteins on root-analogue surfaces of rabbit permanent incisor teeth. Calcif Tissue Res 1977; 24:223-9.

[23] Eastoe JE. Enamel protein chemistry- past, present and future. J Dent Res 1979; 58: 753-63.

[24] Sacerodotti C, Frattin G. Factors of osteogenesis and the secretory function of transitional epithelium. Arch Path Anat u Physiol u Klin Med 1902; 168:431-43.

[25] Pearce RM. Notes on the later stages of the repair of kidney tissue (dog) with special reference to the proliferation of the pelvic epithelium and heteroplastic bone formation. J Med Res 1909; 20 (111): 53-65.

[26] Huggins CB. Influence of Urinary Tract Mucosa on the Experimental Formation of Bone. Arch Surg 1931; 22: 377

[27] Huggins CB, Mccarroll HR and Dahlberg AA. Transplantation of tooth germ elements and the experimental heterotypic formation of dentin and enamel. J. Exp. Med. 1934; 60:199-210.

[28] Rawles ME. Tissue unteractions in scale and feather development as studied in dermal-epidermal recombinations. J Embryol Exp Morphol 1963; 11:765-789.

[29] Kollar EJ and Baird GR. The influence of the dental papilla on the development of tooth shape in embryonic mouse tooth germs. J Embryol Exp Morphol 1968; 21:131-48.

[30] Kollar EJ and Baird GR. Tissue interactions in embryonic mouse tooth germs. I. Reorganization of the dental epithelium during tooth germ reconstruction. J Embryol Exp Morphol 1970; 24:159-71.

[31] Kollar EJ and Baird GR. Tissue interactions in embryonic mouse tooth germs. II. The inductive role of the dental papilla. J Embryol Exp Morphol 1970; 24:173-86.

[32] Urist MR. Bone: formation by autoinduction. Science 1965; 150:893-9.

[33] Urist MR, Granstein R, Nogami H, *et al.* Transmembrane bone morphogenesis across multiple-walled diffusion chambers: New evidence for a diffusible bone morphogenetic property. Arch Surg 1977; 112:612-9.

[34] Urist MR, Chang JJ, Lietze A, *et al.* Preparation and bioassay of bone morphogenetic protein and polypeptide fragments. Methods Enzymol 1987; 146:294-312.

[35] Zussman WV. Osteogenic activity of odontoblasts in transplanted tooth pulps. J Dent Res 1966; 45:144-51.

[36] Bang G, Urist M R. Bone induction in excavation chambers in matrix of decalcified dentin. Arch Surg 1967; 94:781-9.

[37] Urist MR Bone histogenesis and morphogenesis in implants of demineralized enamel and dentin. J Oral Surg. 1971; (2):88-102.
[38] Tsay T-G, Veis A. The Preparation, Detection and Characterization of an Antibody to Rat α-Phosphophoryn. Biochemistry 1985; 24: 6363-9.
[39] Koskinen KP, Kanwar YS, Sires B *et al.* An Electron Microscopic Demonstration of Induction of Chondrogenesis in Neo-natal Rat Muscle Outgrowth Cells in Monolayer Cultures. Connect Tissue Res 1985; 14:141-58.
[40] Veis A, Sires B, and Clohisy J. A search for the osteogenic factor in dentin. Rat incisor dentin contains a factor stimulating rat muscle cells in vitro to incorporate sulfate into altered proteoglycan. Connect Tissue Res 1989; 23:37-44.
[41] Veis A., Sires B, Clohisy J,. *et al.* Rat incisor dentin contains a factor which alters the phenotypic expression and stimulates chondrogenesis in fibroblast-like cells in Vitro. Biomaterials 1990; 11:16-8.
[42] Amar S, Sires B, Sabsay B, *et al.* The Isolation and partial characterization of a rat incisor dentin matrix polypeptide with in vitro chondrogenic activity. J. Biol. Chem. 1991; 266:8609-18.
[43] Bi W, Deng JM, Zhang Z, *et al.* Sox9 is required for cartilage formation. Nat Genet 1999; 22:85-9.
[44] Ducy P, Zhang R, Geoffroy V, *et al.* Osf2/Cbfa1: a transcriptional activator of osteoblast differentiation. Cell 1997; 89:747-754.
[45] Veis A, Tompkins K, Goldberg M. Amelogenin peptides have unique milieu-dependent roles in morphogenic path determination. Proceedings of a Conference: "The Many Faces of Osteoarthritis". June 2001. V. Hascall and H. Reddi, Eds. Birkhäuser Verlag, Basel, Switzerland, 2002; pp 101-5.
[46] Begue-Kirn C, Smith AJ, Ruch JV, *et al.* Effects of dentin proteins, transforming growth factor beta 1 (TGF beta 1) and bone morphogenetic protein 2 (BMP2) on the differentiation of odontoblast in vitro. Int J Dev Biol 1992; 36:491-503.
[47] Tompkins K. Veis A. Polypeptides translated from alternatively spliced transcripts of the amelogenin gene, devoid of the exon 6a,b,c region, have specific effects on tooth germ development in culture. Connect Tissue Res 2002; 43:224-31.
[48] Tompkins K, Veis A. Small amelogenin splice products have different effects on tooth germ differentiation in vitro International Association for Dental Research, San Diego: USA 2002
[49] Veis A. Amelogenin gene splice products: potential signaling molecules. CMLS, Cell Mol Life Sci 2003; 60: 38-55.
[50] Tompkins K, Alvares K, George A, *et al.* Two related low molecular mass polypeptide isoforms of amelogenin have distinct activities in mouse tooth germ differentiation in vitro. J Bone Miner Res 2005; 20:341-9.
[51] Six M, Goldberg M, LasFargues J-J, *et al.* Effet de Molécules Ostéogéniques sur la Minéralization Pulpaire. Les Cahiers de L'ADF 2002 ; 5:12-7.
[52] Six N, Tompkins K, Lasfarges J-J, *et al.* Bioengineering of Reparative Dentin and Pulp Mineralization, In: Proceedings of the International Conference on Dentin/Pulp Complex 2001. Ishikawa T, Takahashi K, Maeda T, Suda H, Shimono M, Inoue T, Eds.) Quintessence Publishing Co., Chicago, 2002; p 52-9.
[53] Goldberg M, Six N, Decup F, *et al.* Bioactive molecules and the future of pulp therapy. American Journal of Dentistry 2003; 16: 66-76.
[54] Six N, Tompkins K, Septier D, *et al.* Recruitment and characterization of the cells involved in reparative dentin formation in the exposed rat molar pulp after implantation of the amelogenin gene splice products A+4 and A-4. Oral Biosci Med 2004; 1: 35-44.
[55] Lacerda-Pinheiro S, Jegat N, Septier D, *et al.* Early in vivo and in vitro effects of amelogenin gene splice products on pulp cells. Eur J Oral Sci 2006; 114 (Suppl 1): 232-238.
[56] Goldberg M, Lacerda-Pinheiro S, Jegat N, *et al.* The impact of bioactive molecules to stimulate tooth repair and regeneration as part of restorative dentistry. Dent Clin North Am. 2006; 50(2):277-98.
[57] Lacerda-Pinheiro S, Septier D, Tompkins K, *et al.* Amelogenin gene splice products A+4 and A-4 implanted in soft tissue determine the reorientation of CD45-positive cells to an osteo-chrondrogenic lineage. J Biomed Materials Res. Part A. 2006; 79(4):1015-22.
[58] Jegat N, Septier D, Veis A, *et al.* Short-term effects of amelogenin gene splice products A+4 and A-4 implanted in the exposed rat molar pulp. Head and Face Medicine 2007; 3: 40.
[59] Goldberg M , Lacerda-Pinheiro S, Priam F, *et al.* Matricellular molecules and odontoblast progenitors as tools for dentin repair and regeneration. Clinical Oral Investigations 2008; 12: 109-12.

[60] Heijl L, Heden G, Svärdström G, *et al.* Enamel matrix derivative (EMDOGAIN) in the treatment of intrabony periodontal defects. J Clin Periodontol. 1997; S;24(9 Pt 2):705-14.
[61] Jepsen S, Heinz B, Jepsen K, *et al.* A randomized clinical trial comparing enamel matrix derivative and membrane treatment of buccal Class II furcation involvement in mandibular molars. Part 1: Study design and results for primary outcomes. J Periodontol 2004; 75:1150-60.
[62] Sculean A, Donos N, Schwarz F, *et al.* Five-year results following treatment of intrabony defects with enamel matrix proteins and guided tissue regeneration. J Clin Periodontol 2004; 31:545-9.
[63] Schwarz F, Rothamel D, Herten M, *et al.* Effect of enamel matrix protein derivative on the attachment, proliferation, and viability of human SaOs(2) osteoblasts on titanium implants. Clin Oral Investig 2004; 8:165-71.
[64] Crea A, Dassatti L, Hoffmann O, *et al.* Treatment of intrabony defects using guided tissue regeneration or enamel matrix derivative: a 3-year prospective randomized clinical study. J Periodontol . 2008; 79(12):2281-9.
[65] Sculean A, Kiss A, Miliauskaite A, *et al.* Ten-year results following treatment of intra-bony defects with enamel matrix proteins and guided tissue regeneration. J Periodontol 2008; 79(10):1991-9.
[66] Sculean A, Windisch P, Szendröi-Kiss D, *et al.* Clinical and histologic evaluation of an enamel matrix derivative combined with a biphasic calcium phosphate for the treatment of human intrabony periodontal defects. J Clin Periodontol 2008; 35(9):817-24.
[67] Hammarström L. Enamel matrix, cementum development and regeneration. J Clin Periodontol 1997; 24(9 Pt 2):669-677
[68] Hammarström L, Heijl L, Gestrelius S. Periodontal regeneration in a buccal dehiscence model in monkeys after application of enamel matrix proteins. J Clin Periodontol 1997; 24(9 Pt 2):669-77
[69] Gestrelius S, Andersson C, Johansson AC, *et al.* Formulation of enamel matrix derivative for surface coating. Kinetics and cell colonization. J Clin Periodontol. 1997; 24(9 Pt 2):678-84
[70] Maycock J, Wood SR, Brookes SJ, *et al.* Characterization of a porcine amelogenin preparation, EMDOGAIN, a biological treatment for periodontal disease. Connect Tissue Res 2002; 43:472-6.
[71] Viswanathan HL, Berry JE, Foster BL, *et al.* Amelogenin: a potential regulator of cementum-associated genes. J Periodontol 2003; 74(10):1423-31.
[72] Boabaid, F., Gibson, C. W., Kuehl, M. A., *et al.* Leucine-rich amelogenin peptide: a candidate signaling molecule during cementogenesis. J Periodontol 2004; 75:1126-36.
[73] Hatakeyama J, Philp D, Hatakeyama Y, *et al.* Amelogenin-mediated regulation of osteoclastogenesis, and periodontal cell proliferation and migration. J Dent Res. 2006; 85(2):144-9.
[74] Nishiguchi M, Yuasa K, Saito K, *et al.* Amelogenin is a negative regulator of osteoclastogenesis via downregulation of RANKL, M-CSF and fibronectin expression in osteoblasts. Arch Oral Biol. 2007; 52(3):237-43.
[75] Yagi Y, Suda N, Yamakoshi Y, *et al.* In vivo application of amelogenin suppresses root reorption J Dent Res. 2009; 88(2):176-181.
[76] Haze A, Taylor AL, Haegewald S, *et al.* Regeneration of bone and periodontal ligament induced by Recombinant amelogenin after periodontitis. J Cell Mol Med. 2009 Feb 17. [Epub ahead of print].
[77] Warotayanont R, Zhu D, Snead ML, *et al.* Leucine-rich amelogenin peptide induces osteogenesis in mouse embryonic cells. Biochem Biophys Res Commun 2008; 367(1):1-6.
[78] Warotayanont R, Frenkel B, Snead ML, *et al.* Leucine-rich amelogenin peptide induces osteogenesis by activation of the Wnt pathway. Biochem Biophys Res Commun 2009; 387(3):558-63.
[79] Matsuzawa M, Sheu TJ, Lee YJ, *et al.* Putative signaling action of amelogenin utilizes the Wnt/beta-catenin pathway. J Periodontal Res 2009; 44(3):289-96.
[80] Tompkins K, George A, Veis A. Characterization of a mouse amelogenin [A-4]/M59 cell surfaced receptor. Bone 2006; 38:172-80.
[81] Wang HJ, Tannukit S, Shapiro JL, *et al.* Using the yeast two-hybrid assay to discover protein partners for for the leucine-rich amelogenin peptide (LRAP) and for tuftelin-interacting protein 11 (TFIP11). Eur J Oral Sci 2006; 114 Suppl1:276-9
[82] Zou Y, Wang H, Shapiro JL, *et al.* Determination of protein regions responsible for interactions of amelogenin with CD63 and LAMP1 Biochem J 2007; 408(3):347-54.
[83] Xu L, Harada H, Yokahama-Tamaki T, *et al.* Reuptake of extracellular amelogenin by dental epithelial cells results in increased levels of amelogenin mRNA through enhanced mRNA stabilization. J Biol Chem 2006; 281(4):2257-62.

[84] Xu L, Harada H, Taniguchi A. The exon 6ABC region of amelogenin mRNA contribute to increased levels of amelogenin mRNA through amelogenin protein-enhanced mRNA stabilization. J Biol Chem 2006;281(43):32439-44

[85] Xu L, Harada H, Taniguchi A. The Effects of LAMP1 and LAMP3 on M180 amelogenenin uptake, localization and amelogenin mRNA induction by amelogenin protein. J Biochem 2008; 144(4):531-37.

[86] Renugopalakrishnan V, Strawich ES, Horowitz PM, *et al.* Studies of the Secondary Structures of Amelogenin from Bovine Tooth Enamel. Biochemistry, 1986; 25:4879-4887.

[87] Goto Y, Kogure E, Takagi T, *et al.* Molecular conformation of porcine amelogenin in solution: three folding units at the N-terminal, central, and C-terminal regions. J Biochem 1993; 113:55-60.

[88] Matsushima N, Izumi Y, Aoba T. Small-angle X-ray scattering and computer-aided molecular modeling studies of 20 kDa fragment of porcine amelogenin: does amelogenin adopt an elongated bundle structure? J Biochem. 1998; 123:150-6.

[89] Lakshminarayanan R, Fan D, Du C, *et al.* The role of secondary structure in the entropically driven amelogenin self-assembly. Biophys J 2007; 93(10):3664-74

[90] Lakshminarayanan R, Yoon I, Hegde BG, *et al.* Analysis of secondary structure and self-assembly of amelogenin by variable temperature circular dichroism and isothermal titration calorimetry. Proteins 2009; 76(3):560-9.

[91] Delak K, Harcup C, Lakshminarayanan R, *et al.* The Tooth Enamel Protein, Porcine Amelogenin, Is an Intrinsically Disordered Protein with an Extended Molecular Conformation in the Monomeric Form. Biochemistry 2009; 48(10):2272-81.

[92] Tompa P. Intrinsically unstructured proteins. Trends Biochem Sci, 2002; 27(10):527-33.

[93] Dunker AK, Silman I, Uversky VN, *et al.* Function and structure of inherently disordered proteins. Curr Opin Struct Biol 2008; 18(6):756-64.

[94] Wright PE, Dyson HJ. Linking folding and binding. Curr Opin Struct Biol 2009; 19(1):31-8.

[95] Fisher LW, Torchia DA, Fohr B, *et al.* Flexible structures of SIBLING proteins, bone sialoprotein, and osteopontin. Biochem Biophys Res Commun 2001; 280(2):460-5.

[96] Uversky VN. Natively unfolded proteins: a point where biology waits for physics. Protein Sci 2002; 11(4):739-56.

[97] Wright PE, Dyson HJ. Intrinsically unstructured proteins: re-assessing the protein structure function paradigm J Mol Biol 1999; 293(2):321-31.

[98] Smock RG, Gierasch LM. Sending signals dynamically. Science 2009; 354(5924):198-203.

[99] Lakshminarayanan R, Yoon I, Hegde BG, *et al.* Analysis of secondary structure and self-assembly of amelogenin by variable temperature circular dichroism and isothermal titration calorimetry. Proteins. 2009; 76(3):560-9.

[100] Du C, Falini G, Fermani S, *et al.* Supramolecular assembly of amelogenin nanospheres into birefringent microribbons. Science. 2005; 307(5714):1450-4.

[101] Sharpe PT. Homeobox genes and orofacial development. Connect Tissue Res 1995 32: 17-25.

[102] Cobourne MT, Sharpe PT. Tooth and jaw: molecular mechanisms of patterning in the first branchial arch. Arch Oral Biol. 2003; 48(1):1-14.

[103] Smith CE, Nanci A. Overview of morphological changes in enamel organ cells associated with major events in amelogenesis. Int J Dev Biol 1995 39: 153-61.

[104] Smith CE. Cellular and chemical events during enamel maturation. Crit Rev Oral Biol Med 1998; 9:128-61.

[105] Sasaki T, Takagi M, Yanagisawa T. Structure and function of secretory ameloblasts in enamel formation. Ciba Found Symp 1997; 205: 32-46 (discussion: 46-50).

[106] Brookes SJ, Robinson C, Kirkham J, *et al.* Biochemistry and molecular biology of amelogenin proteins of developing dental enamel. Arch Oral Biol 1995; 40(1): 1-14.

[107] Fincham A.G., Moradian-Oldak J. Recent advances in amelogenin biochemistry. Connect Tissue Res 1995; 32(1-4): 119-24.

[108] Moradian-Oldak J. Amelogenin assembly, processing, and control of crystal morphology. Matrix Biol. 2001; 20: 293-306.

[109] Lau EC, Simmer JP, Bringas P Jr, *et al.* Alternative splicing of the mouse amelogenin primary RNA transcript contributes to amelogenin heterogeneity. Biochem Biophys Res Comm 1992; 188(3): 1253-60.

[110] Hu CC, Ryu QQ, Qian Q, *et al.* Cloning, characterization and heterologous expression of exon-4-containing amelogenin mRNAs. J Dental Res 1997; 76(2): 641-7.

[111] Fincham AG, Hu Y, Lau EC, *et al.* Amelogenin post-secretory processing during biomineralization in the postnatal mouse molar tooth. Arch Oral Biol 1991; 36(4): 305-17.

[112] Nishikawa S., Takagi T., Sasa S. Immunocytochemical localization of amelogenin in rat incisor ameloblasts using ultrathin frozen sections. J Elec Microsc 1990; 39(5): 404-7.

[113] Gibson CW, Kucich U, Collier P, *et al.* Analysis of amelogenin proteins using monospecific antibodies to defined sequences. Connect Tissue Res. 1995; 32: 109-14.

[114] Wurtz T, Lundmark C, Christersson C, *et al.* Expression of amelogenin mRNA sequences during the development of rat molars. J Bone Min Res 1996; 125-131.

[115] Iacob S., Veis A. Identification of temporal and spatial expression patterns of amelogenin isoforms during mouse molar development. Eur J Oral Sci 2006; 114(S1): 194-200.

[116] Hu J.C-C., Sun X., Zhang C., *et al.* A comparison of enamelin and amelogenin expression in developing mouse molars. Eur J. Oral Sci 2001; 109: 125-32.

[117] Gibson CW, Li Y, Daly B, *et al.* The leucine-rich amelogenin peptide alters the amelogenin null enamel phenotype. Cells Tiss Org 2009; 189: 169-74.

[118] Ravindranath RM, Devarajan A, Bringas P Jr. Enamel formation *in vitro* in mouse molar explants exposed to amelogenin polypeptides ATMP and LRAP on enamel development. Arch Oral Biol 2007; 52: 1161-71.

[119] Andrei C, Dazzi C, Lotti L, *et al.* The secretory route of the leaderless protein interleukin 1 ß involves exocytosis of endolysosome-related vesicles. Mol Biol Cell 1999; 110: 1463-75.

[120] Kannan K, Stewart RM, Bounds W, *et al.* Lysosome-associated membrane proteins h-LAMP1 (CD107a) and h-LAMP2 (CD107b) are activation-dependent cell surface glycoproteins in human peripheral blood mononuclear cells which mediate cell adhesion to vascular endothelium. Cell Immunol 1996; 171: 10-9.

[121] Kawase T, Okuda K, Momose M, *et al.* Enamel matrix derivative (EMDOGAIN) rapidly stimulates phosphorylation of the MAP kinase family and nuclear accumulation of smad2 in both oral epithelial and fibroblastic human cells. J Periodont Res 2001; 36: 367-76.

[122] Wight PA, Dobretsova A. Where, when and how much: regulation of myelin proteolipid protein gene expression. Cell Mol Life Sci 2004; 61: 810-21.

[123] Moncada S, Higgs A. The L-arginine-nitric oxide pathway. N Engl J Med 1993; 329: 2002-12.

[124] Stasiv Y, Kuzin B, Regulski M, *et al.* Regulation of multimers via truncated isoforms: a novel mechanism to control nitric-oxide signaling. Genes Dev 2004; 18: 1812-1823.

[125] Ignarro IJ, Buga GM, Wood KS, *et al.* Endothelium-derived relaxing factor produced and released from artery and vein is nitric oxide. PNAS USA 1987; 84: 9265-9.

[126] Wang G, Moniri NH, Ozawa K, *et al.* Nitric oxide regulates endocytosis by S-nitrosylation of dynamin. PNAS USA 2006; 103(5): 1295-1390.

[127] Mukherjee S, Tessema M, Wandinger-Ness A. Vesicular trafficking of tyrosine kinase receptors and associated proteins in the regulation of signaling and vascular function. Circ. Res. 2006; 98(6): 743-56.

[128] Thuringer D, Maulon L, Frelin C. Rapid transactivation of the vascular endothelial growth factor receptor KDK/Flk-1 by the bradykinin B2 receptor contributes to endothelial nitric-oxide synthase activation in cardiac capillary endothelial cells. J Biol Chem 2002; 277: 2028-32.

[129] Kondo T, Kobayashi K, Murohara T. Nitric oxide signaling during myocardial angiogenesis. Mol Cell Biochem 2004; 264: 25-34.

[130] Gratton JP, Bernatchez P, Sessa WC. Caveolae and caveolins in the cardiovascular system. Circ Res 2004; 94: 1408-17.

[131] Tatemichi M, Ogura T, Nagata H, *et al.* Enhanced expression of inducible nitric oxide synthase in chronic gastritis with intestinal metaplasia. J Clin Gastroent 1998; 27: 240-5.

[132] Stein CS, Fabry Z, Murphy S, *et al.* Involvement of nitric oxide in IFN-□-mediated reduction of microvessel smooth muscle cell proliferation. Mol Immun 1995; 32: 965-73.

[133] Kolodziejski PJ, Koo S, Eissa NT. Regulation of inducible nitric oxide synthase by rapid cellular turnover and cotranslational down-regulation by dimerization inhibitors. PNAS USA 2004; 101(52): 18141-6.

[134] Navarro-Lerida I., Martinez-Morenao M., Ventoso I., *et al.* Binding of CAP70 to inducible nitric oxide synthase and implications for the vectorial; release of nitric oxide in polarized cells. Mol. Biol. Cell 2007; 18(7): 2768-77.

[135] Bratt A., Birot O., Sinha I., *et al.* Angiomotin regulates endothelial cell-cell junctions and cell motility. J Biol Chem 2005; 280(41): 34859-69.

[136] Rumbo M, Courjault-Gautier F, Sierro F, *et al.* Polarized distribution of inducible nitric oxide synthase regulates activity in intestinal epithelial cells. FEBS J 2005; 272(2): 444-53.
[137] Iacob S, Veis A. Identification of the functional activity of the [A-4] amelogenin gene splice product in newborn mouse ameloblasts. Bone 2008; 42(6): 1072-9.

CHAPTER 13

Amelogenin Exons 8 and 9

Wu Li[1], Jean Yves-Sire[2], Yoshiro Takano[3], Mary MacDougall[4], Michel Goldberg[5] and Pamela DenBesten[1] *

[1]Department of Orofacial Sciences, University of California at San Francisco, PO 0422, San Francisco, CA 94143-0422, USA; [2]UMR 7138, Université Pierre et Marie Curie, Quai Saint-Bernard, 75005 Paris, France; [3]Department of Hard Tissue Engineering, Tokyo Medical and Dental University Graduate School, 1-5-45, Yushima, Bunkyo-ku, Tokyo 113-8549 Japan; [4]Institute of Oral Health Research, University of Alabama, SDB 702, 1530 3rd Ave. S. Birmingham, AL 35294-0007 and [5]Laboratoire Différenciation de Cellules Souches et Prions, U747, Université Paris Descartes, rue des Saints Pères, 75006 Paris, France.

Abstract: Exons 8 and 9 are two novel exons found in several transcripts of rodent amelogenin gene. These transcripts result from alternative splicing, in which exon 7 is replaced by exons 8 and 9, and they add a unique 3' terminus to amelogenin isoforms. Therefore, the alternatively spliced amelogenins end either at exon 7, encoding a single aspartic acid, or at exons 8 and 9, coding for 14 amino acids. So far, a total of seven alternatively spliced amelogenin mRNAs ending at exons 8 and 9 have been identified in rodents. The formation of these two exons results from a duplication of a DNA region containing exon 5, followed by its translocation dowstream exon 7. This event occurred during evolution of the rodent lineage at a period that postdates the divergence of the squirrel lineage, around 50 millions years ago. Therefore, exon 8 is homolog to exon 5. The amelogenins carrying the region encoded by exons 8 and 9 locate not only in ameloblasts and the enamel matrix but also in odontoblasts and dentin. The replacement of exon 7 by exons 8 and 9 leads to an additional hydrophilic domain, the function of which is not known, but may in part be related to the uniquely different rod and interrod structure seen in rodent enamel as compared to human enamel. The function of the amelogenins with exons 8 and 9 terminal peptides has been preliminarily investigated. They were found to enhance the proliferation of mesenchymal cells.

Key Words: Tooth Enamel, Amelogenin, mRNA Alternative Splicing, Novel Exons

INTRODUCTION

The mature enamel matrix is made up of more than 95% mineral [1-3], formed in a self-assembled protein matrix secreted by a layer of epithelially derived ameloblasts [5]. In the early developing enamel, the matrix is over 80% organic, comprised primarily of amelogenins, which are known to modulate enamel crystal growth [6-8]. Amelogenins are hydrophobic proteins that contain high concentrations of proline, glutamine, leucine and histidine, and a single phosphorylation at serine 16 [9, 10]. They are alternatively spliced from a single gene, resulting in heterogeneous combinations of different sized amelogenin proteins and peptides in the matrix [11-18]. The alternatively spliced isoforms for mouse [15, 16], rat [18], bovine [14] and human [13] amelogenins have shown remarkable similarity, suggesting that the alternatively spliced amelogenins have a long evolutionary story and an important role in enamel formation.

Amelogenins are transcribed from a single gene on the X chromosome (mouse and rat) [20] or from two genes on the X and Y chromosomes (human and bovine) [13, 14, 21-23]. The pro-mRNA isolated from mice was initially reported to contain seven exons [11, 21], and the predominant splice isoforms were reported as lacking exon 4. This exon is absent in non-mammalian amelogenins and was created early in mammalian evolution, which means that the ancestral amelogenin was composed of six exons (see chapter 1 of this book). Splice patterns include deletion of the small exons (exons 3, 4 and 5) and a reduction in the size of exon 6 by internal splicing [11, 20]. Amelogenins synthesized by these alternatively spliced mRNAs can be categorized into high molecular weight amelogenins, derived from mRNAs spliced with an intact exon 6 or most of the exon 6, and low molecular weight amelogenins with most or all exon 6 spliced out.

Michel Goldberg (ED)

In 1995, our group used a modified PCR strategy to amplify the 5' and 3' ends of mRNA of amelogenins from rat ameloblasts and discovered a unique 3' terminus in several amelogenin spliced mRNAs [17]. We determined that this unique end was derived from 2 additional exons, 8 and 9 [24].

DISCOVERY OF AMELOGENIN EXONS 8 AND 9

Rapid amplification of 5' and 3' complimentary DNA ends (5' and 3' RACE) was used to identify rat amelogenin sequences [17]. The advantage of RACE is that this method is highly sensitive for the transcripts at low quantity. Following amplification by RACE, individual PCR products were dissected from agarose separating gels and cloned for sequencing. Surprising to us at that time was that in addition to several transcripts identical to alternatively spliced patterns reported previously in the mouse and other species, we also found a novel sequence at the 3' termini of splice fragments, which replaced the original exon 7. Exon 7 has 155 nucleotides, including a short coding sequence of only 6 nucleotides in length, which code for a single aspartic acid and a stop codon, followed by a non-coding region. The newly identified 3' end included 156 nucleotides, coding for 19 amino acids. At that time, rodent genome databases were not available, so to determine whether this unique end was a result of alternative splicing, we designed primers to amplify potential intron regions. A forward primer located in the non-coding region of exon 7 and several reverse primers derived from the unique 3' terminal sequence were used for long PCR amplification of mouse and rat genomic DNA [24]. The results showed that this unique sequence included two exons, which we then named exons 8 and 9 (Figure 1).

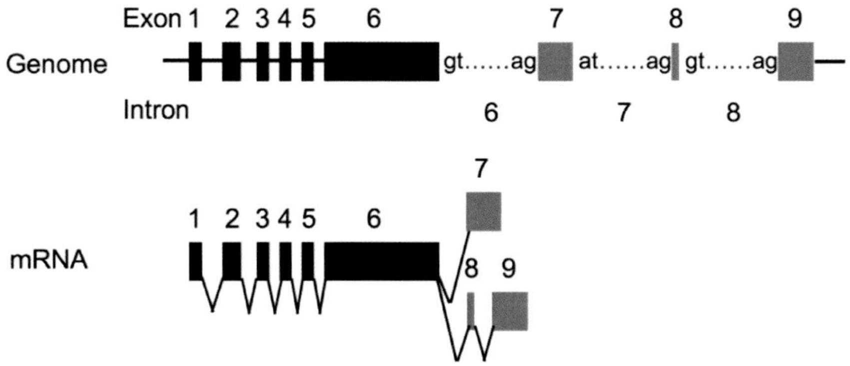

Figure 1: Alternative 3' ends of amelogenins with either exon 7 or exons 8 and 9. The upper picture shows the structure of exons and introns of rat (or mouse) genomic amelogenin. The introns between exons 6 and 7, exons 6 and 8, and exons 8 and 9 follow the rule of "GU-AG", while the sequence between exons 7 and 8 does not. Splicing will either exclude intron 6 to end with exon 7 or splice out intron 6, exon 7 and intron 8, to form a terminal mRNA sequence consisting of exons 8 and 9 (lower picture).

Exons 8 and 9 have 45 and 111 base pairs (bp), coding 15 and 9 residues and a stop codon, respectively. These two exons are separated by a 2 kb intron in the genomic sequence. They replace exon 7 at the 3' end of amelogenin. Therefore, amelogenin has two different C termini, coded by either exon 7 or by exons 8 and 9. The sequence between exon 7 and exon 8 is a 1.5 kb sequence. This sequence is not identified as an intron, as the boundary nucleotides in the sequence between exons 7 and 8 do not follow the splicing rule of "GU-AG" of 5' donor site and 3' acceptor site of typical introns. When exon 7 is not transcribed, the region between exons 6 and 8 is considered as intron 6. However, there is no doubt that the DNA sequence between exons 8 and 9 is spliced, resulting in mRNA sequences containing these exons [24].

As shown in figure 2, the alternatively spliced products with the alternate 3' sequence (derived from exons 8 and 9) show the same splicing patterns as those previously found in mouse transcripts ending in exon 7. We identified four of these alternatively spliced sequences in our 3' RACE studies of rat amelogenin [17, 24] and later another three alternatively spliced patterns were identified in mice [25]. So far seven alternatively spliced fragments containing exons 8 and 9 in rodents have been reported. It is interesting that a splicing pattern with a completely spliced-out exon 6 (R57) was found only in the transcripts carrying exons 8 and 9.

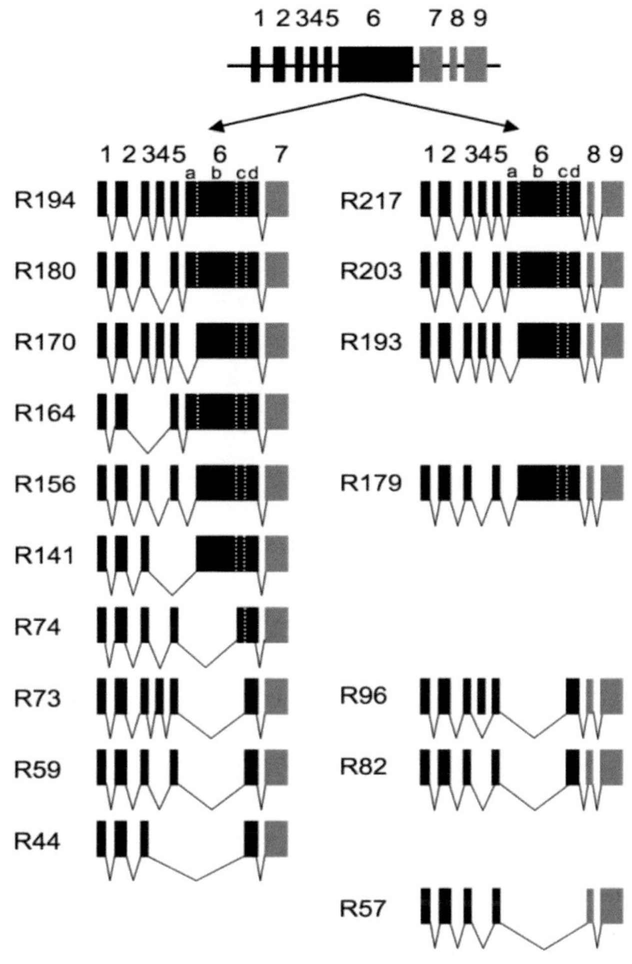

Figure 2: Amelogenin alternative splicing patterns in rodents. Internal spliced fragments of exon 6 are indicated by a, b, c and d. R57 has the entire exon 6 spliced out. Each splicing pattern is named by R (indicating rodents, mice or rats) followed by the numbers of amino acids without signal peptides. The number 1-9 above the splicing patterns indicates the corresponding exons.

It is interesting to notice that exons 8 and 9 always co-exist with both exons 3 and 5. Exon 8 is highly similar to exon 5 and part of the sequence upstream exon 8 is highly homologous to exon 4, indicating that this region, including exon 8, results from a duplication of the exon 4-exon 5 region and its translocation downstream exon 7 [25]. This translocation may also trigger the activation of its downstream sequence, resulting in the expression of exon 9[25]. It is unusual that duplicated exons such as exons 8 and 5 co-exist in the same isoforms as this would duplicate the function of the encoded amino acid sequence. In general, they are alternatively spliced. Considering the high conservation of these isoforms between species and their existence for millions of years, this duplication should be useful and functional in tooth enamel development.

CHARACTERISTICS OF AMELOGENIN EXONS 8 AND 9

Amelogenins are hydrophobic proteins, consisting of many neutral and uncharged residues, and have an extremely hydrophilic C termini. Among the 24 last amino acids at the C terminal ending with exon 7, there are eight charged residues, including four glutamic acids, two aspartic acids, two lysines and one arginine. The C terminal ending with exons 8 and 9 adds an extra relatively hydrophilic end to amelogenin and its alternatively spliced proteins. In the 24 residue short peptide encoded by exons 8 and 9, there are six charged amino acids containing two lysines, two aspartic acids, one arginine and one histidine. These residues change the hydrophobicity of the alternatively spliced amelogenins as shown in the hydrophobicity plots in figure 3.

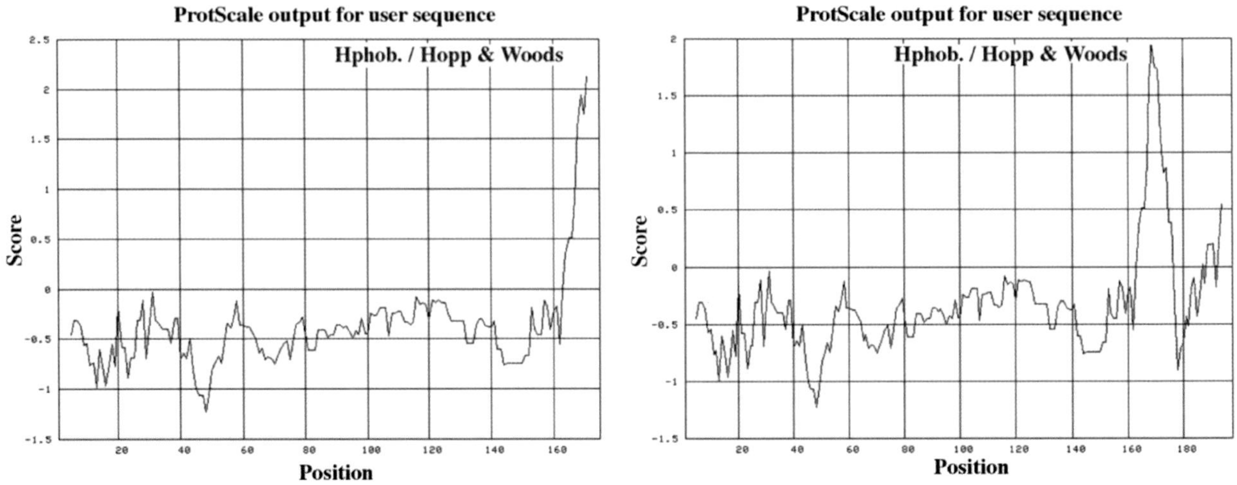

Figure 3: Hydrophobicity analysis of amelogenins with exon 7 (left, R180) and with exons 8 and 9 (right, R203) by Hopp and Woods scale using an online software Protscale in Expasy website (http://ca.expasy.org). Note the extra hydrophilic tail resulted from exons 8 and 9 after the original hydrophilic peak in right panel.

The effects of this change in hydrophobicity on amelogenin function and self-assembly are not clear. However, it is interesting that the structure of rodent enamel is uniquely different by its extreme prism decussation and characteristic division of two distinct layers [26-30] as compared to human. The unique structure of rodent enamel has lead us to speculate that structural changes in amelogenins, related to the presence of alternatively spliced amelogenins ending in exons 8 and 9, could have a role in altering the enamel structure.

Amelogenin assembly in an aqueous environment results in the C terminal ends forming a hydrophilic shell outside of the hydrophobic core[31, 32]. This hydrophilic outer layer is important for amelogenin interactions with inorganic mineral crystal hydroxyapatite and organic components such as other enamel matrix proteins and proteinases. The addition of the extra hydrophilic domain at the amelogenin C termini encoded by exons 8 and 9 decreases the hydrophobicity of the proteins and also changes their PI to relatively more neutral as compared to the amelogenins with exon 7 (Table. 1).

Table 1: Structures, base pairs, molecular weights (Mr) and PIs of amelogenins with exon 7 or exons 8 and 9.

Amelogenins with exon 7					Amelogenins with exons 8 and 9				
Name	**Exons (w/signal peptide)**	**Base pairs**	**Mr (Da)**	**PI**	**Name**	**Exons (w/signal peptide)**	**Base pairs**	**Mr (Da)**	**PI**
R194	1-7	582	21816	6.72	R217	1-6. 8-9	651	24554	7.32
R180	1-3, 5-6, 7	540	20292	6.51	R203	1-3, 5-6, 8-9	609	23031	6.95
R170	1-5, 6b-6d, 7	510	19033	6.89	R193	1-5, 6b-6d, 8-9	579	21771	8.18
R164	1-2. 5-6, 7	492	18569	6.65					
R156	1-3, 5, 6b-6d, 7	468	17509	6.62	R179	1-3, 5, 6b-6d, 8-9	537	20247	7.26
R141	1-3, 6b-6d, 7,	423	15667	6.27					
R75	1-3, 5, 6c-6d, 7	222	8482	5.16	R98	1-3, 5, 6c-6d, 8-9	288	11220	6.72
R73	1-5, 6d, 7	219	8262	6.05					
R59	1-3, 5, 6d, 7	177	6739	5.16	R82	1-3, 5, 6d, 8-9	246	9477	6.72
R44	1-3, 6d, 7	132	4897	4.59					
					R57	1-3, 5, 8-9	171	6665	9.22

The estimated mass and isoelectric points for alternatively spliced amelogenins with either exon 7 or exons 8 and 9 are summarized in Table 1. The addition of exon 8 and 9 coded sequences at the 3' ends of amelogenins increases both molecular weight and the isoelectric point (PI) of the proteins from alternatively spliced RNAs.

IDENTIFICATION OF EXONS 8 AND 9, AND THEIR ORIGIN AND EVOLUTION

Following our identification of amelogenin exons 8 and 9 in rats [17, 24], Takano and co-workers [19] subsequently demonstrated their presence in ameloblasts using *in situ* hybridization and localized the encoded proteins in the rat enamel matrix by immunohistochemistry.

MacDougall's group [4] then identified exon 8 and 9 containing transcripts in a mouse tooth cDNA library and cDNA from an enamel organ epithelial (MEOE-3M) cell line. They used forward primers derived from mouse amelogenin sequences located in either exon 2 or exon 5 and a reverse primer located in exon 9 of the rat amelogenin sequence for PCR amplification. They found two major amplicons containing exons 8 and 9 at sizes of approximately 350-bp and 750-bp in the mRNA samples extracted from newborn and four-day-old Swiss mouse mandible. The length of mouse amelogenin encoded by exons 8 and 9 is 24 amino acids, identical to that of rat. They also performed immunocytochemical staining using the antibody against the exon 9 peptide sequence, which further confirmed the existence of these unique exons in mouse dental mesenchyme. The sequences are highly conserved between mouse and rat, with only 11 nucleotide differences, showing 93% identity (Figure 4). Three residues, Met, Thr and Ser, were found to differ from the sequence of mouse amelogenin exons 8 and 9, as compared to the rat.

Our group analyzed cDNA extracted from human fetal primary incisors using a forward primer located at exon 8 and reverse primer located in exon 9 [24]. Though a 2 kb amplicon could be detected in mouse gDNA, PCR products of exons 8 and 9 from human gDNA samples could not be amplified. Furthermore, we used a P^{32} labeled oligonucleotide probe to detect exons 8 and 9 in EcoR I digested mouse and human gDNA. A 4.2 kb band and a 4.7 kb band were detected from both mouse and human gDNA samples. However, although intensive *in silico* searches were performed in the National Center of Biotechnology Information database (http://www.ncbi.nlm.nih.gov/) no similar sequences of exons 8 and 9 could be identified in the downstream region of human amelogenin exon 7, indicating that exons 8 and 9 may be unique in rodent enamel formation. In retrospect, it was likely that the positive southern blots in our previous report [24] were in fact recognizing exon 5, which has high similarity with exon 8.

This sequence similarity between exon 5 and 8 was found by Bartlett et al., using a BLASTN alignment against mouse genome [25]. A 3907 bp sequence from downstream of exon 7 to the end of exon 9 of mouse amelogenin gene had an extra Blast hit in addition to the query sequence, and had 91% (191/209) homology to another region of the mouse amelogenin X chromosome. The highly homologous sequence contained exons 4 and 5. Exon 4 was aligned with a downstream sequence of exon 7 showing an identical sequence, which was referred to as exon 4b. Exon 5 is highly homologous to exon 8 with only seven amino acids difference. This seven amino acid difference arises from just eight different nucleotides. This interesting discovery suggests that exon 8 was generated from exon 5 by the duplication of a 200- to 300-bp segment, containing exons 4 and 5 in the amelogenin X chromosome, translocated downstream exon 7. Furthermore, Bartlett and co-workers[25] speculate that expression of the downstream exon 9 is activated by the translocation of this segment. They did not identify these unique exons 8 and 9 in human and bovine amelogenin gDNA sequences downstream exon 7 and concluded that the duplication occurred in an ancestral rodent.

Using *in silico* analyses we provide new data on the evolutionary story of these unique exons in mammals. We have explored the amelogenin gDNA region (10 kb) downstream exon 7 in 26 species representatives of the main mammalian lineages in order to find exons 8 and 9. The results can be summarized as follows: Exon 8 was not identified in primates (5 amelogenin sequences analyzed), tree shrew (1), leurasiatherians (10), afrotherians (3), marsupials (1) and monotremes (1), but was only found in rodents (Figure 4). Out of the six rodent sequences screened in the study, only squirrel amelogenin lacked exon 8.

```
   exon 4                              exon 5
 Mouse          agAAGTCACATTCTCAGGCTATCAATACTGACAGGACTGCATTAgt...agGTGCTTACCCCTTTGAAGTGGTA

 exon 4b                               exon 8
 Mouse          agAAGTCACATTCTCAGGCTATCAATACTGACAGGACTGCATTAgt...agGCGTTTTCTCCTATGAAGTGGTA
 Rat            agAACTCACACTCTCAGGCTATCAATACTGACAGGACTGCATTAgt...agGCATTTTCTCCTATGAAGTGGTA
 Deer mouse     agAAGTCACATTCTCAGGCTATCAATACTGACAGGACTGCATTAgt...agGTGTTTTCTCCTAAGAAGTGGTA
 Kangaroo rat   agAACTCACAGTCTCAGATTGTCACTACTGACAGAACTGTTTTAat...agGTGGTTGCCCCTACAAAGTGGTA
 Guinea pig     agAAGTCACATATTCAGGCTATCAATATTGACAGGACTACATTAgt...agGTGCATACTCCTTTGAAGTGGTA
                  ## #####   #### #  ### ## ###### ###   ###       #    # # ###   ########

 exon 5
 Mouse          CCAGAGCATGATAAGGCAGCCGgt

 exon 8                                 exon 9
 Mouse          CCAGGGCATGACAAGGCATCCGgt...agCTTAACATGGAAAGCACAACAGAAAAATGATTCCAACCACTCTCC
 Rat            CCAGGGCACGGCAAGGCATCCGgt...agCTTAACATGGAAACCACAACAGAAAAATGATT-CAACCACTCTCC
 Deer mouse     CCAGAGCATGACAAGGCATCCGgt...agCTTAACATGGAAAGCACACCAGAAAAATGATTTCAACCTGTCTCC
 Kangaroo rat   CCAGAACATGCTAAGGCAGCCGgt...ggATTAATATAGGAACCACATGGAAAACATGATTTCAACCAAG-TCC
 Guinea pig     CCAGAAT---GCAAGGCAGCAGgt...agCTTAATTTAGGGAATTAGAACAGAAAAACAGT--AA--AATTTC
                ####        ###### # #        ####  # #  #             ## #  # #  ##      # #

 exon 9
 Mouse          TACCTTCCCAGAACATAA-TGGCATGTAGTAGTGTTCAATATTGCCTT-AATAAAATTCTCATCGGCTTA
 Rat            TACCCTTGCAGAACACAA-TGGCATGTAGTAGTATTCAATATTGCTTT-AATAAAATCTCACTGGCTTA
 Deer mouse     TACCTTTCCAGAACATAA-TGGCATGTAGTAGTGTTCAATATTGCTTT-AATAAAATTCTCATCGGCTTA
 Kangaroo rat   TATAT---CAGAATAGAGGTGGCATATAGTAATGTCCAG-AT-GTT---AATAAAGATA--ATCGGCTGT
 Guinea pig     TACATTTCTTGGACATAGCAGG-ATCTAGTAGTATTTCACATTGTCTTCACTAAA-TACTCATCAACCTA
                ##          # # # #   ## ## ##### # #      ## #      # ####        #    #

 exon 4         exon 5
 Mouse          KSHSQAINTDRTAL VLTPLKWYQSMIRQP

 exon 4b        exon 8       exon 9
 Mouse          KSHSQAINTDRTAL AFSPMKWYQGMTRHP LNMESTTEK*
 Rat            NSHSQAINTDRTAL AFSPMKWYQGTARHP LNMETTTEK*
 Deer mouse     KSHSQAINTDRTAL VFSPKKWYQSMTRHP LNMESTPEK*
 Kangaroo rat   NSQSQIVTTDRTVL VVAPTKWYQNMLRQP INIGTTWKT*
 Guinea pig     KSHIQAINIDRTTL VHTPLKWYQN-ARQQ LNLGN*
                 #  #    #### #    # ####  #    #
```

Figrue 4: Alignment of the nucleotide (top) and protein (bottom) sequences of five rodent amelogenin exons 4b, 8 and 9 found in the gDNA using *in silico* approaches (NCBI database). Mouse amelogenin sequences of exons 4 and 5 are copied on top of the alignments in order to show the high conservation of the derived exons 4b and 8. Note that the exon 4b has not been found as an exon in the currently known amelogenin transcripts.

In kangaroo rat amelogenin, the intronic splice acceptor site downstream exon 4b and the splice donor site upstream exon 9 are not correct which suggests this amelogenin region is not coding. In guinea pig, the signal of polyadenylation (squared) is located 100 bp downstream. # indicates unchanged positions. (-) were inserted for a correct alignment.

Deer mouse = Peromyscus maniculatus; Kangaroo rat: Dipodomys ordii; Guinea pig = Cavia porcellus; Squirrel = Spermophilus tridecemlineatus.

We confirm that exon 8 arose from a duplication of an amelogenin gDNA segment containing exons 4 and 5, followed by a translocation of the copy downstream of exon 7. Exon 8 is the copy of exon 5. Exon 4, duplicated and translocated upstream in the same segment as exon 5, is clearly identified upstream exon 8 [25]. The alignment of the two regions (original with exons 4 and 5 and the copy with exons 4b and 8) from the five rodent amelogenins reveals that the duplicated segment comprised approximately 900 bp: including circa 350 bp of intron 3, exon 4 (42 bp), intron 4 (96), exon 5 (45), intron 5 (269), and beginning of exon 6 (100) (Figure 4).

Exon 9 was identified in all rodent amelogenins possessing exons 4b and 8. However, in many mammalian amelogenins, a similar region with high percentage of nucleotide identity was also identified in the 10 kb gDNA explored downstream exon 7 (e.g., 78% in human, 81% in dog, 82% in bovine amelogenin). Most of these homologous regions possess a correct splice donor site at their 5' side and a polyadenylation signal at the right place. We have currently no reason to claim that this region is a coding exon as no alternative spliced transcripts including this region was reported in non-rodent mammalian amelogenins. Moreover in some sequences the splice donor site is mutated. We believe that this region, which is highly conserved for an unknown reason yet, was a good target to become exon 9 when the duplicated segment was translocated downstream exon 7.

The detailed analysis of the five rodent sequences possessing exons 4b, 8 and 9 reveals that exon 4b is extremely well conserved in all amelogenins (Figure 4). It is therefore surprising that previous studies have not identified this exon in some transcripts because such a high conservation during tens of millions years should indicate a functional importance. If not, the only explanation is an error in genome assembly provoked by the presence of similar sequence related to the segment duplication. Sequencing this region of gDNA would answer the question of the origin of exon 4b.

Our analysis also points to wrong intronic splice sites in the kangaroo rat sequence, and in particular the splice donor site upstream exon 9, which suggests that this region is no longer coding (Figure 4). In guinea pig exon 9, the stop codon is located after five codons instead of nine in the other sequences, and the polyadenylation signal is mutated. However, another polyadenylation signal is located downstream (not shown).

To summarize this evolutionary analysis, the duplication event that led to the creation of exon 8 and the recruitment of exon 9 occurred in an ancestral rodent, after the divergence of the squirrel lineage, around 50 millions years ago (Figure 5).

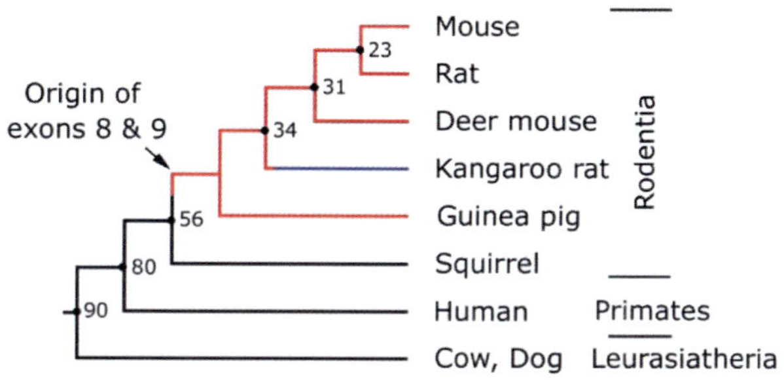

Figure 5: Schematical rodent phylogeny with the location of the duplication event that led to the creation of amelogenin exon 8. The gDNA segment containing amelogenin exon 4 and 5 was duplicated in an ancestral rodent, after the squirrel-related lineage diverged around 50 million years ago. These exons were conserved during evolution of this group (red lines) and are still present in mouse-related and caviomorph species. However, it seems that this coding sequence was invalidated in kangaroo rat (blue line). Exon 8 was neither found functional nor invalidated in Primates and Leurasiatheria. Numbers at the nodes refer to estimated times of divergence.

Divergence times from Adkins et al. [33] and Huchon et al. [34]; Rodent phylogeny simplified from Blanga-Kanfi et al.[35].

Fifty millions years is a relatively short time (at the geological level) but this is a long enough period for accumulating mutations at random, except when the region is subjected to functional constraints. These exons were most likely conserved in most subsequent rodent lineages because they have functional importance. However, it seems that this region is probably no longer useful in kangaroo rat. Two questions remain to be answered: is the duplicated exon 4b a coding exon or an artifact of genome assembly? What is the meaning of the homologous region of exon 9 in non-rodent mammalian amelogenins?

DISTRIBUTION AND EXPRESSION OF EXONS 8 AND 9 IN RODENT TEETH

The distribution of exons 8 and 9 has been studied by several investigators [4, 19, 24]. Immunohistochemical staining using an antibody against an exon 9-coded 12-mer peptide (including three residues at N terminal from exon 8), shows strong staining in enamel matrix, ameloblasts and papillary layer [19]. In the cells of the papillary layer, staining is primarily in the nuclear region, while staining in the ameloblasts is cytoplasmic, located in the distal portion of the cell near the enamel matrix. Within undifferentiated inner enamel epithelium of developing mouse tissues, little or no immunohistochemical staining of amelogenins containing exons 8 and 9 coded peptide is observed (Figure 6) [19].

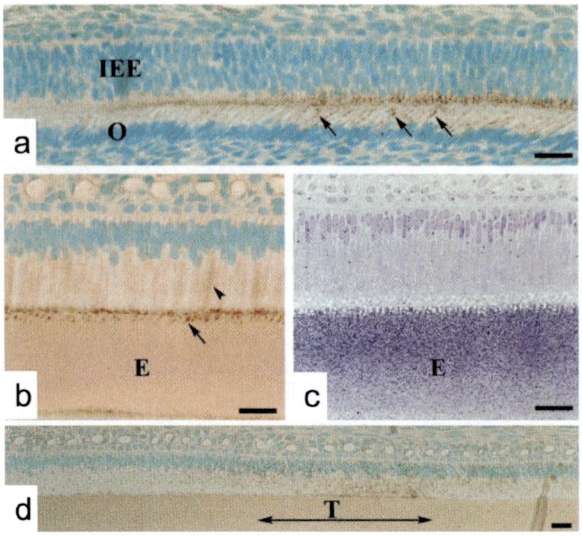

Figure 6: Immunostaining of amelogenin exons 8 and 9 coded proteins. a) The target proteins are located in the distal ends of inner enamel epithelium (IEE). Extracellular immunoreactions (arrows) are also detected in the preodontoblasts. b) The exons 8 and 9 coded proteins are found in secretory ameloblasts with moderate staining in the supranuclear and Golgi regions (arrowhead) and intense reactions in the Tome's process regions at the distal cell end (arrow). Enamel matrix is lightly stained and showed a biphasic pattern. c) Immunostaining of exons 8 and 9 coded proteins in GMA section. The whole thickness of secretory enamel layers is evenly stained with the antibody. No significant reaction is seen in the cytoplasm of ameloblasts. d) Immunostaining of exons 8 and 9 coded proteins in longitudinal sections of a rat incisor from late secretory to early maturation stages. Arrow indicates incisal direction. The granular immunoreactions were shown in the intercellular regions of ameloblasts at the transitional stage (T). O, odontoblasts; E, enamel matrix; Bars = 20 µm. (Baba et al. [19] with permission).

Amelogenins ending with peptides coded by exon 9 are immunolocalized in a pattern similar to that of other amelogenins ending with exon 7, expressed in pre-ameloblasts, differentiated ameloblasts and post-secretory ameloblasts, but not in maturation stage ameloblasts. Stratum intermedium cell staining is also observed. The similarity of the localization patterns of immunoreactions using these two antibodies indicates the co-synthesis, co-secretion and co-existence of the amelogenin with or without exons 8 and 9 coded proteins and their possible co-function (Figure 6) [19].

Intracellularly, in the rat incisor, immunoreactions for the amelogenins ending with exons 8 and 9 coded sequence can be first identified in the distal cytoplasm as well as distal intercellular spaces of the cells of the inner enamel epithelium or in early presecretory ameloblasts. The cytoplasmic reactions are stronger in the more incisally located preameloblasts, where supranuclear cytoplasm (Golgi regions) began to show some immunoreactivity. The Golgi regions in the tall secretory ameloblasts throughout the secretory stage is moderately stained and the Tome's processes inserting in the newly formed enamel matrix show clear immunoreactions to exons 8 and 9, confirming the secretion of the amelogenins carrying these two exons coded ends. Towards the end of the secretory stage, the reactions at the distal cytoplasm of ameloblasts gradually diminishes and finally disappears by the end of the transitional stage (Figure 6) [19].

The enamel matrix is stained in both rat and mouse. When a thin layer of enamel starts to form immediately after the formation of a distinct layer of mineralized dentin, strong reactions for the amelogenin exons 8 and 9 coded protein are observed. The positive staining shows a biphasic pattern as the strong positive signals are shown predominantly at dentinoenamel junction and the area close to the ameloblast cell layer (Figure 6 and 7) [4, 19].

A possible explanation for this biphasic distribution is due to the poor antibody penetration resulted from the effects of paraffin embedding on the immature enamel matrix [36]. The immunoreactivity of the remaining enamel matrix gradually intensifies until the late maturation stage, when the entire matrix disappears during sample decalcification processing. The existence of amelogenin exons 8 and 9 coded proteins was further confirmed by Western blot studies [4, 19].

Immunohistochemical analysis of mouse incisors showed similar positive immunostaining of the ameloblasts and developing enamel matrix as compared to those of the rat (see Figure 7) [4]. Further analyses showed immunohistochemical localization of exon 8 and 9 coded peptides in both odontoblasts and dentin matrix. Extracellular immuno-reactions are observed in the fibrous matrix of future mantle dentin. Amelogenin exon 8 and 9 coded proteins are strongly and clearly immunolocalized in young odontoblasts but not in preodontoblasts and mature odontoblasts. When using the mouse MO6-G3 odontoblast cell lines, clear granule-like positive strainings are observed in the cytoplasm of these immobilized cells. These findings indicate the possible functional role of the amelogenin isoforms including exons 8 and 9 encoded regions in early dentin development (Figure 7) [4].

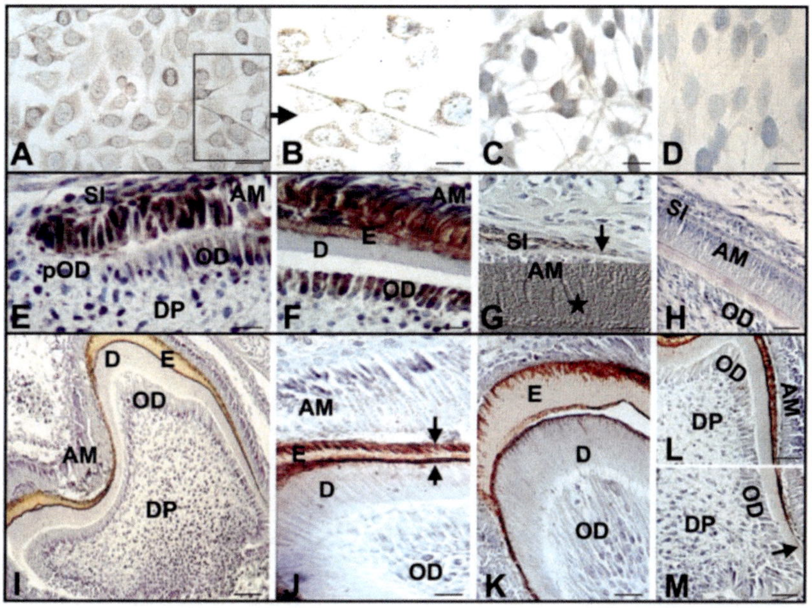

Figure 7: Immunohistochemistry of the mouse dental cell lines with amelogenin exons 9 antibody. Panels A and B show low (A) and high (B) magnification of ameloblast cells MEOE-3M. Panel C shows low magnification of odontoblast cells MO6-G3. Panel D shows negative control in MO6-G3 cells. Bars: 62.5 μm (A); 31.25 μm (C); 15.625 μm (B, D). Immunohistochemistry of mouse developing tooth organs showed the developmental pattern of amelogenin exons 8 and 9 encoded peptide. Panels E-G show positive staining within the ameloblast (AM), odontoblasts (OD), and stratum intermedium cells (SI). Pre-odontoblasts (pOD; panel E) and mature odontoblasts (panels I-M) were devoid of staining. SI staining was down-regulated (panel G, black arrow) concomitant with the maturation stage of ameloblasts (G). Note the high expression of amelogenin in secretory ameloblasts (F), in contrast to the negative expression in maturation ameloblasts (I-M). Panels I-M show intense biphasic positive staining in the enamel (E). Enamel staining is mainly observed near the dentinoenamel junction and in the newly formed matrix (panel J, black arrows). Enamel staining is clearly diminished near the cementoenamel junction (M; black arrow). No staining was seen within the dentin (D) or dental pulp cells (DP). Bars: 62.5 μm (I); 25 μm (H,L,M); 15.625 μm (E-G); 12.5 μm (J, K). Panel H shows negative control after primary antibody omission. (Papagerakis et al. [4] with permission).

RELATIVE AMOUNTS OF AMELOGENIN EXONS 8 AND 9 CODED PROTEINS

Quantitative PCR analyses of amelogenins ending in exon 7 as compared to those ending with exons 8 and 9 were done by Barlett et al. [25] using total RNA from first molars extracted from mice at different developing stages, including secretory stage (days 3 and 5), secretory-early maturation stage (day 7) and maturation stages (days 9 and 11). The expression of both types of amelogenin transcripts (with exon 7 or with exons 8 and 9) decreased from secretory to maturation stage. As compared to the expression level of amelogenin with exon 7, the expression of amelogenins containing exons 8 and 9 were five-fold-lower in these developmental stages [25].

THE POSSIBLE FUNCTIONAL ROLES OF EXONS 8 AND 9 CODED AMELOGENINS

In preliminary studies we have used cells from the dentin pulp complex to explore possible differences in cell signaling by low molecular weight amelogenins, specifically leucine rich amelogenin peptides (LRAP) with and without exons 8 and 9 coded sequences. These studies have shown that LRAP ending with exons 8 and 9

(LRAP+89) enhanced the dental pulp cell proliferations *in vivo* and *in vitro* as did LRAP alone. Furthermore, *in vivo* data showed that LRAP+89 enhanced dentin formation following a direct pulp exposure. Neither of the full-length amelogenin plus exons 8 and 9 nor peptide exons 8 and 9 alone showed any effects on cell proliferation *in vitro*. The mechanisms and long-term effects of these molecules are still in investigation.

In summary, alternatively spliced rodent amelogenins have two different 3' termini, which end either at exon 7 with a single amino acid (aspartic acid) or at exons 8 and 9 (24 residues), resulting from alternative splicing of RNA. A total of seven alternatively spliced amelogenins ending at exons 8 and 9 have been identified in rodents. The formation of these two exons is the result of a duplication of the DNA region containing exons 4 and 5, and its translocation downstream exon 7. This event occurred during evolution of the rodent lineage at a period that postdates the divergence of the squirrel lineage, around 50 millions years ago. The replacement of exon 7 by exons 8 and 9 results in an additional hydrophilic domain, which may in part be related to the uniquely different rod and interrod structure seen in rodent enamel as compared to human enamel.

REFERENCES

[1] Fincham AG, Simmer JP. Amelogenin proteins of developing dental enamel. Ciba Found Symp 1997; 205: 118-30; discussion 30-4.
[2] Fincham AG, Moradian-Oldak J, Simmer JP. The structural biology of the developing dental enamel matrix. J Struct Biol 1999; 126(3): 270-99.
[3] Robinson C, Brookes SJ, Shore RC, *et al.* The developing enamel matrix: nature and function. Eur J Oral Sci 1998; 106 Suppl 1: 282-91.
[4] Papagerakis P, Ibarra JM, Inozentseva N, *et al.* Mouse amelogenin exons 8 and 9: sequence analysis and protein distribution. J Dent Res 2005; 84(7): 613-7.
[5] Moradian-Oldak J. Amelogenins: assembly, processing and control of crystal morphology. Matrix Biol 2001; 20(5-6): 293-305.
[6] Robinson C, Brookes SJ, Kirkham J, *et al.* Crystal growth in dental enamel: the role of amelogenins and albumin. Adv Dent Res 1996; 10(2): 173-9; discussion 9-80.
[7] Beniash E, Simmer JP, Margolis HC. The effect of recombinant mouse amelogenins on the formation and organization of hydroxyapatite crystals in vitro. J Struct Biol 2005; 149(2): 182-90.
[8] Margolis HC, Beniash E, Fowler CE. Role of macromolecular assembly of enamel matrix proteins in enamel formation. J Dent Res 2006; 85(9): 775-93.
[9] Fincham AG, Moradian-Oldak J. Amelogenin post-translational modifications: carboxy-terminal processing and the phosphorylation of bovine and porcine "TRAP" and "LRAP" amelogenins. Biochem Biophys Res Comm 1993; 197(1): 248-55.
[10] Fincham AG, Moradian-Oldak J, Sarte PE. Mass-spectrographic analysis of a porcine amelogenin identifies a single phosphorylated locus. Calcif Tissue Int 1994; 55(5): 398-400.
[11] Simmer JP. Alternative splicing of amelogenins. Connect Tissue Res 1995; 32(1-4): 131-6.
[12] Gibson CW, Golub E, Ding WD, *et al.* Identification of the leucine-rich amelogenin peptide (LRAP) as the translation product of an alternatively spliced transcript. Biochem Biophys Res Comm 1991; 174(3): 1306-12.
[13] Salido EC, Yen PH, Koprivnikar K, *et al.* The human enamel protein gene amelogenin is expressed from both the X and the Y chromosomes. Amer J Human Genet 1992; 50(2): 303-16.
[14] Gibson CW, Golub EE, Abrams WR, *et al.* Bovine amelogenin message heterogeneity: alternative splicing and Y-chromosomal gene transcription. Biochemistry. 1992; 31(35): 8384-8.
[15] Lau EC, Simmer JP, Bringas P, Jr., *et al.* Alternative splicing of the mouse amelogenin primary RNA transcript contributes to amelogenin heterogeneity. Biochem Biophys Res Comm 1992; 188(3): 1253-60.
[16] Simmer JP, Hu CC, Lau EC, *et al.* Alternative splicing of the mouse amelogenin primary RNA transcript. Calcif Tissue Int 1994; 55(4): 302-10.
[17] Li R, Li W, DenBesten PK. Alternative splicing of amelogenin mRNA from rat incisor ameloblasts. J Dent Res 1995; 74(12): 1880-5.
[18] Bonass WA, Brookes SJ, Kirkham J, *et al.* The rat amelogenin gene--some aspects of evolution and expression. Adv Dent Res 1996 Nov;10(2):182-6.

[19] Baba O, Takahashi N, Terashima T, Li W, DenBesten PK, Takano Y. Expression of alternatively spliced RNA transcripts of amelogenin gene exons 8 and 9 and its end products in the rat incisor. J Histochem Cytochem 2002; 50(9): 1229-36.
[20] Sasaki S, Shimokawa H. The amelogenin gene. Int J Dev Biol 1995; 39(1): 127-33.
[21] Shimokawa H, Ogata Y, Sasaki S, *et al.* Molecular cloning of bovine amelogenin cDNA. Adv Dent Res 1987; 1(2): 293-7.
[22] Nakahori Y, Takenaka O, Nakagome Y. A human X-Y homologous region encodes "amelogenin". Genomics 1991; 9(2): 264-9.
[23] Gibson C, Golub E, Herold R, *et al.* Structure and expression of the bovine amelogenin gene. Biochemistry 1991; 30(4) :1075-9.
[24] Li W, Mathews C, Gao C, *et al.* Identification of two additional exons at the 3' end of the amelogenin gene. Arch Oral Biol 1998; 43(6): 497-504.
[25] Bartlett JD, Ball RL, Kawai T, *et al.* Origin, splicing, and expression of rodent amelogenin exon 8. J Dent Res 2006; 85(10): 894-9.
[26] Lyngstadaas SP, Moinichen CB, Risnes S. Crown morphology, enamel distribution, and enamel structure in mouse molars. Anat Rec 1998; 250(3): 268-80.
[27] Risnes S. The prism pattern of rat molar enamel: a scanning electron microscope study. Amer J Anat 1979; 155(2): 245-57.
[28] Risnes S. A scanning electron microscope study of aberrations in the prism pattern of rat incisor inner enamel. Amer J Anat 1979; 154(3): 419-36.
[29] Risnes S. Multiplane sectioning and scanning electron microscopy as a method for studying the three-dimensional structure of mature dental enamel. Scanning Microsc 1987; 1(4): 1893-902.
[30] Risnes S, Peterkova R, Lesot H. Distribution and structure of dental enamel in incisors of Tabby mice. Arch Oral Biol 2005; 50(2): 181-4.
[31] Branden C, Tooze J. Introduction of Protein Structure. 2nd ed. New York: Garland Publishing 1999.
[32] Murphy KP. The Hydrophobic Effect. In: Murphy KP, Ed. Protein Structure, Stability, and Folding. New Jersy: Hamana Press 2001: 5.
[33] Adkins RM, Gelke EL, Rowe D, *et al.* Molecular phylogeny and divergence time estimates for major rodent groups: evidence from multiple genes. Mol Biol Evol 2001; 18(5): 777-91.
[34] Huchon D, Madsen O, Sibbald MJ, *et al.* Rodent phylogeny and a timescale for the evolution of Glires: evidence from an extensive taxon sampling using three nuclear genes. Mol Biol Evol 2002; 19(7): 1053-65.
[35] Blanga-Kanfi S, Miranda H, Penn O, *et al.* Rodent phylogeny revised: analysis of six nuclear genes from all major rodent clades. BMC Evol Biol 2009; 9: e71.
[36] Uchida T, Tanabe T, Fukae M, *et al.* Immunochemical and immunohistochemical studies, using antisera against porcine 25 kDa amelogenin, 89 kDa enamelin and the 13-17 kDa nonamelogenins, on immature enamel of the pig and rat. Histochemistry 1991; 96(2): 129-38.

CHAPTER 14

In Vivo Effects of Amelogenins on Reparative Dentin Formation

Yassine Harichane[1], Sasha Dimitrova-Nakov[1], Anne Poliard[2], Arthur Veis[3], Pamela DenBesten[4], Odile Kellermann[1] and Michel Goldberg[1]*

[1]Laboratoire Différenciation de Cellules Souches et Prions, U747, Université Paris Descartes, rue des Saints Pères, 75006 Paris, France; [2]EA2496 Faculté de Chirurgie Dentaire, Université Paris Descartes, Montrouge, France. [3]Cell & Molecular Biology, Feinberg School of Medicine, Northwestern University, Chicago, IL, 60611, USA and [4] Department of Orofacial Sciences, University of California at San Francisco, POB 0422, San Francisco, CA 94143-0422, USA.

Abstract: Two low molecular weight amelogenin gene splice products (A+4 and A-4), used for pulp capping after surgical pulp exposure in the rat first maxillary molars, have been shown to induce the formation of a reparative dentinal bridge. A-4 can induce mineralization of the atubular orthodentinal type to totally fill the root pulp canal with a homogeneous mineralized structure. The two molecules recruit latent adult pulp progenitors to form actively dividing cells, which differentiated into cells bearing an osteoblast-odontoblast phenotype to produce an extracellular matrix implemented in reparative mineralization. We conclude that pulp capping with bioactive molecules will direct new approaches in biodentistry.

Key Words: Dental Pulp, Progenitor Cells, Amelogenin Splice Products, Pulp Capping, Biodentistry.

INTRODUCTION: TOWARD A BIODENTISTRY

Pulpitis, pulpal necrosis, and apical periodontitis, which are frequent consequences of deep carious lesions, constitute public health problems and contribute dramatically to the cost of dental treatments after endodontic therapies. In addition, the failure rate of root canal treatments is rather high, despite improvements that have been noted during the last two decades. The percentage of failures has decreased from 38% to 23% [1, 2]. However, it is still too high, and many teeth are lost and consequently the quality of life diminishes.

It is well documented that the dental pulp contains cells that demonstrate potential for regeneration and repair. Up to now, the most frequently used treatment aiming to preserve pulp vitality is the calcium hydroxide pulp-capping therapy. However, this approach has had only limited successes in the retention of residual pulp vitality, and in preventing the occurrence of sealing defects leading to bacterial re-colonization. Published clinical evaluations show high rates of failure: about 40-44.5% 5 years post surgery; and 79.7% after 10 years [3, 4].

Therefore, there is a strong need to develop new strategies for stimulating the emergence of resident pulp stem cells, to mimic the natural healing properties of the dental pulp. Currently experimental cell therapies are under consideration for many dental and non-dental tissues. Concepts derived from tissue engineering studies are now applied experimentally to clinical dentistry and dental pulp treatments. These new tools may pave the way toward what may be named a *biodentistry.* In parallel, implantation of pulp stem cells may enhance the regeneration of the dentin and/or pulp tissues, and may be further enhanced through the use of bioactive molecules. However, further work is required to address some of the questions that arise from the data already obtained, and they have to be answered before moving to clinical application in humans.

In the adult human tooth, the location and the elements of the presumptive niche(s) providing the physiological environment supporting pulpal stem cells homeostatic self-renewal and odontogenic differentiation are not known. Whatever the biological tools that are used, cells or molecules, trends in pulp engineering are oriented toward three key points focused on the identification of molecules initiating the signaling cascades that: 1) control the proliferation potential of precursor cells; 2) direct their differentiation towards osteoblast or odontoblast lineages, and 3) drive the cells to the end-stage of differentiation by sustaining the formation of a mineralized matrix. Two

Michel Goldberg (ED)

different targets for pulp biodentistry are currently under investigation; either the dental pulp regenerates and heals, or its mineralization provides the best biological filling of the tooth.

PULP RESPONSE TO INJURY AND THERAPIES

Following moderate carious tooth decay, odontoblasts are able to produce a reactionary dentin layer located beneath a calciotraumatic line. Tubular or atubular orthodentin or osteodentin protect the pulp from a new injury. As odontoblasts are post-mitotic cells, they are not renewed, and the formation of reactionary dentin is limited. Subjacent cells located in the Höehl's layer have the potential to replace irreversibly altered odontoblasts, but the numbers of available cells are limited. [5, 6].

Odontoblasts are polarized cells that align in a layer between dentin and pulp. In response to stimulus, developing processes protruding from odontoblasts cell bodies located at the periphery of the pulp are detectable within the newly formed mineralized matrix of tubular **orthodentin**. Atubular reactionary dentin may be also observed, resulting from the merging of calcospheritic structures. As a third possibility, an **osteodentin** is formed, with a bone-like structure, cells being trapped in lacuna, as is the case for osteocytes. Because reactionary dentin is unstained by the "stains all" method and by antibodies raised against dentin phosphoprotein, it is assumed that either phosphorylated proteins are lacking, or that the proteins are present but not phosphorylated [7-9]. Such differences in matrix composition at a molecular level reflect differential biomechanical properties between preformed dentin and reactionary dentin which whatever the type (tubular, atubular orthodentin or osteodentin) is always less resistant to further decay.

More severe dental injuries such as rapidly progressing deep carious lesions display rapid progress, affect the odontoblasts viability as well as the underlying cells of the Höehl layer, preventing the formation of any reactionary dentin. At a still reversible stage of the pathology, odontoblast-like or osteoblast-like cells arise from the traumatized dental pulp and synthesize a reparative dentinal bridge leading to the closure of the pulp exposure. A layer of osteodentin is formed, characterized by an atubular mineralized matrix embedding the cells within lacunae, reminiscent of a bone matrix surrounding osteocytes. Of note, the differentiating osteo-odontogenic cells responsible for reparative dentin formation, are thought to be derived from resident pulpal stem cells. Distinct cell populations displaying progenitor/stem cells properties have been described within the post-natal dental pulp [10-13] supporting the idea that the pulp may represent a promising source of stem cells. Indeed, it contains not only cells that behave as precursors of mineralized tissues which participate to the natural regenerative processes, but also, a subset of cells that exhibit multilineage differentiation potential towards an odonto-osteogenic, chondrogenic, adipogenic, myogenic, and even neurogenic fate following implantation at ectopic sites.

From an embryological point of view, pulp stem cells have a mesodermal or mesectodermal (neural crest) origin. Normally present in adult teeth at a quiescent state within the stroma and in the perivascular regions of the healthy pulp, they are thought to be mobilized upon severe tooth injury to replace the loss of odontoblasts and provide an ultimate support for a restorative response. Nevertheless, in the absence of selective criteria to characterize stem cells, the identity and mechanisms sustaining the regenerative capacity of the pulp progenitors remain largely unknown. In particular, how the autocrine stem cell microenvironmments (niches), paracrine inflammatory factors or blood supply may cooperate to provide signals ensuring the recruitment and differentiation of these dormant odontogenic cells remains to be clarified.

It must also be taken under consideration that if the pulp inflammation and degeneration progresses too rapidly, pulp healing cannot be achieved. This is followed by endodontic therapies. Early treatment to slow these processes, to reduce pulp inflammation must be developed as a part of future engineered pulp treatments. In this context, it is important to recall that cell-matrix-mineral interactions play a crucial role in the formation and in homeostasis of mineralized tissues i.e. bone and teeth. Clearly, the onset, progression and maintenance of programmed osteo-odontoblastic differentiation depends on regulatory processes related to matrix assembly as well as to the nature and concentration of signaling molecules sequestered within the dentin matrix. As soon as the matrix is formed, mineral deposition may also participate in the implementation of a functional odontoblastic phenotype. Investigations are currently in progress to test the power of mineral compounds, extracellular matrix (ECM) proteins, cytokines in directing the odontogenic fate of odontoblast precursors contained within the dental pulp, which consequently contribute to reparative processes.

PULP THERAPIES: EFFECTS OF CALCIUM HYDROXIDE AS PULP CAPPING AGENT

Since the introduction of calcium hydroxide, Ca(OH)2, as capping agent by Hermann in 1930 [14], the mechanisms involved in the healing process have been largely clarified [15-18]. Due to a pH of 12, an initial caustic effect occurs, leading to superficial necrosis of the exposed pulp. Inflammatory cells migrate in the wounded area, followed by the recruitment of mesenchymal cells or odontoblast/osteoblast progenitors near the lesion. These cells synthesize a collagen-rich ECM that subsequently undergoes mineralization, forming a reparative dentinal bridge. Cell inclusions as debris and pulp remnants contribute to the formation of tunnels, lacunae and other defects, resulting in a lack of homogeneity of the resultant dentinal bridge. This lack of homogeneity in dentinal bridge formation frequently results in secondary bacteria colonization, thus accounting for the numerous failures occurring after such therapies (Figure 1). Use of mineral compounds such as Mineral Trioxide Aggregate (MTA), recently put on the market and consequently evaluated only short periods of time, may contribute to the formation of a much more resistant barrier. Nevertheless, the formation of a dentinal bridge in response to these agents suggests that pulp-capping procedures, in concert with therapies to enhance cellular responsiveness, could significantly improve the effectiveness of dentin repair.

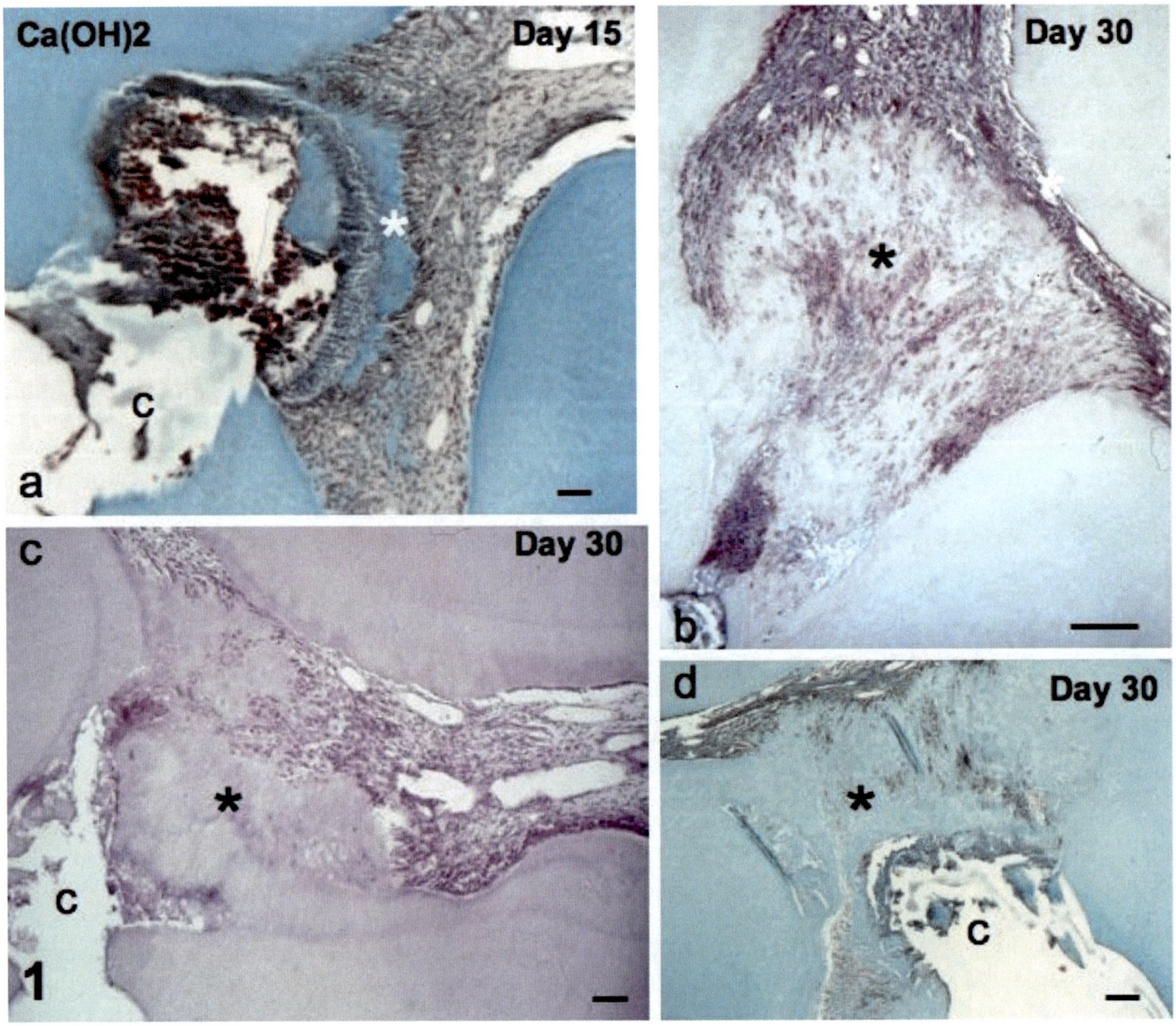

Figure 1: Effects of Ca(OH)2 capping on the exposed pulp of the first rat maxillary molar. (a): 15 days after capping, the formation of a thin reparative dentinal bridge is seen (white asterisk), located between the cavity (c) and the pulp surface. (b, c and d): after 30days a thick reparative dentinal bridge is formed (asterisk). Tunnels and cell debris inclusions cross the reparative bridge formed by an osteodentin-like structure.

Bar= 100 mm

BIOACTIVE MOLECULES FOR PULP REPAIR

Type 1 collagen is the predominant component of the dentin ECM. It provides the protein scaffold for the architecture of teeth into which the hydroxyapatite mineral crystals are accumulated. In conjunction, numerous dentine-associated non-collagenous proteins (Table 1) such as proteoglycans, Small Integrin-Binding Ligand N-linked Glycoproteins (SIBLINGs), maintain the structural and functional integrity of the dentin tissue. Since some of these ECM-associated biomolecules may influence stem cell recruitment, they may be potential tools for tissue engineering and pulp therapies.

Table 1: Non collagenous dentin extracellular matrix proteins. At this time,the effects of DMP-1, BSP, MEPE, A+/-4, ILGF I, TGFb and BMPs have been investigated as pulp capping agent.

Phosphorylated proteins	SIBLINGs	*Dentin sialophosphoprotein (DSPP), hydrolyzed immediately after secretion into: Dentin phosphoprotein (DPP) Dentin glycoprotein (DGP) Dentin sialoprotein (DSP) *Dentin matrix protein-1 (DMP-1) *Bone sialoprotein (BSP) *Osteopontin *Matrix extracellular phosphorylated glycoprotein (MEPE)
	Amelogenin	A+4 / A-4 (LRAP)
	Decorin (DCN)	
Lipoproteins and phospholipids		ECM associated phospholipids: acidic phospholipids, phosphatidylcholine, sphingomyelin, phosphatidylethanolamine
Non-phosphorylated proteins	Osteocalcin & Gla proteins Osteonectin (SPARC)	
	*Small leucine-rich proteoglycans (SLRPs) *Large proteoglycans	*CSPG (chondroitin sulfate proteoglycans): biglycan, decorin *KSPG (keratan sulfate proteoglycans): fibromodulin, lumican, osteoadherin *Versican
	Serum proteins	* Albumin □□a_2-HS glycoprotein
	Growth factors	BMPs, TGFβ, FGF-2, ILGF I & II, PDGF
	Enzymes and enzyme inhibitors	Acid & alkaline phosphatases MMPs and other proteases, TIMPs
	Polyamines	Putrescine and cadaverine Spermidine and spermine

These ECM-associated molecules perform many roles essential for dentin formation and control of odontoblast functions. Among them, some provide the dentin framework for mineralization, or regulate matrix calcification by controlling the pool of calcium and inorganic phosphate available for hydroxyapatite crystal formation. Others act as signaling molecules and participate in cell-matrix interactions or ~~to~~ intercellular communications. They likely act in concert, since adequate mechanical support may have a critical role in the presentation or adequate concentrations of signaling biomolecules.

Needless to say, even if each of these proteins exerts a specialized function, it does not act alone and is often multifunctional through its interactions with distinct extracellular target complexes. For example, adhesion molecules or integrins by interacting with partners in microdomains at the cell surface, can ensure connections between the cytoskeleton and the external ECM, and at the same time may regulate the recruitment of signaling cascades.

The experimental use of ECM molecules as pulp capping agents derives from the observation that dentin fragments or chips from rabbit incisor implanted in dog dental pulps display dentinogenetic effects [19]. Interestingly, soluble dentin extracts promote the same response indicating that biologically active molecules of the matrix fraction are responsible for induction of cell differentiation [20]. Since that time, the effects of DMP-1, BSP, MEPE, A+/-4, ILGF I, TGFβ and BMPs on dental repair have been investigated. The dentinogenic nature of the pulpal responses to these molecules were highly variable, ranging from no significant effects to beneficial healing, restorative mineralization, or uncontrolled pulp obstruction. Even~~,~~ for promising candidates such as BMPs (see below), several shortcomings have been seen which give rise to many conceptual and technical pertinent questions. Moreover, the changes in methodology for each individual study (differences between species, implantation designs, growth factor dose applications, time-dependency of the events, carrier systems…) bring some confusion regarding how more adequate responsiveness should be achieved. An accurate knowledge of the cause-effect~~s~~ relationships between ECM biomolecules and odontogenic differentiation must still be determined prior to therapeutic use. Except for amelogenin (see the references related to enamel matrix derivative [EMD] put on the market as Emdogain), the translation of these studies into a clinical application for dental repair is not yet a reality.

As an example, Bone Morphogenetic Proteins (BMPs), and in particular the most osteoinductive BMP2 and BMP7, are used in the orthopedic field (clinical approval mostly for spinal fusion procedure and some particular treatment options) but are not approved for dental applications. BMPs-mediated signaling is implicated in odontoblast differentiation during tooth development [21]. Crude allogeneic mixtures of BMPs were first tested by capping an amputated dog dental pulp [22]. After 4 weeks, reparative osteodentin was formed over pulpal tissue. After 8 weeks, a tubular ECM dentin was formed next to the osteodentin layer. Human recombinant BMP-2 and/or BMP-4 also promote the formation of a superficial layer of osteodentin associated with tubular dentin in the deeper part of pulp cavity [23]. The recombinant human BMP-7, also named Osteogenic Protein 1 (OP1) was then used as pulp capping agent in monkeys, and was found to induce a massive filling of the root canal with osteodentine [24, 25].

When implanted in the rat molar, using type I collagen as carrier, we observed that BMP7 induces firstly a moderate inflammatory process 8 days after capping which gradually resolves and could not be detected after 15 days. After one month, the mesial part of the coronal pulp chamber was filled by a heterogeneous osteodentin with poorly merged globular structures and pulp remnants in the interglobular spaces i.e. unable to resist to secondary bacterial recolonization. By contrast, the mesial root was totally filled with a homogeneous mineralized tissue appearing as being of the atubular orthodentin-type occluding the lumen of the root canal [26] representing an alternative to endodontic treatments. These data highlight differential responses to BMP7 relative to the pulp area. This may result from the recruitment of osteo-odontogenic cells with distinct identities reminiscent of their embryonal origin.

The difference between the coronal and root pulp reaction may be also related to amelogenin environment. During odontogenesis, an enamel organ involved in the secretion of amelogenin encloses the coronal pulp. This amelogenin is essential for the differentiation of forming odontoblastic cells of the crown. In contrast, amelogenin may not be necessary to obtain a resistant dentin barrier in the root, since during root formation the dentin forming pulp cells are delimited by the Hertwig's sheath and are thus not exposed to amelogenin. However, in some species, Hertwig's epithelial sheath cells themselves do secrete some enamel-related proteins including amelogenin. Of note, in the rat a weak amelogenin immunostaining is found to be restricted to the most apical part of the Hertwig's sheath but is not detected later during root dentinogenesis or cementogenesis. In addition, the amelogenin mRNA has not been detected by in situ hybridization at theses steps.

Thus, in the absence of significant amelogenin secretion in post-natal pulp, BMP7 treatment may be more efficient in the root. However, other factors may also play a role. In this context, vascular and nerve networks show substantial differences between the crown where large vessels loops are seen, and the root where capillaries are characterized by a fishnet arrangement [27]. These distinct local microenvironments may more or less influence BMP7 inductive action on the responsive cells.

Questions arise concerning the spatio-temporal self-limitation of the process. Further investigations based on dose-dependency action and longer periods of time were conducted in our laboratory, but no difference was detected. Of note, while BMP7 is known for its efficient osteo-inductive action, the mineralization process was exclusively restricted to the dental pulp area and never expand~~s~~ed to the periapical zone. The periodontal ligament remains intact. Hence, BMP7 display promising inductive properties, provided its action on the crown defect repair could be improved by synergy with other(s) biomolecule(s).

BSP mainly synthesized by osteoblasts, but also, to a lesser extent by odontoblasts, has been experimentally used to promote bone repair in critical-size defect of rat calvaria [28, 29] and reparative dentin in the dental pulp [30]. Eight days after BSP implantation in rat molar, we observed an inflammatory process in the mesial part of the coronal pulp [30]. Two weeks after, the inflammation was resolved and reparative dentin formation initiated. Within one month, the mesial pulp chamber is completely filled by a homogeneous orthodentin-like atubular dentin matrix while no effect could be visualized in the root. As compared to $Ca(OH)_2$ capping, the BSP-induced dentin formation seemed to be faster and more homogenous for efficient long-term pulp protection. The ability of BSP to activate a reparative process only in the coronal part of the pulp sustains the idea that this bioactive molecule may be suitable for protective effects in restorative applications without impairing subsequent endodontic treatments.

Among the SIBLINGs, the impact of a peptide of MEPE, also called Dentonin or AC100, on reparative dentin formation in rat molar was also investigated [31]. Eight days after implantation, PCNA labeling revealed the presence of proliferative cells expressing RP59, an early marker of osteogenic differentiation. These cells, which might be osteo-odontogenic precursor cells, also express OPN, but DSP could not be detected by immunolabelling. Reparative osteodentin filled the coronal part of the pulp and some mineralized globular structures also appeared at the junction between the coronal and root parts of the pulp. The reaction was rapidly initiated, but stopped before any actual total mineralization in about 50% of the samples, whereas in the other half, the pulps displayed large mineralized areas. It is possible that future strategies using sequential implantations of AC100 within the pulp, or co-implantation of AC100 with other bioactive molecules could be utilized.

At present, the experiments aiming at deciphering the reparative potential of ECM- derived molecules on dentin repair are still at a pioneering stage. However, they have already provided methodological and conceptual advances highlighting the complexity of the dental pulp, including the mosaic of anatomical and physiological domains bearing individual specificities. These studies highlight the need to obtain better knowledge related to the location and identity of odontogenic precursor cells participating to *de novo* dentin formation. This will allow us to accurately use precise spatial and temporal regulation as the biomolecules are implanted to effectively and reproducibly positively influence the healing processes.

As discussed above, amelogenins are not considered dentin matrix molecules. However, they have shown great promise in promoting healing in the dental pulp. Although a biochemical understanding of amelogenins signaling action is just emerging, we will described below some *in vivo* experimental approaches aimed at filling in this the lack of knowledge. We will focus on the specific action of amelogenin on target cells, the identification of niches of progenitors and the potential role of inflammatory mediators and their direct or indirect involvement in signaling responses of pulp cells.

THE NEED OF AN *IN VIVO* ACCESSIBLE MODEL: THE RAT MOLAR

The impact of ECM-related biomolecules on reparative dentin formation has been tested in monkeys [32], mini-swine [33], dogs [34], ferrets [35], rats [36] and mice [37], leading to debatable interpretations due to species differences. Variations in the shape of the teeth, the type of food, variations of dentin formation during aging potential affect the overall results. To overcome this difficulty, we selected rat maxillary molars as a reliable animal model, and set-up reproducible experimental protocols to accurately evaluate the spatio-temporal action of bioactive agents within the pulp.

The rat molar has been extensively used for pulp repair studies. Indeed, the rat first maxillary molar is a tooth with limited growth, and despite some anatomic specificity, not significantly different from the human tooth. Despite its small size, the surgical procedure is relatively simple, and usual dental instruments are suitable for use. The legal rules on animal care must be followed, but with many fewer controls and regulation as compared with dogs, pigs and monkeys.

Ohshima [38] reported the first protocol allowing an accurate and reproducible preparation of a cavity on the maxillary tooth, with the large diastema providing easy access to the mesial aspect of the molar. We introduced some modifications of this protocol to gain better access to the cervical pulp. For example, gingival electrosurgery was carried out on the mesial aspect, close to the junction between the crown and the root [30]. In doing so, two advantages were obtained: 1) The cervical location of the cavity avoids inadvertent wounding of pulp horns during cavity preparation. This pulp horn-related area is quite different from the rest of the pulp because it is subjected to reactionary dentin formation under the influence of masticatory pressures and abrasion of an enamel-free cusp. 2) Restorations can be placed in the cavity to maintain the carrier in place with or without the bioactive molecules, preventing bacterial contamination of the exposed pulp. The restoration has less exposure to the dislodging effects of occlusal pressures to maintain its protective function.

After anesthesia with a single intraperitoneal injection of Chloral (400 mg/kg body weight), the mesial gingival papilla is removed by electrosurgery (Servotom, Satelec, France). A cavity, 600 μm in diameter, is prepared with a carbide dental bur. The residual dentin wall is pushed with a steel probe, to produce a pulp exposure. This step avoids stretching of the pulp tissue around the bur and the resultant more extensive pulp damage. One draw back of this technique is that dentin fragments may often and inevitably be pushed into the pulp, and thus contribute by themselves to the formation of a reparative dentin structure by releasing some ECM molecules [21].

Therefore, it is important to include a sham group to evaluate the incidence of the surgical preparation on the pulp. A control group to determine the biological effects of the carriers alone (collagen or agarose beads), which are never bioinert, must also be included (Figure 2). Both of these controls are then used to determine the effect of implantation with beads soaked in a solution containing the bioactive agent, thus monitoring the inductive/reparative impact of the biomolecules. The procedure is completed by filling the cavity with a glass-ionomer cement to protect the pulp and avoid bacterial colonization [26, 36, 39].

The use of the rat model provides easily accessible and valuable data. A statistically significant number of rats/teeth is rather easy to reach. It is reliable, of low cost, and presumably the results obtained with studies based on experimental approaches on this animal can reasonably be transferred to the human.

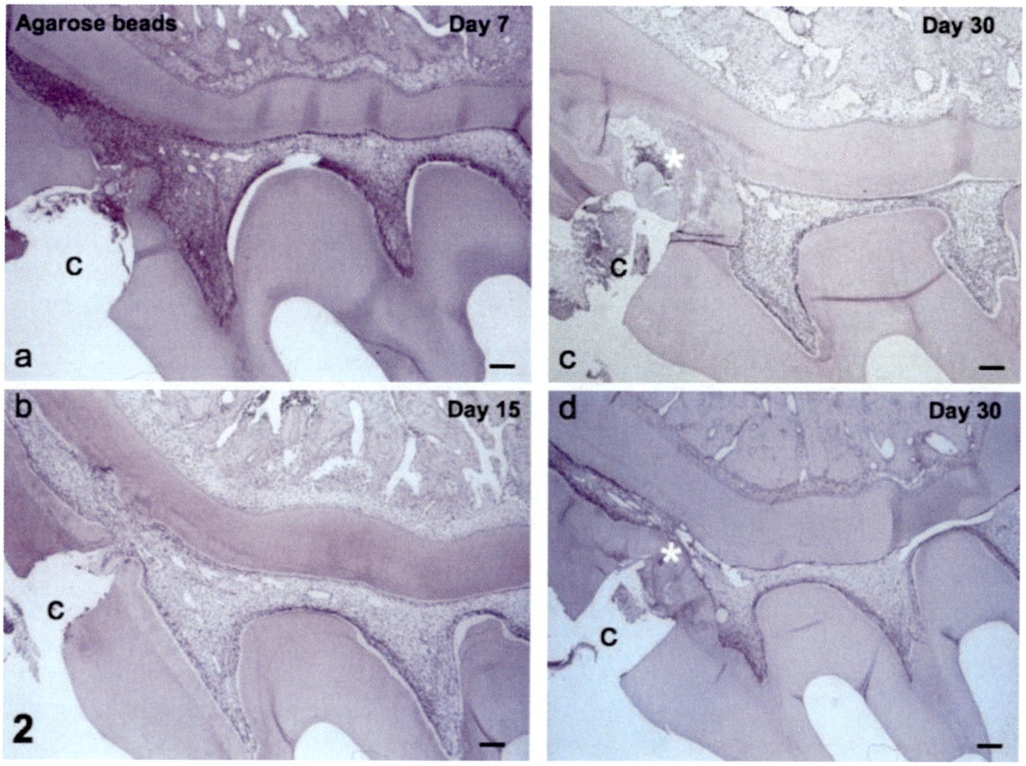

Figure 2: Effects of agarose beads implantation in the dental pulp (control group). (a): after 7 days, an inflammatory process is seen in the mesial pulp chamber. (b): after 15 days the inflammatory process is largely resolved. Apposition of reparative dentin is seen in the coronal mesial part of the pulp and along the root canal. The beginning of a closure process is seen at the exposure site. (c): after 30 days the weak bioactivity of agarose beads contribute to the healing of a few teeth (asterisk), whereas in most of the treated teeth (d) a thin dentinal bridge is formed, concomitantly with some reduction in width of the root canal due to the formation of mineralized layer (asterisk) beneath a calcio-traumatic line.

Bar= 100 mm

AMELOGENINS AS TOOLS FOR PULP CAPPING

A+4, A-4 or LRAP: Amelogenin Gene Splice Products

In previous studies, a low molecular mass (6-10 kDa) amelogenin polypeptide was isolated from the rat incisor dentin matrix. It had the capacity to stimulate *in vitro* embryonic muscle fibroblasts to express sulfated proteoglycans and type II collagen [40, 41]. Two specific cDNAs were identified in the rat incisor tooth odontoblast/pulp library: the first (A+4, 8.1kDa) results from the expression of amelogenin gene exons 2, 3, 4, 5, 6d, and 7; the second (A-4, 6.9kDa) from exons 2, 3, 5, 6d and 7, the expression of exon 4 being omitted [42]. *In vitro*, A+4 stimulates Sox9 expression whereas A-4 stimulated Cbfa1/runx2 mRNA expression [42].

In the mouse enamel organ, the larger full length (M194) and near full length (M180) amelogenin isoforms are the principal products directing the formation of the mineralized enamel. A-4 and the Leucine-Rich Amelogenin Peptide, LRAP (M57), share the same primary sequence containing the carboxy- and amino-termini residues of amelogenin but lacking the central domain[43].

A+4 and A-4 are also synthesized by odontoblasts notably at the perinatal development period just prior dentin mineralization [44, 45]. It has been postulated that, at that time, both peptides may participate to the signaling exchanges between ameloblasts and odontoblasts at the amelo-dentinal junction [46]. Interestingly, both *in vitro* and *in vivo* experiments have provided convincing evidence that these amelogenin gene splice products act as signaling molecules [47-49], though their mechanisms of action at biochemical and cellular levels are still unclear. Many questions remain unresolved: do they act on distinct target cells? do their signaling effects vary according to the cell types or is there an overlap in their expression patterns and in their signaling functions?

On the therapeutic side, many observations led to the proposal that amelogenin derivatives may enhance formation of the dentin mineralized matrix [50]. Nevertheless, a causal link between one specific amelogenin-derived molecule and the implementation of an osteo-odontogenic differentiation cascade not been established. In the context of pulp repair, an important aspect will be the identification of the physiological targets of A+4/A-4 bioactive molecules.

We may be reminded that in the past, the osteoinductive effects of BMPs were first observed at ectopic sites. Khouri et al. [51] were able to transform mesenchymal tissue into bone with BMP3 and demineralized bone matrix. Similarly, when A+4 and A-4 loaded in a biopolymer matrix were implanted in the rat hind muscle [42], the samples were invaded by a vascular network and mineral deposits of calcium phosphate were identified 4 weeks later. This response was accompanied by the positive immunolabeling of two bone-specific matrix proteins, BSP and BAG-75 (a bone molecule similar to DMP-1), within the ECM. Both peptides induced ectopic calcification in hind muscle but A-4 was more efficient that A+4. These observations have provided the first evidence that these amelogenin splice products may each acts as signals to promote mineralization, though their mineralization efficiency was affected by the prescence or absence of exon 4 translated amino acid sequences while not having equivalent properties.

When A+4 or A-4 were investigated in another ectopic site, mice gingiva, there were no parallels reactions to those observed with BMP [52]. At day 3 after implantation with agarose beads as carrier, an inflammatory process was observed in the lamina propria, decreasing at day 8 and not detectectable at day 30. Cells expressing markers representative of the osteo-chondrogenic lineage such as RP 59, Sox9, BSP, OPN and negative for DSP, could be visualized by immunolabelling at the implantation site, but no traces of an initial mineralization process could be detectable. It was hypothesized that these cells may originate from circulating cells or inflammatory cells since PCNA labeling failed to reveal any mitogenic effect of the A+4/A-4 peptides. Thus, it appears that A+4 or A-4 does not mobilize resident precursor cells in oral gingiva and has no mineralizing effects.

Since, an in vitro treatment of rat or human gingival fibroblasts by amelogenin derivatives also fail to induce any mineralization [53, 54], these observations illustrate the need to define the molecules that sustain an A+4/A-4-induced response in mesodermal tissue. In this context, it becomes apparent that such questions could be addressed at least in part, by experiments performed in the dental pulp.

A+4–Mediated Reparative Action Upon Implantation in the Exposed Pulp of Rat Molar

The most natural target sites where A+4 and A-4 may exert their physiological actions likely reside within the dental pulp. Indeed, it has to be underscored that the term "amelogenins" include amelogenins derivatives generated by proteolytic processing whose individual actions on reparative process have never been explored. Thus, to evaluate a biological effect of A+/-4, it was important to avoid the problems associated with the use of uncontrolled amelogenin species and to use purified recombinant A+/-4 amelogenin peptides [42]. We exploited the rat molar model and used agarose beads (75-150 mm in diameter) as a carrier [39, 55]. The bead aggregated, resulting in a total of 3 to 7 beads implanted in each exposed pulp.

Since carriers are never bioinert, first, we checked the bioactivity of this linear sulphated galactan that provides antiviral and anticoagulant properties to the agarose beads.[39, 55-57]. No reportable effect could be visualized in the coronal part of the pulp, but a dentin-like apposition significantly reduced the width of the root canal. This reduction in size of the lumen was limited when compared to the effects of amelogenin peptide implantation (Figure 2).

Upon implantation of beads soaked with A+4 (about 0.2mg absorbed on each bead), in the exposed pulp (Figures 3 and 5), a PCNA immunolabelling revealing a mitogenic effect takes place rapidly in the mesial part of the coronal pulp, reaching a maximum at day 3, and decreasing gradually after day 7. Since, concomitantly, a moderate inflammatory process generally occurs in the same area, it is difficult, at this early stage of the response, to discriminate whether these proliferating cells have an inflammatory origin or are latent osteo-odonto progenitors [61].

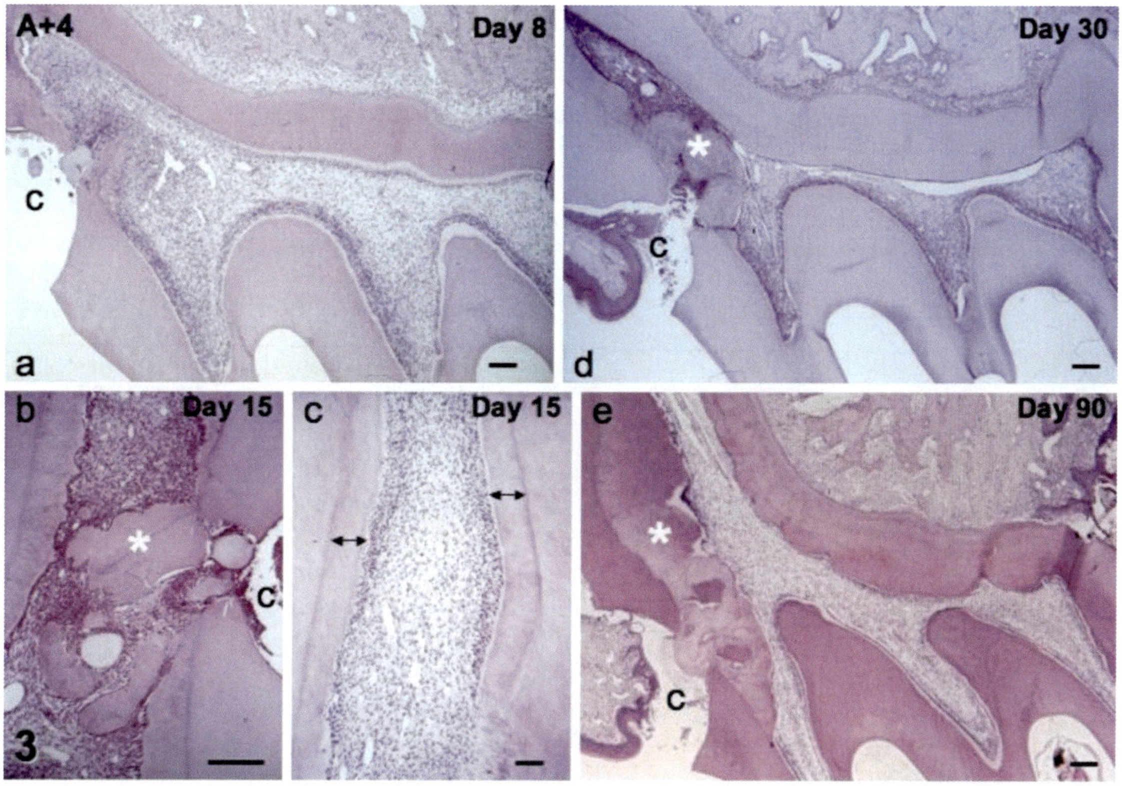

Figure 3: Effects of the implantation of agarose beads loaded with A+4 in the dental pulp. (a) After 8 days, the healing process starts. (b) The formation of a reparative dentinal bridge occluding the pulp exposure is obvious at 15 days (asterisk). (c) In the root at the same period of time the width of the radicular pulp is reduced by dentin apposition (double arrows), seen beneath the calico-traumatic line. After 30 days, a thick reparative dentinal bridge is formed (asterisk). (e)Despite the formation of the bridge closing totally the pulp exposure (asterisk), there is still a living pulp in the root canal.

Bar= 100 mm

After A+4 or A-4 implantation, cell migation is indicated by the temporal location of PCNA positive cells in time-course studies. In the crown, it appears that dividing cells are initially present in the center (day 1 to day 7), and migrate toward the periphery of the pulp, ultimately reaching an area near the implantation site (day 7 to 15). In addition, at day 7, cells positively stained for PCNA are seen near the beads but they are not lining the agarose surface. They constitute a second ring around the beads, a first ring being formed by osteopontin-labeled cells displaying hallmarks of committed osteo-odontogenic cells. In the root, PCNA-labeled cells are located initially (days 1 -3) along the blood vessels. At day 15, dividing cells are still present exclusively in the sub-odontoblastic cell layer, whereas at 30 days PCNA labeling is no more observed [39].

A repertoire of markers representative of osteo-odontogenic cells were used to characterize the recruitment of presumptive dentin forming stem cells in response to A+4. An antibody raised against RP 59, a protein synthesized by hematopoietic precursors, mesenchymal cells, osteoblast and odontoblast progenitors [58], allows to detect positive cells as soon as one day after A+4 implantation. Of interest, at the initial stage of the response, the RP59 expressing cells and PCNA positive cells were detectable in the same area, suggesting that A+4 can recruit precursor cells i.e. exert a mitogenic effect associated to the onset of their differentiation program. At day 15, still dividing cells were not adjacent to the beads. Cells positively immunostained for RP59 and osteopontin (OPN), but negative for DSP formed a ring at the surface of beads (Figure 5).

DSP was used as a marker to trace cells displaying an odontoblast phenotype following A+4 pulp capping. DSP is one of the 3 peptides derived from the proteolytic cleavage of the DSPP full-length protein after its secretion. It is strongly expressed by odontoblasts and to a much lesser extent by osteoblasts [59]. DSP cannot be visualized within the pulp at the initial period after A+4 implantation. From day 8, DSP expressing cells are present in a very restricted area, near the pulp exposure, close to the place where the future dentin bridge will develop.

After one month a homogeneous robust atubular reparative dentinal bridge is formed in the crown, closing the pulp exposure and isolating the mesial pulp chamber from the cavity. In the control group, the formation of a dentinal bridge quite never occurs. In parallel, the lumen of the root canal is gradually occluded by a massive dentin-like deposition occurring along the walls of the radicular pulp. It worth to be noted that A+4 is mostly involved in the closure of the coronal pulp exposure and has more limited effects on the radicular pulp even after 90 days (Figure 3).

Whereas a living pulp is located in the central and distal part of the pulp chamber, a thick dentinal bridge isolated the mesial part from the cavity. The absence of tunnels, lacuna and other defects makes obvious the advantage of A+4 compared with $Ca(OH)_2$.

A-4–Mediated Reparative Action Upon Implantation in the Exposed Pulp of Rat Molar

Upon implantation of beads soaked with A-4 (about 0.2mg absorbed on each bead) in the exposed pulp, the extent of inflammatory phase was very limited, becoming almost undectectable as soon as day 7 (Figure 4). In the crown, PCNA-labeled cells are initially (day 3 to 7) observed in the central part of the pulp, at some distance away from the agarose beads. Afterward, as already observed for A+4, a ring of proliferating cells come closer the beads, but never in intimate contact with their surfaces [55] (Figure 5). Also, in the root, PCNA-positive cells are located exclusively in the subodontoblastic layer, and at day 15, dividing cells are no more detected.

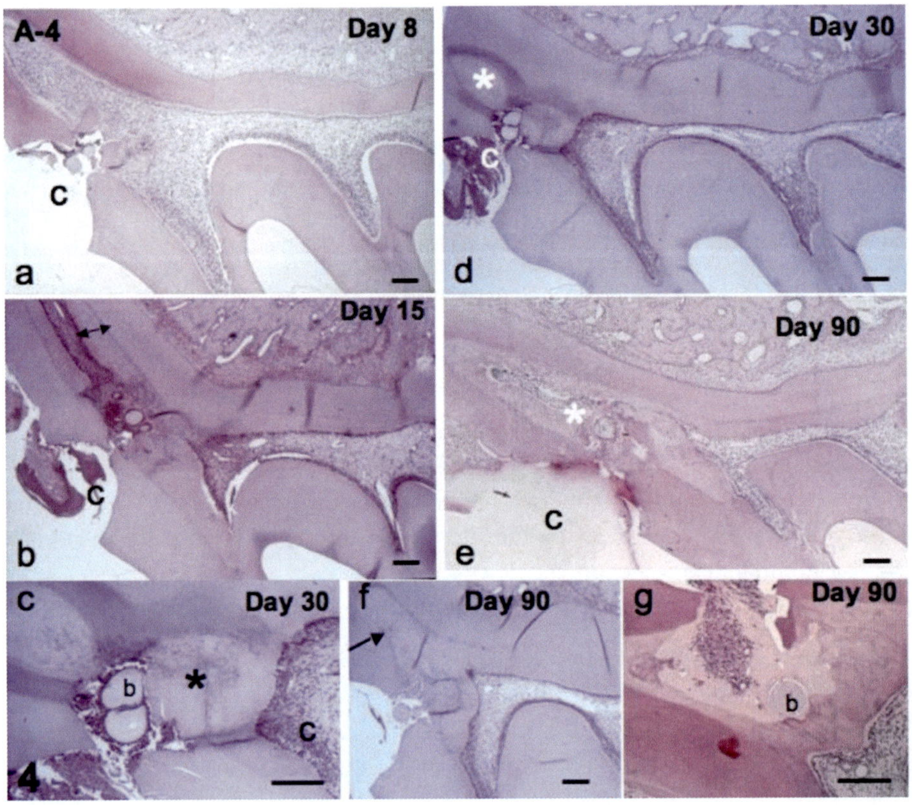

Figure 4: Effects of the implantation of agarose beads loaded with A-4 in the dental pulp. (a) At day 8, the initial inflammatory process is weak, there is no evidence for a reparative process. (b) The formation of reparative dentin is obvious at day 15 both in the pulp chamber and in the root canal. The double arrow indicates the thickness of the dentin layer formed along the lumen of the canal. (c and d): at day 30, a thick reparative dentin layer occludes the pulp exposure and the root canal (asterisks) and remnants of the beads (b) are surrounded by reparative dentin. At day 90 (e, f and g), the pulp responsiveness remains similar than the one observed at day 30. A mineralized ECM of atubular dentin occludes the root canal (seen on undemineralized sections by electron microprobe associated with SEM device, not shown) and the periodontal ligament remains intact (see 4e).

Bar= 100 mm

At this time, the cells in close contact with the surface of the beads are positive for RP59, OPN and BSP, but negative for DSP. This indicates that at this time these cells display an osteoblastic phenotype, but do not undergo an odontoblast differentiation pathway. Cells positive for DSP thus bearing an odontoblasts phenotype are seen far away from the beads and exclusively within the implantation area near the pulp exposure [39].

Of interest, between days 14 and 30, a homogenous atubular mineralized structure of the orthodentin type fills gradually the mesial pulp chamber in the crown, beads becoming embedded in the newly formed mineralized ECM. At the same time, a reparative dentin deposit gradually reduces the width of the root canal. Noteworthily after 90 days, the mineralization process is exclusively restricted to the dental pulp area and never expands to the periapical zone. In all samples, the periodontal ligament remains intact.

Hence, A-4 displays promising inductive properties, either for its action on the crown defect or for root canal therapy.

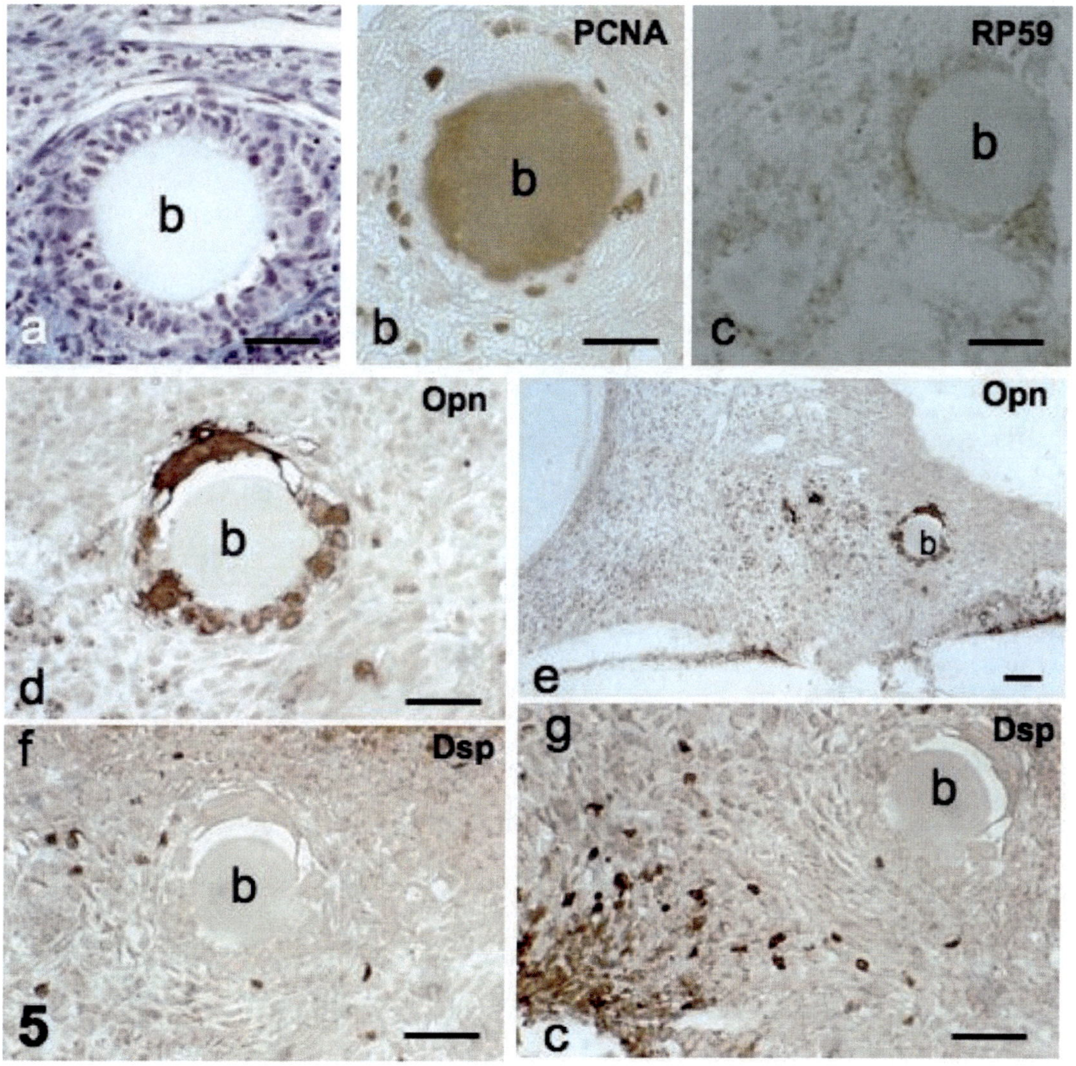

Figure 5: A+4 or A-4 recruit proliferating cells and differentiating cells exhibiting osteoblastic or odontoblastic markers. (a) At day 8, after implantation of A+4 or A-4, the surface of the agarose beads is covered by a ring of cells displaying an osteogenic phenotype, as inferred by their labeling by RP59 (c) and Opn (d,e) antibodies. (b) Cells in mitosis, labeled by PCNA form a second ring at some distance away from the surface. Cells expressing DSP are not detected around the beads (f). DSP positive cells likely correspond to preodontoblasts or odontoblasts accumulating near the pulp exposure, in the area where the future dentinal bridge will be built (g).

Bar= 100 mm

PERSPECTIVES

This new set of experiments aiming to evaluate the reparative potential of A+4 or A-4, used as pure molecules for capping in rat molar, reveal some remarkable effects of these amelogenin splice products on exposed pulp cells. These data add to the network of questions concerning the exciting development of regenerative therapies based on amelogenin -related products, since their launch as clinical devices.

A+4/A-4 impact on another subset of target cells forming a homogeneous robust atubular reparative dentinal bridge at the site of implantation. But it takes several days before the recruitment of such DSP positive cells far from the beads and only near the pulp exposure, are observed. These odontoblastic-like cells appear to arise from the stroma and to migrate to the site for repair, but we also cannot exclude that they could also emanate from the Höehl's layer and result from the lateral sliding of these cells.

One can imagine that their onset at the wound site would require sequential temporally limiting events i.e. the rate of diffusion of A+4/A-4 within the pulpal stroma, the time-dependent migration of the progenies of recruited cells, indirect signaling effects or need to cooperative action of active cytokines. Whatever their mechanisms of action, A+4 and A-4 mobilize odontoblast-like cells and increase their reparative potential.

Enamel matrix derivatives (EMD), a trade product already available in the market under the name of "Emdogain", contains high levels of amelogenin-related proteins (95%), mixed with propylene glycol alginate (PGA) as carrier which may have by itself an anti-bacterial action [60]. Used as capping agent on exposed human pulps, EMD induces pulp healing. There is still a debate on the robustness of the dentinal bridges observed by some clinicians, while others do not consider the beneficial effects of EMD as superior to $Ca(OH)_2$ [61-63]. It is not known whether A+4 and/or A-4 are part of "Emdogain" since the precise molecular identity of the amelogenin derivatives included in this material are not described.

Amelogenin full-length protein (25-23kDa) is able to self-aggregate, thus giving rise to nanospheres, which are recovered in the ECM and becomes substrates of several specific proteases of the matrix [64]. Some of these proteases are also present in "Emdogain" that is extracted from enamel matrix. Thus, diverse polypeptides or peptides are known to derive from the sequential proteolytic processing of amelogenin [65]. They are released from the insoluble amelogenin assemblies. Are they acting as active biomolecules or are they only degradation products? At least one of the amelogenin domains, the tyrosine–rich amelogenin peptide (TRAP, 5kDa) is candidate as functional peptide [66].

Amelogenin is recognized for its positive influence on ECM dentin mineralization, and therefore the questions remain as to whether amelogenins have a role in ECM matrix assembly and mineral deposition, or do they interact, as ligands, on some target cells, stem cells or odontoblasts, and modulate their functions. Thus a major challenge in analyzing the effects of Emdogain is to distinguish the true functional bioactive molecules among various amelogenin derivatives. Certainly, A+4 and A-4, which are not proteolytic amelogenin have been shown by many investigators to have signaling actions [47].

LAMP-1, LAMP-2 or LAMP 3 have been identified as putative receptors of both the full length amelogenin and A-4 splice product [48, 49, 67]. Since these receptors, and in particular LAMP1, have been localized in the Golgi apparatus, this raise the questions of the actual site of action of these amelogenin products and of the mechanisms leading to their putative internalization. The signaling impact and the potential involvement of A+4/A-4 in the intracellular trafficking are presently under investigation by different research groups.

Many questions arise from these experiments focused on the function of A+4 and A-4 on pulp healing, however the data establish unambiguously that these two amelogenin gene splice products could be used as putative biomolecules can promote pulp healing in rat molars.

What remains to be clarified is whether the progenitors that are rapidly recruited byA+4/A-4 (mobilized within 24h cells) and are induced towards an osteogenic fate, are the progenies of dividing stem cells. However, the temporo-spatial distribution of PCNA versus RP59/OPN positive cells suggests that such might be the case. The superimposed rings of recruited mitotic cells and of the osteoblastic cells formed around the beads are puzzling and raise the same questions concerning the affiliation between stem cells and mineralizing cells. Such an encircling of beads was neither observed in the control group (beads alone), or with others biomolecules such as BMP7, and thus suggests that these are precursor cells responsive to A+4/A-4 that exist within the pulp. Moreover, they suggest that the introduction of exogenous A+4/A-4 within the pulp may attract target cells and even exert an influence on their spatial distribution or migration, which may be important for the modeling of the reparative/new, formed mineral scaffold. Still unsolved questions raised by the data concern (i) the niche(s) and the identity of these osteoblastic-like precursor cells which are recruited in the central part of the pulp and (ii) the nature of the signaling mechanisms underlying A+4/A-4-related effects.

In summary, the use of A+4 and A-4 as capping biomolecules in the rat molar has led to promising results for dentin regeneration. For both proteins, the inflammatory reaction was minimal (as in the sham group). The effects on ECM mineralization are restricted to the pulp. As compared with $Ca(OH)_2$ or others biomolecules, the homogeneity of the dentinal bridge predicts a true protective effect against bacteria re-colonization.

Of interest, each protein displays its own specificity to promote an expected responsiveness of pulpal cells depending on the severity of injuries. A+4 may substitute the use of traditional mineral-based capping agents ($Ca(OH)_2$, MTA) by triggering the construction of a reparative dentinal bridge in the coronal pulpal one. Conversely, A-4 may be an alternative to endodontic treatments by sealing the tooth from the crown to the apex, or in case of a necrotic pulp, after eliminating infected pulp remnants within the root canal, the molecule may promote the formation of an engineered new pulp.

A+4 and A-4 have distinct functional properties. They differ by 14 amino acids, which confer a higher polarity and charge density on the [A+4], may interfere in the folding of the proteins or sustain differential post-translational modifications (namely phosphorylation and glycosylation). Up to now, little has been done to characterize the structure-function relationship of the amelogenin isoforms [68].

On the therapeutical side, A+4 and A-4 each contributes to the formation of a thick dentinal bridge in the coronal part. In addition, A-4 induces a more diffuse mineralization in the mesial pulp chamber, and promotes a profuse mineralized ECM formation within the radicular pulp.

A new biodentistry, focused on a better knowledge of these biomolecules, may increase the efficiency of tooth reparation and replace material-based therapies by innovative biomimetical approaches recruiting pulpal resident stem cells.

ACKNOWLEDGEMENTS

We wish to thank our technical staff, especially Dominique Septier, our PhD students (Ngampis Six, Nadège Jegat and Frank Decup), the Fondation de l'Avenir for the financial support attributed in 2007 and 2008, and an INSERM/CNRS grant (Réseau cellules souches adultes).

REFERENCES

[1] Sjogren U, Hagglund B, Sundqvist G, *et al.* Factors affecting the long-term results of endodontic treatment. J Endod 1990;16(10):498-504.

[2] Ng YL, Mann V, Gulabivala K. Outcome of secondary root canal treatment: a systematic review of the literature. Int Endod J 2008;41(12):1026-46.

[3] Barthel CR, Rosenkranz B, Leuenberg A, *et al.* Pulp capping of carious exposures: treatment outcome after 5 and 10 years: a retrospective study. J Endod 2000;26(9):525-8.

[4] Al-Hiyasat AS, Barrieshi-Nusair KM, Al-Omari MA. The radiographic outcomes of direct pulp-capping procedures performed by dental students: a retrospective study. J Am Dent Assoc 2006;137(12):1699-705.

[5] Lesot H, Begue-Kirn C, Kubler MD, *et al.* Experimental induction of odontoblast differentiation and stimulation during reparative processes. Cells Mat 1993(3):201-217.

[6] Goldberg M, Smith AJ. Cells And Extracellular Matrices Of Dentin And Pulp: A Biological Basis For Repair And Tissue Engineering. Crit Rev Oral Biol Med 2004;15(1):13-27.

[7] Takagi Y, Sasaki S. Histological distribution of phosphophoryn in normal and pathological human dentins. J Oral Pathol 1986;15(9):463-7.
[8] Rahima M, Tsay TG, Andujar M, *et al.* Localization of phosphophoryn in rat incisor dentin using immunocytochemical techniques. J Histochem Cytochem 1988;36(2):153-7.
[9] MacDougall M, Slavkin HC, Zeichner-David M. Characteristics of phosphorylated and non-phosphorylated dentine phosphoprotein. Biochem J 1992;287 (Pt 2):651-5.
[10] Gronthos S, Mankani M, Brahim J, *et al.* Postnatal human dental pulp stem cells (DPSCs) in vitro and in vivo. Proc Natl Acad Sci U S A 2000;97(25):13625-30.
[11] Pierdomenico L, Bonsi L, Calvitti M, *et al.* Multipotent mesenchymal stem cells with immunosuppressive activity can be easily isolated from dental pulp. Transplantation 2005;80(6):836-42.
[12] Miura M, Gronthos S, Zhao M, *et al.* SHED: stem cells from human exfoliated deciduous teeth. Proc Natl Acad Sci U S A 2003;100(10):5807-12.
[13] Iohara K, Zheng L, Ito M, *et al.* Side population cells isolated from porcine dental pulp tissue with self-renewal and multipotency for dentinogenesis, chondrogenesis, adipogenesis, and neurogenesis. Stem Cells 2006;24(11):2493-503.
[14] Hermann BW. Dentinobliteration der wurtzelkanale nach behandlung mit calcium. Zahnartzl Rdsch 1930(39):887–899.
[15] Zander HA. Reaction of the pulp to calcium hydroxide. J Dent Res 1939(18):373-9.
[16] Glass RL, Zander HA. Pulp healing. J Dent Res 1949;28(2):97-107.
[17] Schroder U. Effects of calcium hydroxide-containing pulp-capping agents on pulp cell migration, proliferation, and differentiation. J Dent Res 1985;64 Spec No:541-8.
[18] Alliot-Licht B, Jean A, Gregoire M. Comparative effect of calcium hydroxide and hydroxyapatite on the cellular activity of human pulp fibroblasts in vitro. Arch Oral Biol 1994;39(6):481-9.
[19] Tziafas D, Kolokuris I, Alvanou A, *et al.* Short-term dentinogenic response of dog dental pulp tissue after its induction by demineralized or native dentine, or predentine. Arch Oral Biol 1992;37(2):119-28.
[20] Tziafas D, Alvanou A, Panagiotakopoulos N, *et al.* Induction of odontoblast-like cell differentiation in dog dental pulps after in vivo implantation of dentine matrix components. Arch Oral Biol 1995;40(10):883-93.
[21] Heikinheimo K, Begue-Kirn C, Ritvos O, *et al.* Activin and bone morphogenetic protein (BMP) signalling during tooth development. Eur J Oral Sci 1998;106 Suppl 1:167-73.
[22] Nakashima M. The induction of reparative dentine in the amputated dental pulp of the dog by bone morphogenetic protein. Arch Oral Biol 1990;35(7):493-7.
[23] Nakashima M. Induction of dentin formation on canine amputated pulp by recombinant human bone morphogenetic proteins (BMP)-2 and -4. J Dent Res 1994;73(9):1515-22.
[24] Rutherford RB, Spangberg L, Tucker M, *et al.* The time-course of the induction of reparative dentine formation in monkeys by recombinant human osteogenic protein-1. Arch Oral Biol 1994;39(10):833-8.
[25] Rutherford RB, Wahle J, Tucker M, *et al.* Induction of reparative dentine formation in monkeys by recombinant human osteogenic protein-1. Arch Oral Biol 1993;38(7):571-6.
[26] Six N, Lasfargues JJ, Goldberg M. Differential repair responses in the coronal and radicular areas of the exposed rat molar pulp induced by recombinant human bone morphogenetic protein 7 (osteogenic protein 1). Arch Oral Biol 2002;47(3):177-87.
[27] Takahashi K. Vascular architecture of dog pulp using corrosion resin cast examined under a scanning electron microscope. J Dent Res 1985;64 Spec No:579-84.
[28] Wang J, Glimcher MJ, Mah J, *et al.* Expression of bone microsomal casein kinase II, bone sialoprotein, and osteopontin during the repair of calvarial defects. Bone 1998;22(6):621-8.
[29] Wang J, Zhou HY, Salih E, *et al.* Site-specific in vivo calcification and osteogenesis stimulated by bone sialoprotein. Calcif Tissue Int 2006;79(3):179-89.
[30] Decup F, Six N, Palmier B, *et al.* Bone sialoprotein-induced reparative dentinogenesis in the pulp of rat's molar. Clin Oral Investig 2000;4(2):110-9.
[31] Six N, Septier D, Chaussain-Miller C, *et al.* Dentonin, a MEPE fragment, initiates pulp-healing response to injury. J Dent Res 2007;86(8):780-5.
[32] Cox CF, Bergenholtz G, Fitzgerald M, *et al.* Capping of the dental pulp mechanically exposed to the oral microflora -- a 5 week observation of wound healing in the monkey. J Oral Pathol 1982;11(4):327-39.
[33] Oguntebi B, Clark A, Wilson J. Pulp capping with Bioglass and autologous demineralized dentin in miniature swine. J Dent Res 1993;72(2):484-9.

[34] Tziafas D, Alvanou A, Papadimitriou S, *et al.* Effects of recombinant basic fibroblast growth factor, insulin-like growth factor-II and transforming growth factor-beta 1 on dog dental pulp cells in vivo. Arch Oral Biol 1998;43(6):431-44.
[35] Smith AJ, Tobias RS, Cassidy N, *et al.* Odontoblast stimulation in ferrets by dentine matrix components. Arch Oral Biol 1994;39(1):13-22.
[36] Six N, Lasfargues JJ, Goldberg M. In vivo study of the pulp reaction to Fuji IX, a glass ionomer cement. J Dent 2000;28(6):413-22.
[37] Lacerda-Pinheiro S, Marchadier A, Donas P, *et al.* An In vivo Model for Short-Term Evaluation of the Implantation Effects of Biomolecules or Stem Cells in the Dental Pulp. Open Dent J 2008;2:67-72.
[38] Ohshima H. Ultrastructural changes in odontoblasts and pulp capillaries following cavity preparation in rat molars. Arch Histol Cytol 1990;53(4):423-38.
[39] Six N, Tompkins K, Septier D, *et al.* Recruitment and characterization of the cells involved in reparative dentin formation in the exposed rat molar pulp after implantation of amelogenin gene splice products A+4 and A-4. Oral Biosciences & Medicine 2004(1):35-44.
[40] Amar S, Sires B, Sabsay B, *et al.* The isolation and partial characterization of a rat incisor dentin matrix polypeptide with in vitro chondrogenic activity. J Biol Chem 1991;266(13):8609-18.
[41] Nebgen DR, Inoue H, Sabsay B, *et al.* Identification of the chondrogenic-inducing activity from bovine dentin (bCIA) as a low-molecular-mass amelogenin polypeptide. J Dent Res 1999;78(9):1484-94.
[42] Veis A, Tompkins K, Alvares K, *et al.* Specific amelogenin gene splice products have signaling effects on cells in culture and in implants in vivo. J Biol Chem 2000;275(52):41263-72.
[43] Fincham AG, Moradian-Oldak J, Simmer JP. The structural biology of the developing dental enamel matrix. J Struct Biol 1999;126(3):270-99.
[44] Tompkins K, Veis A. Polypeptides translated from alternatively spliced transcripts of the amelogenin gene, devoid of the exon 6a, b, c region, have specific effects on tooth germ development in culture. Connect Tissue Res 2002;43(2-3):224-31.
[45] Iacob S, Veis A. Identification of temporal and spatial expression patterns of amelogenin isoforms during mouse molar development. Eur J Oral Sci 2006;114 Suppl 1:194-200; discussion 201-2, 381.
[46] Bourd-Boittin K, Septier D, Hall R, *et al.* Immunolocalization of enamelysin (matrix metalloproteinase-20) in the forming rat incisor. J Histochem Cytochem 2004;52(4):437-45.
[47] Veis A. Amelogenin gene splice products: potential signaling molecules. Cell Mol Life Sci 2003;60(1):38-55.
[48] Tompkins K, George A, Veis A. Characterization of a mouse amelogenin [A-4]/M59 cell surface receptor. Bone 2006;38(2):172-80.
[49] Shapiro JL, Wen X, Okamoto CT, *et al.* Cellular uptake of amelogenin, and its localization to CD63, and Lamp1-positive vesicles. Cell Mol Life Sci 2007;64(2):244-56.
[50] Foster BL, Somerman MJ. Regenerating the periodontium: is there a magic formula? Orthod Craniofac Res 2005;8(4):285-91.
[51] Khouri RK, Koudsi B, Reddi H. Tissue transformation into bone in vivo. A potential practical application. Jama 1991;266(14):1953-5.
[52] Lacerda-Pinheiro S, Septier D, Tompkins K, *et al.* Amelogenin gene splice products A+4 and A-4 implanted in soft tissue determine the reorientation of CD45-positive cells to an osteo-chondrogenic lineage. J Biomed Mater Res A 2006;79(4):1015-22.
[53] Keila S, Nemcovsky CE, Moses O, *et al.* In vitro effects of enamel matrix proteins on rat bone marrow cells and gingival fibroblasts. J Dent Res 2004;83(2):134-8.
[54] Van der Pauw MT, Van den Bos T, Everts V, *et al.* Enamel matrix-derived protein stimulates attachment of periodontal ligament fibroblasts and enhances alkaline phosphatase activity and transforming growth factor beta1 release of periodontal ligament and gingival fibroblasts. J Periodontol 2000;71(1):31-43.
[55] Jegat N, Septier D, Veis A, *et al.* Short-term effects of amelogenin gene splice products A+4 and A-4 implanted in the exposed rat molar pulp. Head Face Med 2007;3:40.
[56] Carlucci MJ, Scolaro LA, Errea MI, *et al.* Antiviral activity of natural sulphated galactans on herpes virus multiplication in cell culture. Planta Med 1997;63(5):429-32.
[57] Melo FR, Pereira MS, Foguel D, *et al.* Antithrombin-mediated anticoagulant activity of sulfated polysaccharides: different mechanisms for heparin and sulfated galactans. J Biol Chem 2004;279(20):20824-35.

[58] Kruger A, Ellerstrom C, Lundmark C, *et al.* RP59, a marker for osteoblast recruitment, is also detected in primitive mesenchymal cells, erythroid cells, and megakaryocytes. Dev Dyn 2002;223(3):414-8.

[59] Ogbureke KU, Fisher LW. Renal expression of SIBLING proteins and their partner matrix metalloproteinases (MMPs). Kidney Int 2005;68(1):155-66.

[60] Arweiler NB, Auschill TM, Donos N, *et al.* Antibacterial effect of an enamel matrix protein derivative on in vivo dental biofilm vitality. Clin Oral Investig 2002;6(4):205-9.

[61] Nakamura Y, Hammarstrom L, Lundberg E, *et al.* Enamel matrix derivative promotes reparative processes in the dental pulp. Adv Dent Res 2001;15:105-7.

[62] Igarashi R, Sahara T, Shimizu-Ishiura M, *et al.* Porcine enamel matrix derivative enhances the formation of reparative dentine and dentine bridges during wound healing of amputated rat molars. J Electron Microsc (Tokyo) 2003;52(2):227-36.

[63] Olsson H, Davies JR, Holst KE, *et al.* Dental pulp capping: effect of Emdogain Gel on experimentally exposed human pulps. Int Endod J 2005;38(3):186-94.

[64] Moradian-Oldak J, Jimenez I, Maltby D, *et al.* Controlled proteolysis of amelogenins reveals exposure of both carboxy- and amino-terminal regions. Biopolymers 2001;58(7):606-16.

[65] Robinson C, Brookes SJ, Shore RC, *et al.* The developing enamel matrix: nature and function. Eur J Oral Sci 1998;106 Suppl 1:282-91.

[66] Dunglas C, Septier D, Paine ML, *et al.* Ultrastructure of forming enamel in mouse bearing a transgene that disrupts the amelogenin self-assembly domains. Calcif Tissue Int 2002;71(2):155-66.

[67] Gruenbaum-Cohen Y, Tucker AS, Haze A, *et al.* Amelogenin in cranio-facial development: the tooth as a model to study the role of amelogenin during embryogenesis. J Exp Zool B Mol Dev Evol 2009;312B(5):445-57.

[68] Uversky VN. Protein folding revisited. A polypeptide chain at the folding-misfolding-nonfolding cross-roads: which way to go? Cell Mol Life Sci 2003;60(9):1852-71.

CHAPTER 15

Cell to Matrix Interactions Suggests a Pathway for Enamel Regeneration Using Artificial Matrices

M.L. Snead[1], Z. Huang[1], C.J. Newcomb[3], M.L. Paine[1], S.N. White [2]Y. Xu[1], Y. Zhou[1], R. S. Lacruz[1] and S.I. Stupp[3,4,5].

[1]*The Center for Craniofacial Molecular Biology, University of Southern California, Los Angeles CA;* [2]*University of California, School of Dentistry, Los Angeles, CA;* [3]*Department of Materials Science and Engineering, Institute for BioNanotechnology in Medicine, Northwestern University, Chicago, IL;* [4]*Department of Chemistry, Northwestern University, Evanston, IL and* [5]*Department of Medicine, Northwestern University, Chicago, IL.*

Abstract: The developing tooth is a well-recognized model for epithelial-mesenchyme organ formation. It is also a model for biomineralization, in which the formation of several unique bioceramic tissues, dentine, enamel and cementum are formed by the influence exerted by the protein matrix on their mineral habit. Enamel is the only ectodermal derived tissue to biomineralize and demonstrates several informative strategies to meet the requirement to produce a tissue that last a lifetime in a wet, bacterial laden environment subjected to the stresses associated with food ingestion. Enamel formation is dependent upon protein self-assembly to fabricate a precursor protein matrix to direct the mineral phase. Cell to matrix interactions are used to continuously monitor matrix fabrication and the mineral conversion process. We demonstrate the use of an artificial matrix created by nanotechology in which peptide amphiphiles undergo self-assembly into nanofibers that support cell proliferation and whose surfaces can be engineered to present biological signals to direct ameloblast differentiation. This biologically inspired technology may be used for regeneration of enamel tissue, offering a biomimetic alternative to traditional dental materials.

Key Words: Biomineralization, Bioceramic, Enamel, Protein Self-Assembly, Nanotechnology, Nanofibers, Enamel Regeneréation.

INTRODUCTION

The developing tooth is a well-recognized model for epithelial-mesenchyme organ formation that has been used to identify reciprocal-signals exchanged between the ectoderm-derived epithelia (ameloblasts) and the neuroectoderm-derived mesenchyme (odontoblasts) that determine cell fate, morphogenesis and terminal differentiation [1-3]. Here, our attention is focused on signals that are maintained during late stages of development, occurring at or near birth and continuing into postnatal life, a time when cell to matrix interactions dominate the fabrication of the enamel bioceramic material. For this reason, we will focus on the matrix and upon amelogenin, the most abundant protein found in the developing enamel matrix. We examine how disruptions in cell to matrix interactions can be leveraged to provide a pathway for enamel regeneration using a nanofabricated artificial matrix. Based on the use of an instructional artificial matrix to achieve either a cell-based or a cell-free enamel biomimetic we provide a translational avenue for enamel regeneration.

Amelogenin has been shown to be essential for control over enamel biomineral habit [4]. The tissue covering vertebrate teeth is enamel. Enamel is the only ectoderm-derived bioceramic tissue in the mammalian body. Enamel contains no collagen and initially consists of a self-organizing protein matrix that guides the mineral phase. Enamel tissue does not remodel and errors made in protein matrix assembly are converted into uncorrectable errors in the mineral phase with consequential loss of material properties. Enamel formation occurs in the extracellular space, a physical location making direct cellular intervention difficult. As a consequence, unique cell strategies have evolved to control the quality and quantity of the proteins that contribute to the self-assembly of the matrix. It has become clear that a poorly formed protein matrix can only give rise to a poorly formed mineral phase that fails prematurely with severe consequences to feeding. Enamel is a hierarchical tissue dependent upon the integration of scale features, from protein-to-protein interaction at the nanoscale, upward to the scale feature of cells and tissue formation. The sum of errors in matrix biosynthesis and conversion to biomineral can be measured by evaluating changes in the material properties of the mature enamel tissue [5-7]. We propose to use the hierarchical feature of enamel to our advantage by regenerating enamel through the application of a self-assembling artificial matrix that mimics the properties of the native matrix and in turn, influences cell behavior.

Mature enamel is the hardest tissue in the vertebrate body, but during its formation, it is a typical living tissue composed of cells that secrete a complex extracellular matrix and with the need for cell to matrix interactions to operationalize cellular functions [8,9]. Enamel begins as a 100% protein extracellular matrix, with amelogenin being the most abundant protein (Figure 1). Self-assembly of the enamel proteins serves to create a matrix that can guide its own replacement by the hydroxyapatite mineral phase [4, 10-12]. In a matter of only days, the enamel covered rodent tooth erupts into the oral cavity, only now the enamel contains less than 0.5% protein [13]. Upon eruption, the ameloblast cells have completed their function to synthesize, assemble and convert the protein matrix into a tissue capable of withstanding a lifetime of mastication. Unlike bone, enamel cannot remodel and the ameloblasts cease to exist upon eruption so there are no second chances to correct defects inherent to matrix production or to cell to matrix interactions.

At the start of enamel formation, the ameloblasts exit the cell cycle and soon thereafter express enamel matrix proteins, such as amelogenin, ameloblastin and other structural proteins [10, 12]. Ameloblasts also serve to regulate the mineral phase by expressing several ion transporters [14]. Along with these biosynthetic processes, the ameloblasts are simultaneously responsible for the re-absorption of degraded enamel matrix protein during mineral replacement [15-17]. These complicated production steps require the ameloblasts to remain precisely orchestrated with a specific segment of the forming matrix [8]. Cell to matrix interactions are accomplished by linking one ameloblast to one enamel rod (aka, prism), the basic subunit of enamel (Figure 1 & 2) [18]. Each rod is the product of a single ameloblast, directed in movement by its secretion of matrix proteins outward from its initial position where it lay on top of the dentine tissue. The cell stays in contact with its specific cylinder of assembled matrix proteins during a migration of a thousand and more micrometers. Exactly how ameloblasts remain in perfect registration over a single rod of newly formed enamel matrix while simultaneously synthesizing, degrading and converting the protein matrix into mineral is poorly understood, but represents an essential function needed to produce enamel.

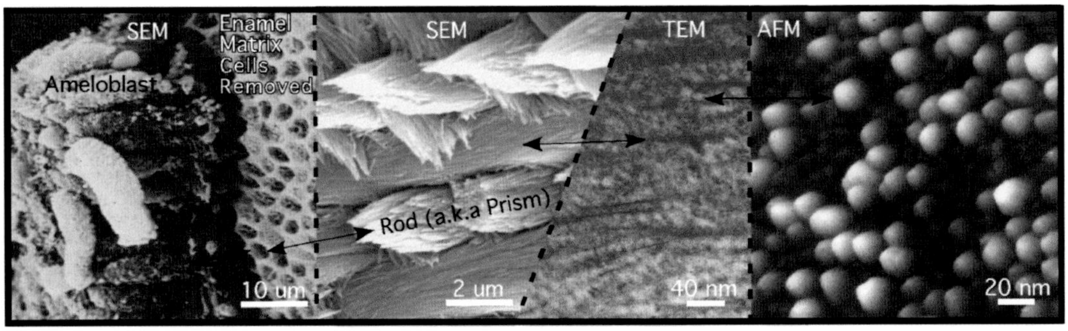

Figure 1: Enamel is a scale-dependent, hierarchically constructed tissue. Ameloblast cells control each step of amelogenesis, from synthesis of proteins that self-assemble at the nanoscale (two right panels) to organizing these molecules into a matrix cylinder at the mesoscale (two left panels). The cylinder of matrix is responsible for guiding mineral replacement and gives rise to the structure of the final enamel tissue known as an enamel rod. The bi-directional arrows denote connections between distinct structures or subscale structures of the hierarchical tissue. Abbreviations: SEM, scanning electron microscopy; TEM, transmission electron microscopy; AFM, atomic force microscopy). Corresponding scale bars are shown.

ENAMEL MATRIX FORMATION: CELL TO MATRIX INTERACTIONS

Enamel is the remarkable bioceramic composite covering the vertebrate tooth. Differentiated ameloblast cells synthesize the protein mixture that guides mineral formation. The enamel extracellular matrix is composed principally of amelogenin protein, with modest contributions from ameloblastin, enamelin, tuftelin, amelotin [20,21] and sulfated proteins [22]. Ameloblast differentiation requires that the inner enamel epithelia receive a cascade of signals that take the form of growth factors, cell adhesion molecules, and extracellular matrix molecules. These instructive signals culminate in activating transcription factors that initiate enamel gene expression [23,24]. Polarized ameloblasts synthesize and secrete the enamel matrix into the space previously occupied by the basement membrane, moving away from the basement membrane [25]. The first wave of enamel matrix protein biosynthesis constitutes the dentine enamel junction (DEJ), a "specialized" enamel that links two dissimilar bioceramic tissues, enamel and dentine [6, 26]. These interactions occur during late embryonic and early postnatal development, at a developmental time well-after ameloblast determination and differentiation. In this review, we focus on the molecular pathways used by the ameloblasts to retain their physical location over the sea of enamel matrix proteins. Changes to the ability of the ameloblast to interact with the matrix can disrupt enamel formation. The consequence of such disruptions are observed in apparently unrelated human diseases such as epidermolysis bullosa [27, 28], hypofunction of integrin subunits [29, 30] or hypofunction of the cognate ligands of integrins such as ameloblastin [31] or laminin [32], as well as by design using genetically altered mice [32-34].

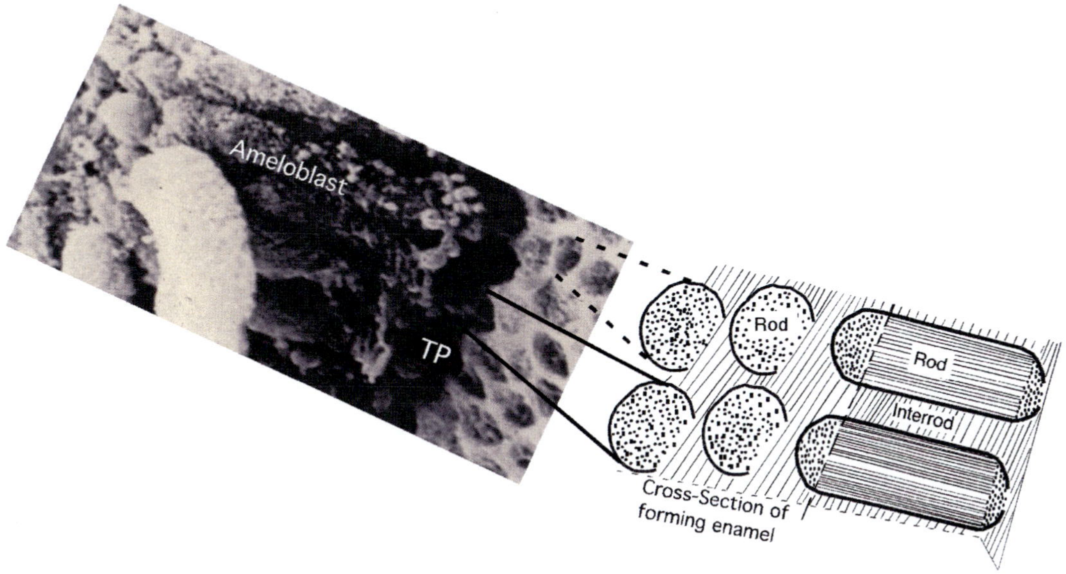

Figure 2: Cell to matrix interactions. The SEM image of ameloblasts and newly formed enamel matrix (with selected cells removed to reveal the underlying extracellular enamel matrix) show Tomes' processes (TP) embedded in a pit formed by the enamel matrix accumulated between adjacent Tomes' processes. The pit and the matrix surrounding each pit correspond to the enamel rod. The specialized cell membrane comprising Tomes' processes secrete and reabsorb the enamel matrix proteins. Tomes processes and receptors embedded therein are responsible for maintaining cell to matrix interactions with the underlying proteins assembled in the enamel extracellular matrix.

Ameloblasts secrete the enamel matrix through a specialized segment of their membrane termed the Tomes' process, with one ameloblast cell responsible for the formation of one enamel rod (Figure 2). One can envision the ameloblast secreting a cylinder of enamel matrix, approximately the same diameter as the ameloblast, starting at dentine and extending outward towards the future chewing surface of the enamel, like a tube of toothpaste being squeezed. A precise cell to matrix registration is preserved over the entire path of secretion, a distance measuring hundreds to thousands of micrometers in length. The design of enamel revolves around the spatial organization of these matrix cylinders one to another. The ameloblasts weave cylinders of enamel matrix proteins so that they coalesce on their inferior surface, producing a linkage between each rod of matrix, called by some, the interrod enamel. The unique biomechanical properties of the final mineralized enamel are believed to be dependent upon the weaving of these matrix cylinders and their coalescence to form the interrod enamel [5, 35]. Within each rod, thousands of substituted hydroxyapatite crystallites form, first as thin crystallites surrounded by amelogenin nanospheres that promote growth along the crystal ends increasing their length (Figure 1) [36, 37]. With time, enamel matrix proteinases degrade the matrix while the crystallites grow in thickness. Eventually, the crystallites lie adjacent to one another in the space previously occupied by the enamel matrix proteins [16, 38, 39].

Amelogenin undergoes self-assembly to form nanospheres and, along with other enamel proteins, self-organizes outside of the ameloblasts as an extracellular matrix. If assembled properly, this matrix is competent to orchestrate its own replacement by the mineral phase. The ameloblast first creates a 100% organic enamel extracellular matrix that initiates enamel formation, although ultimately this extracellular matrix is converted to greater than 99.5% inorganic hydroxyapatite crystals [10, 12, 13, 40]. This metamorphosis is not achieved in a single step, but rather by a continuum of incremental steps in which amelogenin undergoes precisely regulated proteolytic degradation and is almost fully removed during mineral replacement and maturation. The resultant approximation of the nanoscale crystallites at the mesoscale produces the enamel rod. In rodents, the rod "threads" are woven in a continuum by ameloblast movement (see figures 1 and 2). This coalescence of hierarchical structure is the principal reasons for the unique materials properties of enamel that allows it to last a lifetime [5]. To achieve this integration, ameloblasts use incremental steps of matrix production [24], followed by protein degradation coupled to mineral growth. The delay between the soft matrix precursor conversion to mineral product allows the cells to guide the weaving of the mineral phase [5]. This production process implies the necessity to maintain a linkage between the ameloblast with the enamel matrix throughout its creation.

AMELOGENIN DOMAINS

The evolutionary analysis by Sire and colleagues [41] and Kawasaki and Weiss [42, 43] point out the highly conserved amelogenin domains located at the amino- and carboxyl-termini (Figure 3, underline). The putative origin of the amelogenin gene has been traced back 630 million years ago to the Precambrian period [44, 45], with these authors identifying a conserved amino-terminal domain. We have focused on the conserved amino acid sequences, showing that the two conserved domains located at the amino- and carboxyl-terminus of M180 amelogenin (see figure 3) are responsible for molecular self-assembly of the protein into nanospheres [46, 47]. Removal of these self-assembly domains from amelogenin in a genetic knock-in mouse results in profound defects to enamel formation, with the ameloblasts loosing cell to matrix interaction signals, detaching from the matrix and re-entering the cell cycle in animals lacking residues 1-42 of the full length M180 protein [34, 48].

Lyngstadaas [49, 50] used ribozymes to target all amelogenin mRNAs expressed in developing mouse teeth resulting in a transient loss of amelogenin mRNA and protein. During the recovery of the ameloblasts from ribozyme treatment the ameloblasts transiently over-compensated amelogenin mRNA levels to values greater than their non-ribozyme treated counterpart. This finding suggests that ameloblasts maintain interactions with the enamel matrix over time, continuously sampling amelogenin abundance and, in this case, compensate for the loss of amelogenin protein in the enamel matrix by increasing amelogenin transcription.

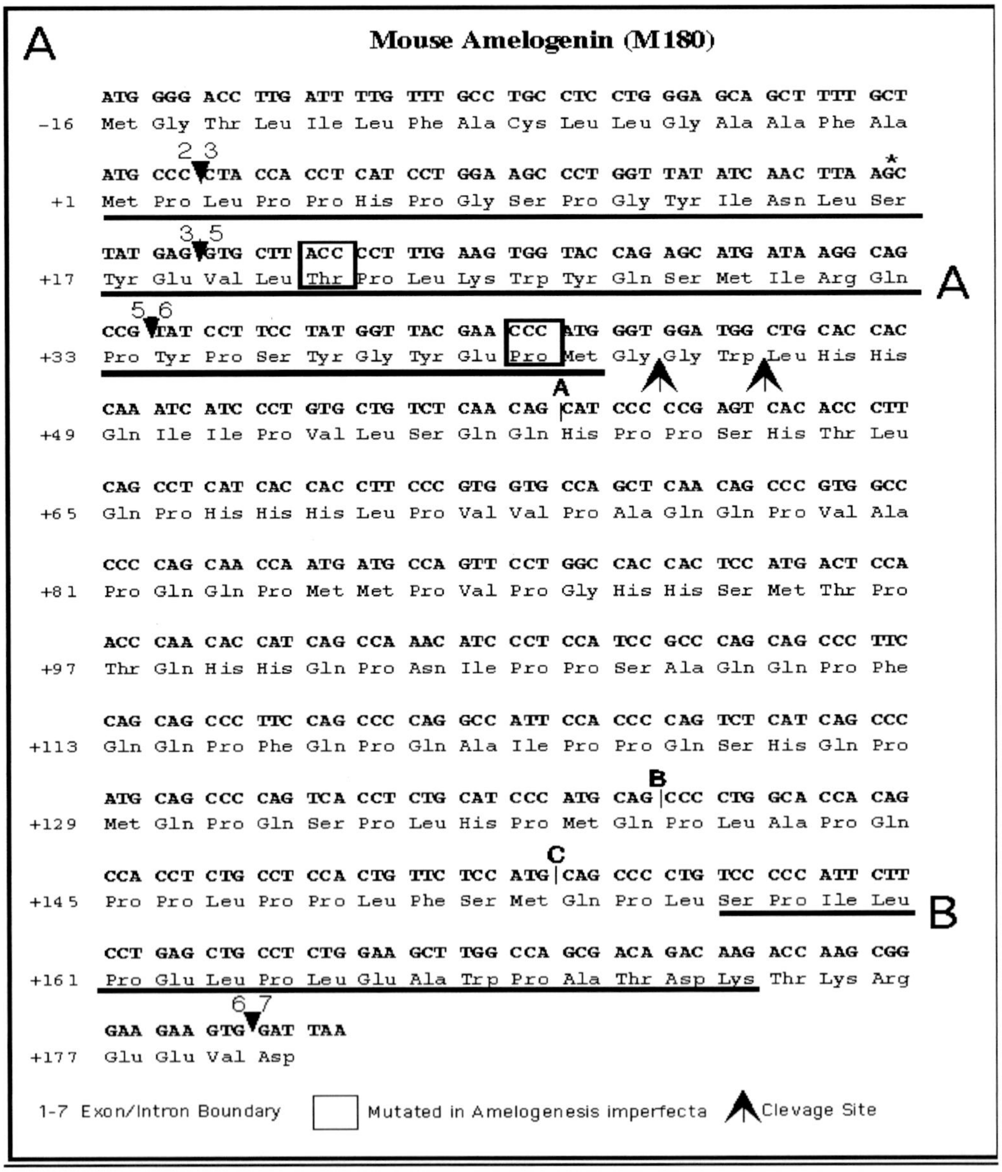

Figure 3: The dominant protein of the forming murine enamel matrix is the 180 amino acids long amelogenin (M180). The highly conserved amino- ("A") and the carboxyl ("B")-terminal domain (underlined) are required for amelogenin self-assembly. Phenocopying the amino acid mutations (boxes) found in *amelogenesis imperfecta* results in amelogenin that also fail to self-assemble into nanospheres. The exon-intron splice junctions (numbered arrowheads) and proteolytic cleavage sites (arrows) are shown. Additional exons and introns have been reported [55].

Enamel thickness is also regulated, stopping at a specific thickness during its development, although the molecular pathway for this regulation is unknown. One potential pathway for generating a signal to "stop" enamel formation is the acquisition by the ameloblasts of the enamel matrix degradation peptides that are reabsorbed by ameloblasts as they interact with the forming matrix [17]. One candidate protein serving as this signal is the tyrosine rich amelogenin peptide (TRAP) that accumulates in maturing enamel [51, 52]. TRAP is similar in sequence to the leucine rich amelogenin peptide (LRAP) except that LRAP is a unique, alternatively spliced mRNA that encodes a separate amelogenin isoform, a fact insightfully suggested by Sasaki in 1984 (see page 201 of reference [53]). This unique origin was latter proven at the molecular level by Gibson and colleagues [54]. LRAP has also been shown to manifests cell-signaling capacity, inducing the differentiation of naïve cells to osteogenic lineage and peridodontal lineage by activating the Wnt signaling pathway [56, 57] (see also the section by Zhou, et. al., this E-book). TRAP has been previously defined as residues 1-45 of the mouse 180 amino acid amelogenin protein [58]. LRAP alone has the ability to alter cell fate and to promote osteogenic fates in other wise naïve cells, but the mechanism(s) responsible for this change in fate was not known [59-65]. Recently, LRAP has been shown to activate the Wnt-signaling pathway, shifting naïve cell fates to osteogenic lineages [56, 66].

Nanci and co-workers found that mineral deposition occurs some distance away from the site of secretion at the Tomes' process of ameloblasts [67]. In this mineral-free zone, enamel matrix proteins undergo assembly into a matrix competent to guide the mineral habit which is as long, thin crystallites aligned along their c'-axis (long axis) parallel to the path of ameloblast movement. Recall that the matrix at this stage is not fully mineralized, but rather it is in the form of a hydrated protein gel. The ameloblasts hover over this gel, with the Tomes' process embedded in the gel. Each ameloblast retains a relationship between one ameloblast and one cylinder of enamel matrix defining the enamel rod (Figures 1, 2 & 4). It is not known what molecules are located on the Tomes' processes that retain the ameloblast over its secreted cylinder of protein matrix, although several candidate proteins for this function are described herein.

AMELOBLASTIN

Ameloblastin is the second most abundant protein in the developing enamel matrix. Fukomoto and colleagues [68] explored the role of ameloblastin in regulating mineral transformation of the matrix by engineering an ameloblastin knock-out mouse. In the absence of ameloblastin they report that ameloblasts lose contact with the matrix mediated through integrin a6, increase their expression levels of Msx2 and p75, reduce their expression of p27, and re-enter the cell cycle to become multi-layered. Recently, Sonoda and colleagues have shown that the carboxyl-terminal end of ameloblastin contains several heparin-binding domains essential for ameloblast proliferation and differentiation [69]. However, an alternative interpretation for their observations on the ameloblastin-null animal includes the reduced abundance of amelogenin protein. Teeth from their ameloblastin knock-out animal confirmed the absence of ameloblastin mRNA but also showed a significantly reduced amelogenin mRNA in 3-day postnatal knock-out molars by RT-PCR analysis [68]. Since amelogenin is more than 90% of the forming matrix, one can suggest that the ameloblastin knock-out enamel matrix also suffers from hypofunction of amelogenin (see Figure 3, Fukumoto et al., [68]) and that the ameloblasts re-enter cell division due to loss of signals generated by cell contact with amelogenin within the matrix. Based on our observations from the D1-42M180 knock-in mouse [34], we propose that the highly conserved amelogenin domain defined by residues 1-42 is required to maintain the differentiation state of the ameloblasts, making the D1-42M180 amelogenin knock-in animal a useful model to study ameloblast to matrix interactions. Wazen and colleagues unexpectedly found that the mouse ameloblastin knock-out animal expresses a truncated form of ameloblastin [70], rather than completely lacking the protein as previously described [68]. It is presently unclear if the truncated ameloblastin serves as a dominant negative, altering assembly of enamel matrix proteins or if another pathogenic mechanism serve to disrupt normal enamel formation as previously observed and reported.

INTEGRINS

Ameloblasts interact with the forming enamel matrix via receptors embedded in their Tomes' processes. Evidence suggests that Tomes' processes express members of the integrin family [30, 71], including a6, b2 and b4. These integrins are candidate molecules that could be used to maintain the registration of the ameloblast over the forming enamel matrix. We have recently shown that ameloblasts can interact with an artificial "RGD" domain found on nanofabricated peptide amphiphiles (RGD-PA) [72]. Here, when primary enamel organ epithelial cells from developing mouse teeth are embedded within a gel of RGD-PAs, we observe enhanced proliferation followed by differentiation demonstrated by increased expression of mRNAs encoding enamel matrix proteins. Similar changes to gene expression are observed among enamel organ epithelial cells at the site of microinjected RGD-PA into developing incisors [72]. We have determined that ameloblast cells grown in the RGD-PA up regulate their expression of a6-, a5- and b4-integrins. These integrins are present but at lower expression levels in the untreated control organs, supporting the notion that integrin mediated interactions between the ameloblast and the matrix occur during enamel formation [30, 71].

Data from Ryan et al., [32] also supports the notion that the integrin a6 expression by secretory ameloblasts is essential to enamel formation. In their defective animals they observed normal incisor development until the onset of enamel secretion, where failure of ameloblast function occurred specifically at the secretory stage of development [32]. Moreover, the observations of Wright and colleagues from their studies on the dentition of patients affected with epidermolysis bullosa similarly serve to support the requirement for cell to matrix interactions during enamel formation [27]. Fukumoto and colleagues examined the requirement for laminin a5 expression during tooth development by using antibodies to block a6b4 expression in E14.5 developing teeth, but they did not extend their studies into newborn stages where amelogenin is first expressed [23]. At this time, it is not possible to separate redundancy between laminin 5 and amelogenin as targets for maintaining ameloblast interactions with the underlying cylinder of matrix.

Nakamura and colleagues reported from their analysis of two unrelated families, that patients suffering from non-Herlitz junctional epidermolysis bullosa manifest skin blisters, skin atrophy and tooth enamel hypoplasia [28]. In the skin, the COL 17A1 protein promotes dermo-epidermal attachment and contributes to hemidesmosome formation and stability, parameters also important in ameloblast cell biology. Mutations in the COL17A1 gene resulted in the creation of premature stop codon resulting in the absence of immuno-detectable COL17A1 protein in the skin. In another patient, a premature stop codon resulted in a carboxyl-terminal truncation with reduced levels of the protein in the skin and a milder phenotype. However, the direct relationship of COL17A1 to ameloblast function remained untested. Studies by Asaka and colleagues directly tested the role of this protein by creating a Col17A1 null mouse using homologous gene targeting [73]. They demonstrated that the absence of Col17A resulted in poorly differentiated ameloblasts, as measured by reduced ameloblastin and amelogenin gene expression, as well as ameloblast failure to maintain a Tomes' process that is essential to proper enamel formation. Here again, the importance of cell to matrix interactions for amelogenesis and the maintenance of ameloblast cell differentiation are underscored.

Huang and colleagues [72] have produced images of integrin a6 localized to the Tomes' processes of wild-type mouse incisors. Here, it was shown that integrin a6 and b4 expression levels increase when either primary ameloblast cells or an ameloblast-like cell line are surrounded by an artificial matrix containing high levels of the "RGD"-domain. These ameloblast cells respond to the artificial matrix by also increasing amelogenin and ameloblastin mRNA expression levels after being grown in the artificial matrix for 24 hours [72]. In contrast, integrin a6b4 expression pattern changes dramatically in the Tomes' processes from D1-42M180 knock-in mice, suggesting that the matrix assembled with amelogenin lacking the amino terminal first 42 amino acids was defective in presenting epitopes that support integrin binding. Taken together, the data suggests that a bioactive artificial matrix could be used to stimulate ameloblast differentiation resulting in enhanced levels of enamel matrix formation.

CD63 AND LAMP1

In addition to integrins, several other proteins have been nominated as candidates for amelogenin receptors, including CD63 and LAMP1 [74]. Both CD63 and LAMP1 are located on the Tomes' process in direct contact with the forming enamel matrix. CD63 is a member of the tetraspanin family characterized by the presence of four transmembrane segments [75, 76]. The tetraspanin proteins mediate signal transduction events that play roles in the regulation of cell development, activation, growth and motility [77]. CD63, and other tetraspanins, are known to complex with integrins and act as organizers of membrane microdomains and signaling complexes [77, 78]. LAMP1 is a transmembrane protein highly expressed in late endosomes and lysosomes and is often used as a marker for these two organelles [79]. LAMP1 immunoreactivity is observed at the plasma membrane of ameloblasts and of organelles in the early endocytotic compartments [17] Zou and colleagues have provided a detailed molecular description for the interaction of LAMP1 with amelogenin and ameloblastin using a combination of recombinant DNA and protein expression techniques, coupled with bioinformatic predictions [80].

ENAMEL MATRIX STIFFNESS

The stiffness of the matrix with which cells interact has been shown to control a variety of functions from gene expression to cell division [81-84]. The self-assembly of amelogenin into nanospheres may be required to maintain a precise stiffness in the enamel extracellular matrix. The loss of amelogenin self-assembly as occurs in the D1-42M180 knock-in mouse may alter the matrix stiffness and serve to influence ameloblast gene expression and the control of cell division. Presently, no investigators have pursued the role of stiffness as an element that controls ameloblast behavior during enamel development. However, Cox has created a multiscale simulation of ameloblast migration during development that predicts the weaving of enamel rods observed in the mature enamel as an outcome dependent on the strain stimulus acting on the ameloblast population [85]. Creating a predictive model for enamel formation, a model in which specific cell behavior parameters can be varied and the resulting enamel architecture observed would be a useful tool for experimentalists interested in developmental and evolutionary biology of the dentition. Along these lines, Jernvall and colleagues have made significant advances in adapting predictive models for tooth formation [86, 87].

EXPRESSION OF ENGINEERED AMELOGENIN PROTEIN IN THE ENAMEL MATRIX

As part of our efforts to better understand enamel matrix formation, we analyzed the role of amelogenin domains in enamel biomineralization [34, 88]. Here, we thought it possible to redesign enamel by limiting the number of amelogenin isoforms expressed during amelogenesis and to engineer the major mouse amelogenin to lack one of its highly conserved domains. For this project, we created a knock-in mouse that expressed exclusively an M180 amelogenin protein lacking residues 1-42 (D1-42M180, e.g. amelogenin containing only residues 43-180) [34]). In all vertebrates, residues 1-42, known as "domain A" (Figure 3), defines a highly conserved amino-terminal domain that controls amelogenin self-assembly. Without this domain, amelogenin cannot form nanospheres [47]. Based on RT-PCR, Northern blot and quantitative real-time PCR we concluded that no other alternatively spliced amelogenin isoforms were expressed from this knock-in gene [34]. We found that ameloblastin levels were unchanged in our amelogenin knock-in animal as assayed by immunodetection of ameloblastin protein in the forming matrix as expression levels were comparable to the control wild type animal. Quantitative real time polymerase chain amplification of ameloblastin mRNAs showed no change to ameloblastin mRNA abundance in ameloblasts from the D1-42 M180 knock-in animal compared to the wild type control animals [34]. As expected, we found significant alterations to the enamel architecture when the matrix is made with amelogenin lacking residues 1-42 due to defective enamel matrix assembly [34].

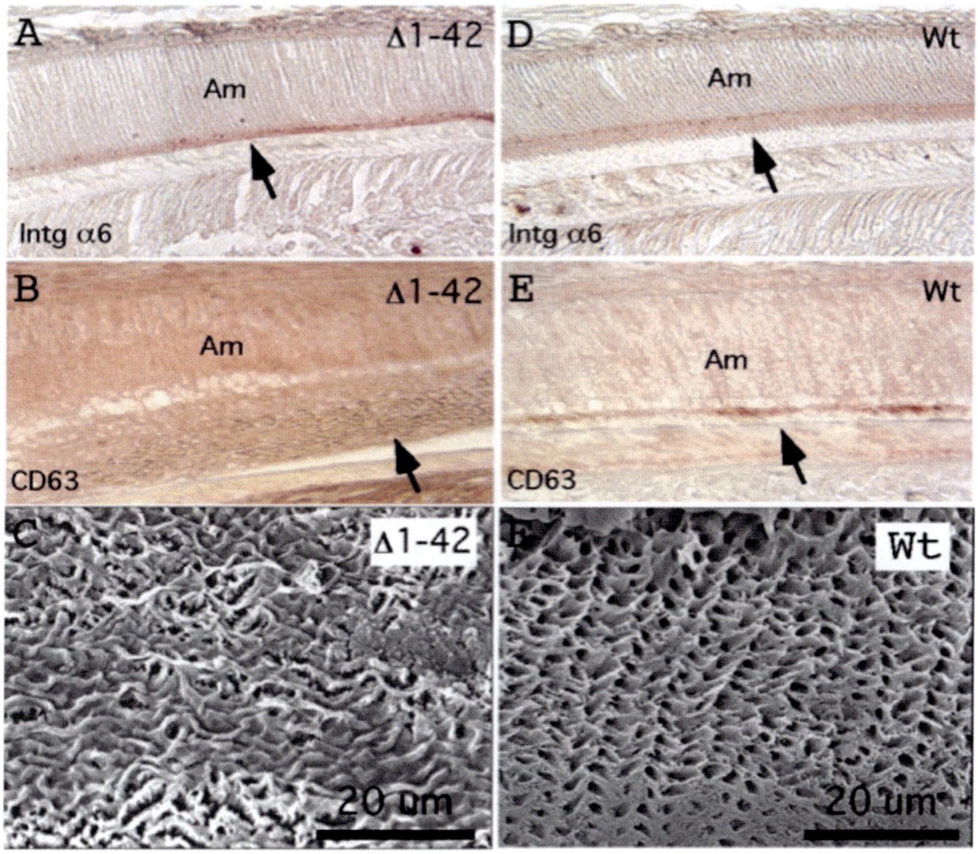

Figure 4: Enamel matrix created from the D1-42 M180 knock-in amelogenin alters Tomes' processes. Changes to proteins a6 integrin (panels A, D) and CD63 (panels B, E) are shown by immunologic examination of Tomes' processes (the apical secretory end piece of ameloblasts). The a6 integrin is localized to the secretory end pieces of ameloblasts (arrow) in the wild-type (Wt) animal shown in panel

D. In the case of enamel matrix homozygous for the D1-42 M180 knock-in (D1-42), the Tomes' processes are blunted, shown in panel A. The candidate receptor for amelogenin, CD63 [74], is localized to Tomes' processes in the wild type enamel (panel E) but is redistributed in the D1-42 M180 knock-in (panel B). The regular outlines corresponding to the regular insertion of Tomes' processes into the forming wild type enamel matrix is shown in panel F. In the case of enamel matrix made with the D1-42 M180 knock-in amelogenin, these outlines are distorted and collapsed, reflecting the altered morphology of Tomes' processes due to the altered interaction between the cell and its cylinder of matrix [89] (see Figure 1 and 2).

An unexpected finding from our work on the D1-42 M180 knock-in mice was the change in morphology of the secretory ends of ameloblasts (also known as "Tomes' process") (Figure 4, panels A, B and C) [89]. For the D1-42 M180 knock-in mice both integrin alpha 6 and CD63 were reduced in their apparent abundance in Tomes' processes (Figure 4, A and B, arrows) compared to their corresponding wild type control (Figure 4, panels D and E, arrows). In the case of ameloblasts from the D1-42 M180 knock-in animal, the Tomes' processes lost their peripheral boundaries and fused into larger domains with a consequential alteration to the interrod enamel (Figure 4, panel C). This is in contrast to the morphology of Tomes' processes from wild type enamel, where we found uniform and repetitive indentations corresponding to the Tomes' processes embedded in the forming wild type enamel (Figure 4, panel F). The images shown in panels C and D of figure 4 were prepared by removing the ameloblasts from the newly formed enamel matrix gel and critical point drying the specimen for visualization by SEM (as was also done to specimens shown in Figures 1 & 2).

Intriguingly, by three days postnatal age the ameloblasts altered their interactions with the enamel matrix, detached from the forming matrix to re-enter the cell cycle and became multilayered. Observing ameloblast detachment and proliferation suggested to us the possibility that the amelogenin domain comprised by residues 1-42 defines the ability of ameloblast to remain linked with the underlying cylinder of matrix via protein-to-membrane receptor interactions. The removal of residues 1-42 has been shown to stop amelogenin from self-assembling into nanospheres [46, 47] suggesting that defective amelogenin nanosphere assembly disrupts the forming matrix by eliminating a critical domain of amelogenin. This in turn alters the ability of the ameloblast to interact with the matrix [9]. We conclude that the domain defined by amelogenin residues 1-42 participates in maintaining ameloblast registration with the underlying sea of matrix via protein-to-membrane interactions and these interactions provide signals to maintain ameloblast differentiation.

Interestingly, the residues 1-42 for amelogenin (Figure 3), also known as TRAP (tyrosine rich amelogenin peptide) is the only amelogenin fragment that is retained in the matrix becoming enriched during enamel maturation [90]. We suggest that the amelogenin domain defined by residues 1-42 are required to maintain cell-matrix interaction until the termination of amelogenesis. Removing the amelogenin domain defined by residues 1-42, as we did in the D1-42 M180 knock-in prematurely removes this essential domain from the forming matrix and results in a loss of signals needed to maintain the differentiation state of the ameloblasts. The ameloblasts interpret the matrix as defective and return to a state of cell division.

We postulate that re-entry to cell division is due to the loss of anti-mitotic activity from C/EBP-alpha and the positive influence of Msx2 on division, essentially, re-patterning the enamel epithelia to a state resembling pre-ameloblasts [91, 92]. Differentiation of ameloblasts is maintained by high levels of C/EBP-alpha and is opposed by Mxs2 and this state of gene expression requires continuous interactions with amelogenin in the enamel matrix [91, 93]. When ameloblasts encounter a defective cylinder of matrix, an increase in Msx2 (proliferation) and the loss of C/EBP-alpha (anti-mitotic) events occur leading to re-entry to the cell cycle, a state similar to that of a pre-ameloblast.

THE NATIVE ENAMEL ECM REDIRECTS AMELOBLAST-LIKE CELLS

As shown in figure 5, we have used a wild type, cell-free-enamel matrix to demonstrate that cell-to-matrix interactions facilitate amelogenin gene expression. This experimental model demonstrates the capacity of ameloblast-like cells to align them selves onto a preformed enamel matrix, suggesting that the matrix contains sufficient information in the form of extracellular matrix proteins to facilitate cell to matrix interactions. We hypothesize that these same cell to matrix interactions are responsible for the ameloblast cells retaining physical registry over a rod of forming enamel. We intend to exploit such cell to matrix interactions to direct enamel gene expression in order to create an enamel biomimetic.

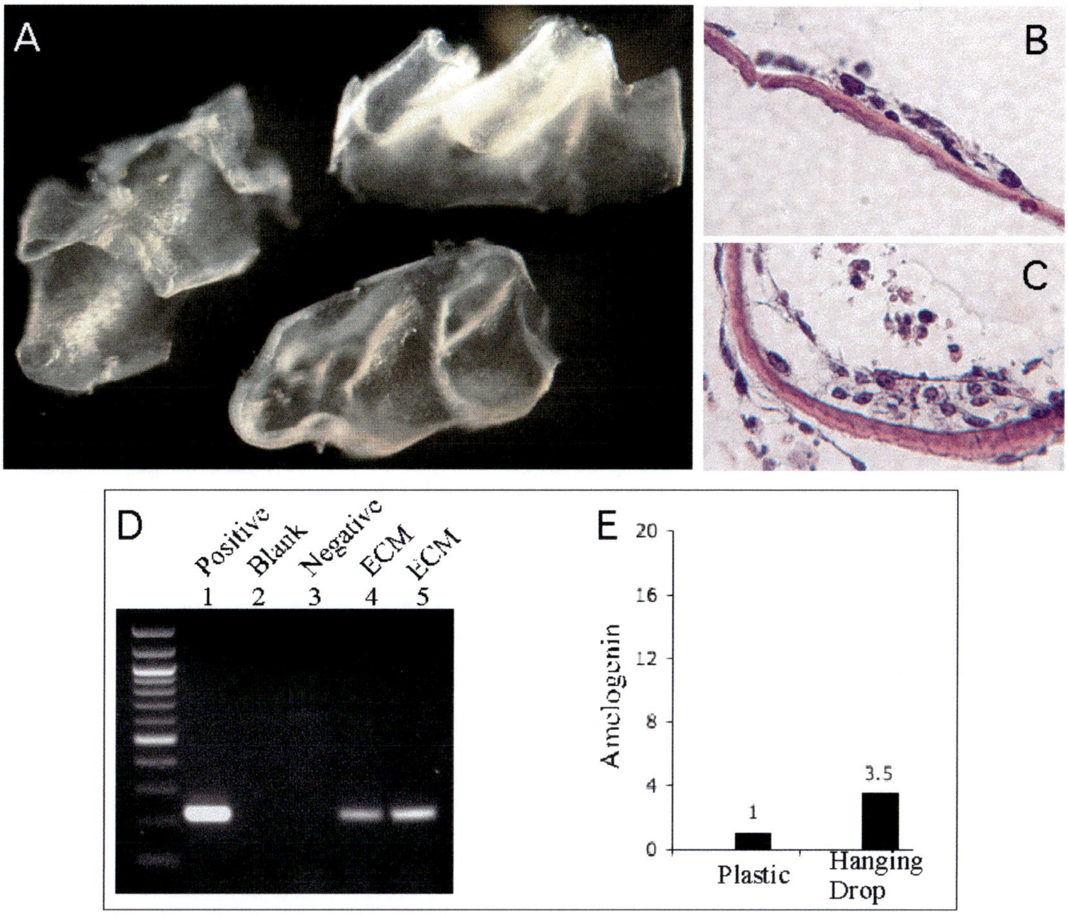

Figure 5: Hanging drop cultures of ameloblast-like LS8 cells were grown on cell-free enamel extracellular matrices (ECM). The enamel ECM from 2-day postnatal molars was isolated by microdissection and made cell-free by several freeze-thaw cycles at -80^{0}C (panel A). LS8 cells (5 x 10^3 cells) were seeded on the enamel-forming surface of the ECM. After 24 hours, the drop of fetal calf serum-free media containing the ECM and cells was flipped over to form a "hanging-drop" culture. Ameloblast-like cells became adherent and grew on the surface of the enamel ECM as shown by histologic sections (panel B and C). RNA was recovered from the matrix-adherent cells for reverse transcription and PCR analysis that revealed amelogenin gene expression by the cells attached to the matrix (panel D) with a 3.5 fold increase in amelogenin gene expression levels (panel E) measured by quantitative RT-PCR for LS8 cells that reattached to the enamel ECM versus LS8 cells grown on plastic as a control. The enhanced amelogenin mRNA expression levels support the importance of cell to matrix interactions on maintaining the ameloblast state of differentiation.

REGENERATIVE MEDICINE

The advances in health care have resulted in a significant increase in the human lifespan generating a growing need for regenerative medicine to enable re-growth of functional tissues lost to injury or degenerative disease. Caries remains the most prevalent infectious disease of mankind [94, 95]. Carious enamel currently must be replaced by an artificial restorative material since regeneration strategies for this mineralized tissue have not yet been realized. Through the application of nanoscience to regenerative medicine, we have designed self-assembling, nanostructured templates to deliver an appropriate substrate and signals for recruitment, matrix remodeling and subsequent mineralization by ameloblast cells. The in vivo requirements for ameloblasts to exert cell to matrix interaction led us to hypothesize that a chemically synthetic nanotechnology for generating bioactive nanofibers could provide clues for cells to fabricate an enamel biomimetic.

BIOMIMETIC SCAFFOLDS

We believe ideal scaffolds for enamel growth should mimic the nanoscale architecture and function of the extracellular matrix in order to interact with cellular receptors and to participate in the formation of oriented apatite nanocrystals. These scaffolds may also be used to deliver proteins that stimulate ameloblast differentiation including signals that enhance expression of the transcription factors that control enamel gene expression such as CEBP-alpha [24, 91]. Although it is clear why factors that enhance gene expression associated with enamel biomineralization are important in tissue regeneration, the need for scaffolds to trigger biomimetic mineralization is less obvious. We hypothesize that a critical but short-lived intermediary composed of mineral deposited on an organic scaffold can serve to evoke subsequent full, phenotypic biomineralization. We predict that an artificial matrix could provide direct or indirect cues for cellular mineralization that are not possible to achieve through proteomics and cell biology alone. Instead, these clues can only be mediated through a biomimetic environment that resembles what cells encounter at the nanoscale. Such scaffolds would be difficult to create with traditional polymers and bioceramics. Instead, in collaboration with the Stupp laboratory, we have turned to a self-assembling supramolecular platform that forms nanostructures resembling the shape and composition of the Natural matrices of biomineralization.

SUPRAMOLECULAR, SELF-ASSEMBLING NANOSTRUCTURES FOR ENAMEL BIOMINERALIZATION

The Stupp laboratory has extensive experience in the design and synthesis of molecules with the capacity to self-assemble into nanostructures under physiologic conditions. These nanostructures have the potential to yield new regenerative materials for dental tissues, based on the principle that Nature utilizes organic templates with nanoscale structure to nucleate and control the orientation of mineral crystals [96-99]. Herein, we have presented evidence that proteins such as amelogenin mediate the growth of long rod-like hydroxyapatite crystals at the nanoscale, while the mesoscale level of organization is responsible for generating the tough, cross-ply structure of enamel, gained through the interaction of cells with the extracellular matrix.

The Stupp laboratory has previously reported on supramolecular systems in which molecules referred to as peptide amphiphiles (Figure 6A) self-assembled into long aspect ratio nanofibers (Figure 6B, C). The chemical structure for a "model" peptide amphiphile (PA) shown in figure 6D [100, 101]. These molecules form fibers with diameters of 6-8 nanometers and lengths of up to several microns. When imaged by transmission electron microscopy (TEM), these nanostructures mimic the architecture of extracellular matrix collagen fibrils as shown in figure 7. The peptide amphiphile molecule undergoes self-assembly with changes in pH or ionic strength. Driven by electrostatic interactions and peptide secondary structure, networks can be formed in physiological fluids such as cell culture media and tissue transudates.

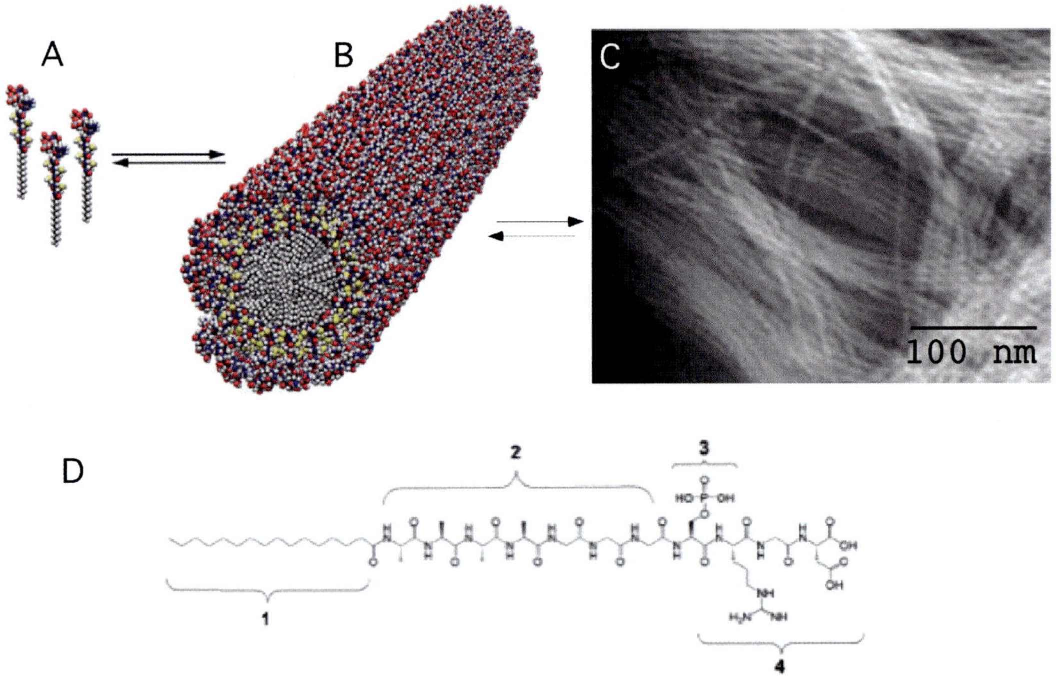

Figure 6: A bioactive self-assembling peptide amphiphile molecule for use as an artificial matrix for regenerative medicine. Upper Panel, graphic representation of peptide amphiphiles (Panel A) undergoing reversible self-assembly into a cylindrical nanofiber (Panel B) and the nanofibers imaged by transmission electron microscopy and negative staining used to show the nanofibers (Panel C). The nanofiber surfaces can be engineered to display high-density peptides to convey biological information for cell adhesion and/or differentiation [102]. The nanofiber is a hierarchical material that can be created to mimic

extracellular matrix molecules by displaying a high density of bioactibe peptides on their surfaces. Panel D, chemical structure for the peptide amphiphile molecule synthesized by the Stupp laboratory highlighting four structural features of the PA. Region 1, is a hydrophobic palmitoyl tail; region 2, is a structural peptide segment consisting of four alanines and three glycines, residues known to promote beta-sheet formation; region 3, is a mineralization-active residue of phosphoserine promoting mineralization of hydroxyapatite crystallites; and region 4 displays the cell adhesion ligand peptide "RGD".

The nanofibers' high aspect ratio leads to network formation at concentrations of 1 wt % or less in solution, creating a highly porous gel (Figure 6C) with aqueous channels for nutrient diffusion and cell migration. One advantage of these ordered, one-dimensional nanostructures is they can present well-defined bioactive epitopes at their surfaces to induce epitaxial mineral nucleation, signal bioactivity or bind proteins in specific conformations. The reversible assembly of the peptide amphiphiles into a self-supporting gel is shown in Figure 7. Furthermore, as biodegradable scaffolds for tissue regeneration, the lability of supramolecular structures is an attractive tool to control the rate of bioerosion and the size of biodegradation products. The small molecules making up the nanofibers should break down into natural amino- and fatty acids, facilitating clearing and avoiding the potential toxicity often associated with the breakdown of larger polymeric materials.

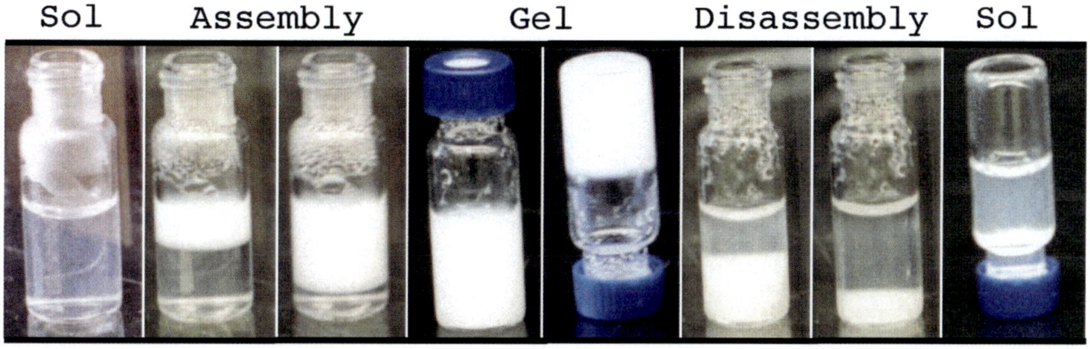

Figure 7: Self-assembly of peptide amphiphiles into self-supporting gel is reversible. This montage depicts a peptide amphiphile self-assembly into a self-supporting gel and reversibly returning with disassembly to a solution state.

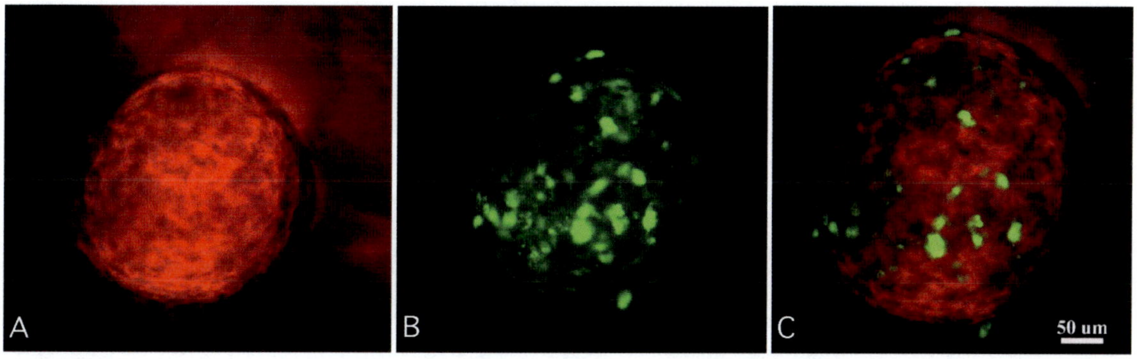

Figure 8: Ameloblast-like LS8 cells enmeshed with the PA nanofiber gel. The branched RGD containing peptide amphiphile was co-assembled with rhodamine derivitized peptide amphiphiles (panel A) and the ameloblast-like LS8 cells were transfected with green fluorescent protein (panel B) in order to permit their identification upon mixing. The cells are suspended and completely enmeshed within the nanofiber supported gel so that the cells encounter the bioactive peptides displayed at high density on the surfaces of the nanofiber [105].

Through changes in the peptide segment of the amphiphile, one can customize the bioactivity of these nanomaterials and their propensity to nucleate specific mineral crystals. The repeated phosphoserine residue on the fibers recreated the function of collagen fibrils in the extracellular matrix, nucleating flat nanocrystals of hydroxyapatite with their c-axis aligned parallel to the nanofiber axis [103, 104] (. In another PA system, one can present biological epitopes such as cell adhesion ligands, for example, the "IKVAV" sequence of amino acids from laminin that can induce unique cellular responses including rapid differentiation of neural progenitor cells into neurons [105]. Additionally, the need for laminin in tooth development [32] motivates the use of this epitope to mediate ameloblast cell to matrix interactions.

NANOFIBER APPLICATIONS TO ENAMEL REGENERATION

In biomineralized tissues crystallite geometry is guided by protein assemblies within an extracellular matrix, yet in vivo, the molecular basis for protein to mineral interactions required to control crystallite geometry and cell to matrix interactions remains vague. Here, we used bioactive artificial matrices as the means to instruct ameloblast-like LS8 cells or primary murine ameloblast cells to express enamel matrix proteins for guiding the mineral habit and the cellular architecture just as they do in the authentic tissue. For this purpose, we used a peptide amphiphile containing the cell adhesion domain comprised by the "RGD" amino acid sequence in a branched configuration [72]. In Figure 8, the LS8 cells and the branched RGD-PA (bRGD-PA) were mixed together to produce a self-supporting nanofiber gel in which the cells are enmeshed. When either LS8 or primary ameloblasts cells were enmeshed in this bioactive bRGD-PA nanofiber network up-regulation of integrin expression and the two most abundant proteins in developing enamel, amelogenin and ameloblastin were observed. The control for this experiment included culture in a peptide amphiphile that mimics charge density and display of a scrambled, non-bioactive peptide domain (Control-PA) [72].

We analyzed the cellular response to the bRGD-PA compared to control-PA using a commercially available quantitative reverse transcription coupled to polymerase chain amplification assay according to the manufacturer's directions (SABioscience). The fold increase in mRNA expression for cells grown in bRGD-PAs compared to values from cells grown in the control PA are shown in Table 1 for selected genes.

Table 1: Gene expression of ameloblast-like LS8 cells enmeshed in branched RGD-peptide amphiphile after 24 hours. Quantitative real time PCR results of reverse transcribed mRNAs encoding proteins critical to enamel formation. The fold enrichment over values obtained from identical cells grown enmeshed in a control non-bioactive peptide amphiphile nanofibers that matches charge density of the branched RGD-peptide amphiphile nanofibers is shown.

Adamts	1.39
Col4a1	1.30
Col4a2	1.21
Itga4	1.97
Lama2	2.11
Hhip	1.64
LEF1	1.24
Atf2	2.39
Cdh1	2.45
FGF4	2.71

The data in Table 1 suggests that the cells respond to the bRGA-PA by expressing a series of extracellular matrix molecules that facilitate cell to bRGD-PA interactions. These are similar to the events that occur when preameloblasts follow their developmental sequence prior to overtly expressing production of the enamel extracellular matrix [106]. We have shown that the bRGD-PA injected into the enamel organ epithelia of neonatal incisors also stimulates the local expression of extracellular matrix molecules, followed by expression of enamel matrix genes, such as amelogenin and ameloblastin. We are pursuing long-term culture of the PA-injected enamel organs to determine if the artificial bioactive self-assembled nanofibers result in recapitulation of enamel formation at the external injection site. Preliminary data suggest that cells are recruited or proliferate locally, contact the self-assembled PA nidus, polarize, develop a Tomes' secretory end piece and assemble the enamel matrix among the PA. Here, long, thin hydroxyapatite crystallites are organized under the control of the ameloblast similar to authentic enamel rods. Based on our in vitro observations, we suggest that the bRGD-PA acts to redirect the developmental cascade for ameloblast differentiation by stimulating proliferation and differentiation of cells from the enamel organ [72]. By using a bioactive artificial matrix that can direct epithelial cell differentiation into functional ameloblasts, we are taking the necessary first steps to create a cell based enamel biomimetic material. We predict this biologically inspired material will provide the requisite mechanical properties by recreating the cell to matrix interactions that serve to create authentic enamel and its inherent materials properties, thus providing a biologically inspired dental restorative material.

ACKNOWLEDGEMENT

Supported by the USPHS, NIH, National Institute of Dental and Craniofacial Research by grants DE06988 (MLS), DE13045 (MLS), DE015920 (SIS), DE14189 (SNW) and DE13404 (MLP). The authors are grateful for the leadership efforts by Dr. Eleni Kousvelari, Dr. Harold C. Slavkin and Dr. Larry Tabak of the National Institute for Dental and Craniofacial Research to bridge chemical, biological, engineering and material science disciplines to the benefit of craniofacial biology and regenerative medicine by promoting transdisciplinary research programs.

REFERENCES

[1] Thesleff I, Vaahtokari A, Partanen AM. Regulation of organogenesis. Common molecular mechanisms regulating the development of teeth and other organs. Int J Dev Biol 1995;39(1):35-50.
[2] Maas R, Bei M. The genetic control of early tooth development. Crit Rev Oral Biol Med 1997;8(1):4-39.
[3] Thesleff I, Sharpe P. Signalling networks regulating dental development. Mech Dev 1997;67(2):111-23.
[4] Gibson CW, Yuan ZA, Hall B, *et al.* Amelogenin-deficient mice display an amelogenesis imperfecta phenotype. J Biol Chem 2001;276(34):31871-5.
[5] White SN, Luo W, Paine ML, *et al.* Biological organization of hydroxyapatite crystallites into a fibrous continuum toughens and controls anisotropy in human enamel. J Dent Res 2001;80(1):321-6.
[6] Fong H, White SN, Paine ML, *et al.* Enamel structure properties controlled by engineered proteins in transgenic mice. J Bone Miner Res 2003;18(11):2052-9.
[7] Bechtle S, Habelitz S, Klocke A, *et al.* The fracture behaviour of dental enamel. Biomaterials 2009.
[8] Sasaki T, Goldberg M, Takuma S, *et al.* Cell biology of tooth enamel formation. Functional electron microscopic monographs. Monogr Oral Sci 1990;14:1-199.
[9] Paine ML, White SN, Luo W, *et al.* Regulated gene expression dictates enamel structure and tooth function. Matrix Biol 2001;20(5-6):273-92.
[10] Fincham AG, Moradian-Oldak J, Simmer JP. The structural biology of the developing dental enamel matrix. J Struct Biol 1999;126(3):270-99.
[11] Du C, Falini G, Fermani S, *et al.* Supramolecular assembly of amelogenin nanospheres into birefringent microribbons. Science 2005;307(5714):1450-4.
[12] Robinson C, Brookes SJ, Shore RC, *et al.* The developing enamel matrix: nature and function. Eur J Oral Sci 1998;106 Suppl 1:282-91.
[13] Smith CE. Cellular and chemical events during enamel maturation. Crit Rev Oral Biol Med 1998;9(2):128-61.
[14] Paine ML, Snead ML, Wang HJ, *et al.* Role of NBCe1 and AE2 in secretory ameloblasts. J Dent Res 2008;87(4):391-5.
[15] Eastoe JE. Enamel protein chemistry--past, present and future. J Dent Res 1979;58(Spec Issue B):753-64.
[16] Simmer JP, Hu JC. Expression, structure, and function of enamel proteinases. Connect Tissue Res 2002;43(2-3):441-9.
[17] Shapiro JL, Wen X, Okamoto CT, *et al.* Cellular uptake of amelogenin, and its localization to CD63, and Lamp1-positive vesicles. Cell Mol Life Sci 2007;64(2):244-56.
[18] Boyde A. Correlation of ameloblast size with enamel prism pattern: use of scanning electron microscope to make surface area measurements. Z Zellforsch Mikrosk Anat 1969;93(4):583-93.
[19] Rauth RJ PK, Ngan AY, Saad DM, *et al.* Dental Enamel: Genes Define Biomechanics. California Deantal Association 2009;37:863-68.
[20] Iwasaki K, Bajenova E, Somogyi-Ganss E, *et al.* Amelotin--a Novel Secreted, Ameloblast-specific Protein. J Dent Res 2005;84(12):1127-32.
[21] Moffatt P, Smith CE, St-Arnaud R, *et al.* Cloning of rat amelotin and localization of the protein to the basal lamina of maturation stage ameloblasts and junctional epithelium. Biochem J 2006;399(1):37-46.

[22] Smith CE, Chen WY, Issid M, *et al.* Enamel matrix protein turnover during amelogenesis: basic biochemical properties of short-lived sulfated enamel proteins. Calcif Tissue Int 1995;57(2):133-44.
[23] Snead ML, Bringas P, Jr., Bessem C, *et al.* De novo gene expression detected by amelogenin gene transcript analysis. Dev Biol 1984;104(1):255-8.
[24] Xu Y, Zhou YL, Luo W, et al. NF-Y and CCAAT/enhancer-binding protein alpha synergistically activate the mouse amelogenin gene. J Biol Chem 2006;281(23):16090-8.
[25] Brownell AG, Slavkin HC. Role of basal lamina in tissue interactions. Ren Physiol 1980;3(1-6):193-204.
[26] White SN, Miklus VG, Chang PP, *et al.* Controlled failure mechanisms toughen the dentino-enamel junction zone. J Prosthet Dent 2005;94(4):330-5.
[27] Wright JT, Hall KI, Deaton TG,*et al.* Structural and compositional alteration of tooth enamel in hereditary epidermolysis bullosa. Connect Tissue Res 1996;34(4):271-9.
[28] Nakamura H, Sawamura D, Goto M, *et al.* Analysis of the COL17A1 in non-Herlitz junctional epidermolysis bullosa and amelogenesis imperfecta. Int J Mol Med 2006;18(2):333-7.
[29] Fukumoto S, Miner JH, Ida H, *et al.* Laminin alpha5 is required for dental epithelium growth and polarity and the development of tooth bud and shape. J Biol Chem 2006;281(8):5008-16.
[30] Salmivirta K, Gullberg D, Hirsch E, *et al.* Integrin subunit expression associated with epithelial-mesenchymal interactions during murine tooth development. Dev Dyn 1996;205(2):104-13.
[31] Cerny R, Slaby I, Hammarstrom L, *et al.* A novel gene expressed in rat ameloblasts codes for proteins with cell binding domains. J Bone Miner Res 1996;11(7):883-91.
[32] Ryan MC, Lee K, Miyashita Y, *et al.* Targeted disruption of the LAMA3 gene in mice reveals abnormalities in survival and late stage differentiation of epithelial cells. J Cell Biol 1999;145(6):1309-23.
[33] Fukumoto S, Yamada A, Nonaka K, *et al.* Essential roles of ameloblastin in maintaining ameloblast differentiation and enamel formation. Cells Tissues Organs 2005;181(3-4):189-95.
[34] Zhu D, Paine ML, Luo W, *et al.* Altering biomineralization by protein design. J Biol Chem 2006;281(30):21173-82.
[35] Boyde A. A 3-D model of enamel development at the scale of one inch to the micron. Adv Dent Res 1987;1(2):135-40.
[36] Fincham AG, Moradian-Oldak J, Diekwisch TG, *et al.* Evidence for amelogenin "nanospheres" as functional components of secretory-stage enamel matrix. J Struct Biol 1995;115(1):50-9.
[37] Wang L, Guan X, Du C, *et al.* Amelogenin promotes the formation of elongated microstructures in a controlled crystallization system. J. Phys. Chem. C. 2007;111:6398-6404.
[38] Smith CE, Chong DL, Bartlett JD, *et al.* Mineral acquisition rates in developing enamel on maxillary and mandibular incisors of rats and mice: implications to extracellular acid loading as apatite crystals mature. J Bone Miner Res 2005;20(2):240-9.
[39] Moradian-Oldak J, Jimenez I, Maltby D, *et al.* Controlled proteolysis of amelogenins reveals exposure of both carboxy- and amino-terminal regions. Biopolymers 2001;58(7):606-16.
[40] Simmer JP, Fincham AG. Molecular mechanisms of dental enamel formation. Crit Rev Oral Biol Med 1995;6(2):84-108.
[41] Sire JY, Delgado S, Fromentin D, *et al.* Amelogenin: lessons from evolution. Arch Oral Biol 2005;50(2):205-12.
[42] Kawasaki K, Suzuki T, Weiss KM. Genetic basis for the evolution of vertebrate mineralized tissue. Proc Natl Acad Sci U S A 2004;101(31):11356-61.
[43] Kawasaki K, Weiss KM. Mineralized tissue and vertebrate evolution: the secretory calcium-binding phosphoprotein gene cluster. Proc Natl Acad Sci U S A 2003;100(7):4060-5.
[44] Delgado S, Girondot M, Sire JY. Molecular evolution of amelogenin in mammals. J Mol Evol 2005;60(1):12-30.
[45] Delgado S, Casane D, Bonnaud L, *et al.* Molecular evidence for precambrian origin of amelogenin, the major protein of vertebrate enamel. Mol Biol Evol 2001;18(12):2146-53.
[46] Paine ML, Snead ML. Protein interactions during assembly of the enamel organic extracellular matrix. J Bone Miner Res 1997;12(2):221-7.
[47] Moradian-Oldak J, Paine ML, Lei YP, *et al.* Self-assembly properties of recombinant engineered amelogenin proteins analyzed by dynamic light scattering and atomic force microscopy. J Struct Biol 2000;131(1):27-37.
[48] Zhu DH, Paine, M.L., Luo, W., *et al.* Engineered amelogenin domains expressed from a genetic knock-in locus: Analysis of herterozygous female incisors. In: Sodek WLJ, editor. 8th Internation Conference on the

Chemistry and Biology of Mineralized Tissues; 2004; Banff, Canada: University of Toronto Press; 2004. p. 99-102.

[49] Lyngstadaas SP. Synthetic hammerhead ribozymes as tools in gene expression. Crit Rev Oral Biol Med 2001;12(6):469-78.

[50] Lyngstadaas SP, Risnes S, Sproat BS, *et al.* A synthetic, chemically modified ribozyme eliminates amelogenin, the major translation product in developing mouse enamel in vivo. Embo J 1995;14(21):5224-9.

[51] Fincham AG, Belcourt AB, Termine JD, *et al.* Dental enamel matrix: sequences of two amelogenin polypeptides. Biosci Rep 1981;1(10):771-8.

[52] Fincham AG, Hu Y, Lau EC, *et al.* Amelogenin post-secretory processing during biomineralization in the postnatal mouse molar tooth. Arch Oral Biol 1991;36(4):305-17.

[53] Sasaki T. Tooth Enamel IV. In: Fearnhead RWaS, S., editor. Proceeding of the Fourth International Symposium on the Composition, Properties and Fundamental Structure of Tooth Enamel; 1984; Asia Center, Odawara, Japan: Elsevier Science Publishers; 1984. p. 1-570.

[54] Gibson CW, Golub E, Ding WD, *et al.* Identification of the leucine-rich amelogenin peptide (LRAP) as the translation product of an alternatively spliced transcript. Biochem Biophys Res Commun 1991;174(3):1306-12.

[55] Papagerakis P, Ibarra JM, Inozentseva N, *et al.* Mouse amelogenin exons 8 and 9: sequence analysis and protein distribution. J Dent Res 2005;84(7):613-7.

[56] Warotayanont R, Frenkel B, Snead ML, *et al.* Leucine-rich amelogenin peptide induces osteogenesis by activation of the Wnt pathway. Biochem Biophys Res Commun 2009.

[57] Matsuzawa M, Sheu TJ, Lee YJ, *et al.* Putative signaling action of amelogenin utilizes the Wnt/beta-catenin pathway. J Periodontal Res 2009;44(3):289-96.

[58] Fincham AG, Belcourt AB, Termine JD, *et al.* Amelogenins. Sequence homologies in enamel-matrix proteins from three mammalian species. Biochem J 1983;211(1):149-54.

[59] Amar S, Sires B, Veis A. A rat incisor dentin matrix protein can induce neonatal rat muscle fibroblasts, in culture, to express phenotypic products of chondroblastic cells. J Biol Buccale 1991;19(1):55-60.

[60] Veis A. Amelogenin gene splice products: potential signaling molecules. Cell Mol Life Sci 2003;60(1):38-55.

[61] Veis A. Procceding of the 7th International Conference on the Composition, Properties and Fundamental Structure of Tooth Enamel. In: Don Layaruu CG, editor. 7th International Conference on the Composition, Properties and Fundamental Structure of Tooth Enamel; 2005; Brewster, MA: European Journal of Oral Science; 2005.

[62] Veis A, Sires B, Clohisy J, *et al.* Rat incisor dentine contains a factor which alters the phenotypic expression and stimulates chondrogenesis in fibroblast-like cells in vitro. Biomaterials 1990;11:35-7.

[63] Veis A, Tompkins K, Alvares K, *et al.* Specific amelogenin gene splice products have signaling effects on cells in culture and in implants in vivo. J Biol Chem 2000;275(52):41263-72.

[64] Goldberg M, Farges JC, Lacerda-Pinheiro S, *et al.* Inflammatory and immunological aspects of dental pulp repair. Pharmacol Res 2008;58(2):137-47.

[65] Goldberg M, Lacerda-Pinheiro S, Priam F, *et al.* Matricellular molecules and odontoblast progenitors as tools for dentin repair and regeneration. Clin Oral Investig 2008;12(2):109-12.

[66] Warotayanont R, Zhu D, Snead ML, *et al.* Leucine-rich amelogenin peptide induces osteogenesis in mouse embryonic stem cells. Biochem Biophys Res Commun 2008;367(1):1-6.

[67] Nanci A, Zalzal S, Lavoie P, *et al.* Comparative immunochemical analyses of the developmental expression and distribution of ameloblastin and amelogenin in rat incisors. J Histochem Cytochem 1998;46(8):911-34.

[68] Fukumoto S, Kiba T, Hall B, *et al.* Ameloblastin is a cell adhesion molecule required for maintaining the differentiation state of ameloblasts. J Cell Biol 2004;167(5):973-83.

[69] Sonoda A, Iwamoto T, Nakamura T, *et al.* Critical role of heparin binding domains of ameloblastin for dental epithelium cell adhesion and ameloblastoma proliferation. J Biol Chem 2009;284(40):27176-84.

[70] Wazen RM, Moffatt P, Zalzal SF, *et al* A mouse model expressing a truncated form of ameloblastin exhibits dental and junctional epithelium defects. Matrix Biol 2009;28(5):292-303.

[71] Fukumoto S, Yamada Y. Review: extracellular matrix regulates tooth morphogenesis. Connect Tissue Res 2005;46(4-5):220-6.

[72] Huang Z, Sargeant T, Hulvat J, *et al.* Bioactive Nanofibers Instruct Cells to Proliferate and Differentiate During Enamel Regeneration. J Bone Miner Res 2008.

[73] Asaka T, Akiyama M, Domon T, *et al.* Type XVII collagen is a key player in tooth enamel formation. Am J Pathol 2009;174(1):91-100.
[74] Tompkins K, George A, Veis A. Characterization of a mouse amelogenin [A-4]/M59 cell surface receptor. Bone 2005.
[75] Stipp CS, Kolesnikova TV, Hemler ME. Functional domains in tetraspanin proteins. Trends Biochem Sci 2003;28(2):106-12.
[76] Bartlett JD, Ganss B, Goldberg M, *et al.* 3. Protein-protein interactions of the developing enamel matrix. Curr Top Dev Biol 2006;74:57-115.
[77] Yunta M, Lazo PA. Tetraspanin proteins as organisers of membrane microdomains and signalling complexes. Cell Signal 2003;15(6):559-64.
[78] Berditchevski F. Complexes of tetraspanins with integrins: more than meets the eye. J Cell Sci 2001;114(Pt 23):4143-51.
[79] Cook NR, Row PE, Davidson HW. Lysosome associated membrane protein 1 (Lamp1) traffics directly from the TGN to early endosomes. Traffic 2004;5(9):685-99.
[80] Zou Y, Wang H, Shapiro JL, *et al.* Determination of protein regions responsible for interactions of amelogenin with CD63 and LAMP1. Biochem J 2007;408(3):347-54.
[81] Rajangam K, Behanna HA, Hui MJ, *et al.* Heparin binding nanostructures to promote growth of blood vessels. Nano Lett 2006;6(9):2086-90.
[82] Stamenovic D, Fredberg JJ, Wang N, *et al.* A microstructural approach to cytoskeletal mechanics based on tensegrity. J Theor Biol 1996;181(2):125-36.
[83] Sims JR, Karp S, Ingber DE. Altering the cellular mechanical force balance results in integrated changes in cell, cytoskeletal and nuclear shape. J Cell Sci 1992;103 (Pt 4):1215-22.
[84] Ingber DE, Folkman J. Mechanochemical switching between growth and differentiation during fibroblast growth factor-stimulated angiogenesis in vitro: role of extracellular matrix. J Cell Biol 1989;109(1):317-30.
[85] Cox B. A multi-scale, discrete-cell simulation of organogenesis: Application to the effects of strain stimulus on collective cell behavior during ameloblast migration. J Theor Biol;262(1):58-72.
[86] Kavanagh KD, Evans AR, Jernvall J. Predicting evolutionary patterns of mammalian teeth from development. Nature 2007;449(7161):427-32.
[87] Salazar-Ciudad I, Jernvall J. A gene network model accounting for development and evolution of mammalian teeth. Proc Natl Acad Sci U S A 2002;99(12):8116-20.
[88] Snead ML. Amelogenin protein exhibits a modular design: implications for form and function. Connect Tissue Res 2003;44 Suppl 1:47-51.
[89] Dunglas C, Septier D, Paine ML, *et al.* Ultrastructure of forming enamel in mouse bearing a transgene that disrupts the amelogenin self-assembly domains. Calcif Tissue Int 2002;71(2):155-66.
[90] Fincham AG, Belcourt, A.B., Termine, J.D. Changing patterns of enamel matrix proteins in the developing bovine tooth. Caries Research 1982;16:64-71.
[91] Zhou YL, Lei Y, Snead ML. Functional antagonism between Msx2 and CCAAT/enhancer-binding protein alpha in regulating the mouse amelogenin gene expression is mediated by protein-protein interaction. J Biol Chem 2000;275(37):29066-75.
[92] Bei M, Stowell S, Maas R. Msx2 controls ameloblast terminal differentiation. Dev Dyn 2004;231(4):758-65.
[93] Zhou YL, Snead ML. Identification of CCAAT/enhancer-binding protein alpha as a transactivator of the mouse amelogenin gene. J Biol Chem 2000;275(16):12273-80.
[94] Caufield PW, Li Y, Dasanayake A. Dental caries: an infectious and transmissible disease. Compend Contin Educ Dent 2005;26(5 Suppl 1):10-6.
[95] Taubman MA, Nash DA. The scientific and public-health imperative for a vaccine against dental caries. Nat Rev Immunol 2006;6(7):555-63.
[96] Mann S, Weiner S. Biomineralization: structural questions at all length scales. J Struct Biol 1999;126(3):179-81.
[97] Lowenstam HA, Weiner S. On biomineralization. New York: Oxford University Press; 1989.
[98] Weiner S, Addadi L. Biomineralization. At the cutting edge. Science 2002;298(5592):375-6.
[99] Weiner S. Organization of extracellularly mineralized tissues: a comparative study of biological crystal growth. CRC Crit Rev Biochem 1986;20(4):365-408.
[100] Stupp SI, LeBonheur VV, Walker K, *et al.* Supramolecular Materials: Self-Organized Nanostructures. Science 1997;276(5311):384-9.

[101] Palmer LC, Newcomb CJ, Kaltz SR, *et al.* Biomimetic systems for hydroxyapatite mineralization inspired by bone and enamel. Chem Rev 2008;108(11):4754-83.

[102] Beniash E, Hartgerink JD, Storrie H, *et al.* Self-assembling peptide amphiphile nanofiber matrices for cell entrapment. Acta Biomater 2005;1(4):387-97.

[103] Hartgerink JD, Beniash E, Stupp SI. Peptide-amphiphile nanofibers: a versatile scaffold for the preparation of self-assembling materials. Proc Natl Acad Sci U S A 2002;99(8):5133-8.

[104] Hartgerink JD, Beniash E, Stupp SI. Self-assembly and mineralization of peptide-amphiphile nanofibers. Science 2001;294(5547):1684-8.

[105] Silva GA, Czeisler C, Niece KL, *et al.* Selective differentiation of neural progenitor cells by high-epitope density nanofibers. Science 2004;303(5662):1352-5.

[106] Wang XP, Suomalainen M, Felszeghy S, *et al.* An integrated gene regulatory network controls stem cell proliferation in teeth. PLoS Biol 2007;5(6):e159.

CHAPTER 16

Signaling Effect of Leucine-Rich Amelogenin Peptide (Lrap) on Bone Regeneration

Yan Zhou[1], Christina. J. Newcomb[2], Rungnapa Warotayanont[3], Malcolm L. Snead[1] and S.I. Stupp[2,4,5].

[1]The Center for Craniofacial Molecular Biology, University of Southern California, Los Angeles CA; [2]Department of Materials Science and Engineering, Institute for BioNanotechnology in Medicine, Northwestern University, Chicago, IL; [3]Department of Orofacial Sciences, University of California, San Francisco School of Dentistry, 513 Parnassus Ave S-704, San Francisco, CA94143; [4]Department of Chemistry, Northwestern University, Evanston, IL and [5]Department of Medicine, Northwestern University, Chicago, IL.

Abstract: Amelogenin is the most abundant protein of the enamel organic matrix and is a structural protein indispensable for enamel formation. A commercial product Emdogain, consisting largely of alternatively spliced and processed amelogenins, could induce new bone, cementum and periodontal ligament formation in the jaws. Using mouse embryonic stem (ES) cells as a model system, we demonstrate that one of the amelogenin splicing isoforms, Leucine-rich Amelogenin Peptide (LRAP) activates the canonical Wnt signaling pathway to induce osteogenic differentiation of mouse ES cells through the concerted regulation of Wnt agonists and antagonists. Furthermore, LRAP stimulates bone regeneration in a rat femoral critical size defect model.

Key Words: LRAP, Leucine-rich Amelogenin Peptide, Wnt Signaling Pathway, ES Cell, Osteogenic Differentiation, Osteogenesis, Bone Regeneration

INTRODUCTION

Amelogenin is the most abundant protein of the enamel organic matrix and is a structural protein indispensable for enamel formation via self-assembly [1-8]. The structural functions for amelogenin are becoming better known and have been previously reviewed [9]. Accumulating evidence suggests that amelogenin, especially Leucine-rich amelogenin peptide (LRAP), an alternatively spliced amelogenin protein, also functions as a signaling molecule. Readers are also directed towards the reviews by Giannobile and Somerman [10], Veis [11], and Goldberg [12].

OVERVIEW

Low molecular weight amelogenin-related polypeptides extracted from mineralized dentin have been shown to induce chondrogenesis in cultures of embryonic muscle-derived fibroblasts (EMF) in vitro and lead to the formation of mineralized matrix in in invo implants [13, 14]. Furthermore, two splicing products of rat amelogenin ([A+4] and [A-4]) have shown signaling capacity, inducing chondrogenic and osteogenic differentiation both in vitro and in vivo [15]. Both products at nanomolar (nM) level enhance in vitro sulfate incorporation into proteoglycan and induce the expression of type II collagen, a chondrocyte marker. However, the inductive activity on osteogenic differentiation is restricted to [A-4], evidenced by the upregulation of Cbfa1 expression in [A-4]-treated rat embryonic muscle fibroblasts (EMF) but not in [A+4]-treated cells. In vivo implant assays further demonstrate that both [A+4] and [A-4], each to a different extent, are active in inducing cellular ingrowth into the implants, followed by extracellular matrix production, vascularization and mineralization. The [A-4] fraction induces a more copious and diffuse mineral deposition than [A+4], which produces more focal and more highly vascularized mineralized areas.

When two splicing products of rat amelogenin ([A+4] and [A-4]) were identified by a molecular screening of a rat pulp-odontoblast cDNA library [15], Veis et al tested the hypothesis that the two amelogenin molecules exert signaling effects on ameloblast and odontoblast development. When lower first molars from postnatal days 1 and 2 CD1 mice were cultured in vitro, exogenous [A-4] induced the expression of cementum attachment protein (CAP) in the mesenchymal cells of the dental follicle, whereas [A+4] induced the expression of dentin matrix protein 2 (DMP2) in the odontoblasts [16]. In a related study, E15/E16 tooth germs were used to better examine the development of the enamel organ. Tooth germs cultured with [A+4] had well-polarized odontoblasts with robust dentin production and concomitant ameloblast polarization. On the other hand, cultures with [A-4] gave rise to a disorganized pre-ameloblast layer and non-polarized ameloblasts along the dentin surface, and odontoblast polarization and dentin production were reduced compared with [A+4]-treated samples [17]. The conclusion drawn was that [A-4] had an inhibitory effect on ameloblast development, whereas [A+4] strongly stimulated odontoblast development. The observation also led to the hypothesis that [A-4] produced in the developing odontoblasts delayed pre-ameloblast maturation until the dentin layer is adequately formed. These seminal observations are clouded by some questions regarding experimental design. For example, in the tooth germ culture setting, whether the target tissue (ameloblasts), is accessible to exogenous [A-4] remains unclear. Tight junctions seal the enamel organ and the peptides would have to find an access route to influence the ameloblasts if a direct effect of the peptide is anticipated. Alternatively, another population of cells in the enamel organ could have been the target and these cells then generated the signal that induced the changes observed in the ameloblast population.

The molecular pathway by which the alternatively spliced amelogenin peptides exert their activity has also been undertaken by members of the Veis group and others. The lysosomal-associated membrane protein 1 (LAMP-1) has been identified as a cell surface receptor for LRAP in a mouse fetal myoblast cell line C2C12 [18]. LAMP-1 is ubiquitously expressed and has been shown to mediate amelogenin intake through endocytosis [19]. The [A-4] peptide stimulates M180 expression partly through the activation of the nitric oxide (NO) signaling pathway in ameloblast-like LS8 cells [20]. LAMP1 participates in the intracellular traffic of [A-4], evidenced by the co-localization of Internalized [A-4] with LAMP1 in late endosomal/lysosomal compartments [20]. While enticing observations, the precise pathway(s) that modify gene expression in responding cells has remained difficult to penetrate and fully characterize.

When implanted in the pulp, recombinant amelogenins that correspond to the alternatively spliced amelogenin gene products [A+4] and [A-4] induce the recruitment, proliferation, and differentiation of reparative cells. The signaling effects of the amelogenin peptides [A+4] and [A-4] appear to depend on the type of target cells, their stage of differentiation, the time of treatment, and the type of amelogenin peptide ([A+4] or [A-4]). However, the mechanisms mediating the signaling effects of the amelogenin peptides remain unclear [21].

STEM CELL INDUCTION

The [A+4] and [A-4] proteins are orthologs of murine amelogenin isoform M73 and M59 respectively, with identical amino acid residues shared between the two species (Figure 1).

M59	**MPLPPHPGSPGYINLSYEVLTPLKWYQSMIRQPPLSPILPELPLEAWPATDKTKREEVD**
M73	**MPLPPHPGSPGYINLSYEVLTPLKWYQSMIRQPKSHSQAINTDRTALPLSPILPELPLEAWPATDKTKREEVD**

Figure 1: Sequence of M59 and M73. M59/LRAP is the murine ortholog of rat [A-4] and M73 is the murine ortholog of rat [A+4].

LRAP has been shown to have a direct effect on cementoblast activity and the involvement of MAPK pathway is suggested by inhibitor assays [22]. We detected LRAP expression during osteogenesis

The isoform M59 is best known as LRAP (Leucine Rich Amelogenin Polypeptide).of wild-type (WT) embryonic stem (ES) cells and observed the absence of LRAP expression in amelogenin-null (KO) ES cells. We explored the signaling effect of LRAP on wild-type ES cells, and the ability of LRAP to rescue the impaired osteogenesis phenotype observed in KO ES cells. Our data indicate that LRAP treatment of WT and KO ES cells induces a significant increase in mineral matrix formation, and significant increases in bone sialoprotein and osterix gene expression. In addition, the amelogenin KO phenotype is partially rescued by the addition of exogenous LRAP. These data suggest a unique function of LRAP during ES cell differentiation along osteogenic lineage [23]. We demonstrated that the canonical Wnt/beta-catenin signaling is activated upon LRAP treatment, as evidenced by elevated beta-catenin level and increased Wnt reporter gene activity. Furthermore, a specific Wnt inhibitor sFRP-1 completely blocked the LRAP-mediated Wnt signaling. However, exogenous recombinant Wnt3a alone was less effective at osteogenic induction of mouse ES cells in comparison to LRAP. Using a quantitative real-time PCR array, we discovered that LRAP treatment up-regulated the expression of Wnt agonists and down-regulated the expression of Wnt antagonists. We conclude that LRAP activates the canonical Wnt signaling pathway to induce osteogenic differentiation of mouse ES cells through the concerted regulation of Wnt agonists and antagonists [24]. In addition, Matsuzawa and colleagues [25] showed that cells of the murine periodontal tissues responded to full length 180-amino-acid long recombinant amelogenin protein through the Wnt pathway. Here, a transgenic mouse bearing a construct designed to report on the site of Wnt activation by turning on lacZ under the control of LEF consensus binding sites (Topflash mouse) demonstrated that cells of the periodontium respond to amelogenin via the Wnt signaling pathway.

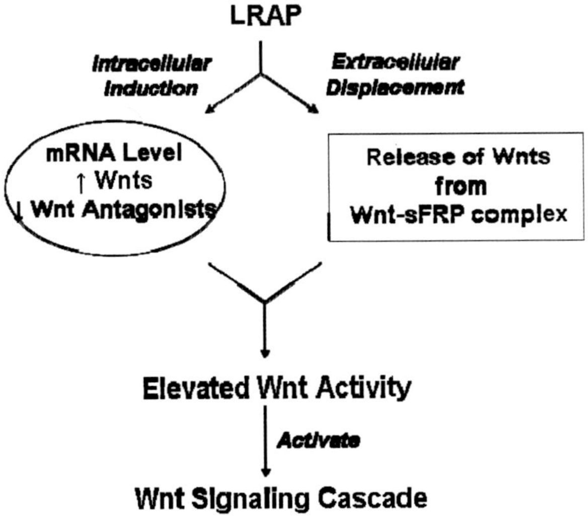

Figure 2: Model of LRAP-Wnt Signaling.

In our model, we propose that LRAP activates Wnt signaling in two distinctive ways. In the cells, LRAP upregulates Wnt expression whereas it simultaneously downregulates the expression of Wnt antagonists. Extracellularly, LRAP is proposed to displace Wnt from its soluble decoy receptor sFRP-1, making Wnt molecules available to bind to canonical membrane receptors. The net effect is to give rise to elevated level of Wnt protein and consequently activated Wnt/b-catenin signaling (Figure 2).

In preliminary studies we sought to determine the effect of LRAP on osteogenesis in vivo. Here, we employed a rat femoral critical size defect model by placing pre-assembled nanofiber artificial matrix gels composed of peptide amphiphiles [26, 27] containing LRAP (50 ng/ml) in a 5-mm gap and analyzed bone formation with micro-computed tomography (microCT). The peptide amphiphile formed nanofiber alone and a scrambled LRAP (50 ng/ml) were used as controls. Preliminary data from microCT analysis demonstrated that animals treated with LRAP had a significantly higher volume of ossified tissues (Figure 3), indicating that LRAP stimulates bone formation effectively in vivo.

PERSPECTIVES

Human genetic studies have implicated Wnt signaling in human bone and metabolic diseases. Loss-of-function mutations in human LRP5, the co-receptor for the Wnt-frizzled receptor, are associated with osteoporosis-pseudoglioma syndrome characterized by low bone mineral density and skeletal fragility [28]. Conversely, mutations in the N terminus of human LRP5 reduce affinity of LRP5 for Dkk1, resulting in high bone mass [29-31]. These human bone phenotypes are largely corroborated independently by animal models with altered expression of LRP5. *Lrp5* null mice exhibit a low bone mass phenotype due to reduced proliferation of precursor cells [32]. Mice overexpressing the G171V LRP5 mutant in osteoblasts have elevated osteoblast activity, reduced osteoblast apoptosis, and a high bone mass phenotype, similar to that observed in humans with this mutation [33].

Interestingly, overexpression of wild-type Lrp5 leads to a more subtle bone phenotype, suggesting that the G171V mutant has a gain-of-function phenotype indicative of a dominant-positive mechanism. Loss of bone mineral density in *Lrp5* null mice is further exacerbated by the loss of an *Lrp6* allele, suggesting that Wnt proteins signal through both the LRP5 and LRP6 coreceptors to influence bone mass [33]. Furthermore, disruption of endogenous LRP inhibitors such as Dkk1 [30] or sclerostin [34] increases the ability of Wnt proteins to stabilize β-catenin and stimulate osteogenesis, demonstrating that signaling from LRP coreceptors is important for bone development. Direct roles for Wnt signaling in the regulation of trabecular bone formation and bone mass were further supported by studies of sFRP-1 null mice [35]. These mice exhibited increased trabecular bone mineral density, volume, and mineral apposition rate when compared with wild-type controls. In addition, deletion of sFRP-1 inhibited osteoblast lineage cell apoptosis while enhancing the proliferation and differentiation of these cells in vitro. Taken together, these studies suggest that endogenous Wnt signaling plays an important role in osteogenesis and bone formation; however, which of the 19 Wnt protein are involved has yet to be delineated. Moreover, it may be difficult to identify a strategy appropriate to deliver the Wnt proteins in therapeutic doses without risking their oncogenic potential in the recipient.

The discovery that LRAP activates Wnt/b-catenin signaling pathway to stimulate osteogenesis makes LRAP amenable to novel therapies and interventions to treat Wnt-related bone disorders. LRAP has the potential to harvest the therapeutic value of Wnt signaling pathways without direct application of Wnt proteins, thereby mitigating the adverse effect on cells of direct Wnt protein exposure. Compared to the glycosylated Wnt proteins (over 40 KDa), LRAP is much smaller (~ 6 KDa), which also gives LRAP a distinct advantage on delivery as a therapeutic agent and may permit other small molecule agonists and antagonists to be identified and delivered via a chemical tether to the self-assembling peptide amphiphiles employed for therapy in human patients.

Emdogain (enamel matrix derivative, EMD) has been used to stimulate regeneration of periodontal tissues lost to periodontal disease. The major (>95%) component of EMD is amelogenins. No other active components have been isolated from EMD, and purified amelogenins have been shown to induce the same effect as the complete EMD (reviewed by [36]. Understanding how LRAP works may shed light on the mechanism by which EMD stimulates periodontal tissue regeneration. Periodontal disease remains one of the most prevalent infectious diseases of mankind. Identifying effective means to simulate periodontal regeneration remains an unfilled reservoir of therapeutic need [37].

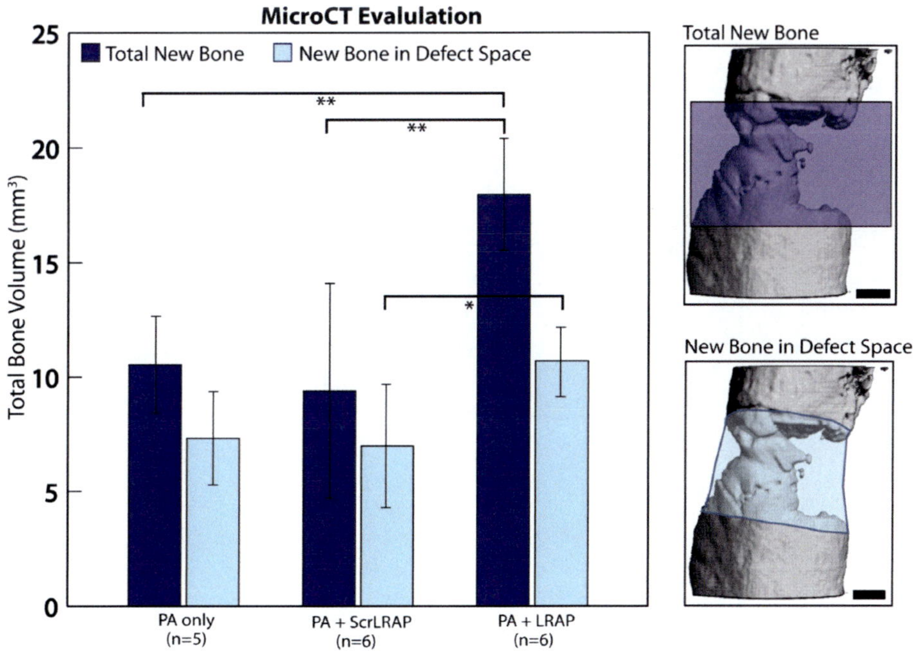

Figure 3: Effect of LRAP on new bone formation in rat femoral critical size defect model. Volumes of total new bone and new bone with defect were quantified by microCT analysis. (* $P<0.05$; ** $P<0.01$).

ACKNOWLEDGEMENT

Supported by the USPHS, NIH, National Institute of Dental and Craniofacial Research by grants DE06988 (MLS), DE13045 (MLS), DE015920 (SIS), and DE017362 (YZ); James H. Zumberge Faculty Research & Innovation Fund, University of Southern California (YZ), and Thammasat University School of Dentistry, Thailand (RW).

REFERENCES

[1] Aldred MJ, Crawford PJM, Roberts E, et al., Identification of a nonsense mutation in the amelogenin gene (AMELX) in a family with X-linked amelogenesis imperfecta (AIH1). Hum Genet 1992. 90(4): 413-6.

[2] Diekwisch T, David S, Bringas P,et al., Antisense inhibition of AMEL translation demonstrates supramolecular controls for enamel HAP crystal growth during embryonic mouse molar development. Development 1993. 117(2): 471-82.

[3] Gibson CW, Yuan ZA, Hall B, et al., Amelogenin-deficient mice display an amelogenesis imperfecta phenotype. J Biol Chem 2001. 276(34): 31871-5.

[4] Lagerstrom M, Dahl N, Nakahori Y, et al., A deletion in the amelogenin gene (AMG) causes X-linked amelogenesis imperfecta (AIH1). Genomics 1991. 10(4): p. 971-5.

[5] Lagerstrom-Fermer M, Nilsson M, Bäckman, et al., Amelogenin signal peptide mutation: correlation between mutations in the amelogenin gene (AMGX) and manifestations of X-linked amelogenesis imperfecta. Genomics 1995. 26(1): 159-62.

[6] Lyngstadaas SP,Risnes S, Sproat BS, et al., A synthetic, chemically modified ribozyme eliminates amelogenin, the major translation product in developing mouse enamel in vivo. Embo J 1995. 14(21): 5224-9.

[7] Paine, M.L. and M.L. Snead, Protein interactions during assembly of the enamel organic extracellular matrix. J Bone Miner Res 1997. 12(2): 221-7.

[8] Paine ML, Zhu DH, Luo W, et al., Enamel biomineralization defects result from alterations to amelogenin self-assembly. J Struct Biol 2000. 132(3): 191-200.

[9] Paine ML,White SN, Luo W, et al., Regulated gene expression dictates enamel structure and tooth function. Matrix Biol 2001. 20(5-6): 273-92.

[10] Giannobile, W.V. and M.J. Somerman, Growth and amelogenin-like factors in periodontal wound healing. A systematic review. Ann Periodontol 2003. 8(1): 193-204.

[11] Veis, A., Amelogenin gene splice products: potential signaling molecules. Cell Mol Life Sci 2003. 60(1): 38-55.

[12] Goldberg M, lacerda-Pinheiro S, Jegat N, et al., The impact of bioactive molecules to stimulate tooth repair and regeneration as part of restorative dentistry. Dent Clin North Am 2006. 50(2): 277-98,

[13] Amar S, Sires B, Sabsay B, et al., The isolation and partial characterization of a rat incisor dentin matrix polypeptide with in vitro chondrogenic activity. J Biol Chem 1991. 266(13): 8609-18.

[14] Nebgen DR, Inoue H, Sabsay B, et al., Identification of the chondrogenic-inducing activity from bovine dentin (bCIA) as a low-molecular-mass amelogenin polypeptide. J Dent Res 1999. 78(9): 1484-94.

[15] Veis A, Tompkins K, Alvares K, et al., Specific amelogenin gene splice products have signaling effects on cells in culture and in implants in vivo. J Biol Chem 2000. 275(52): 41263-72.

[16] Tompkins, K. and A. Veis, Polypeptides translated from alternatively spliced transcripts of the amelogenin gene, devoid of the exon 6a, b, c region, have specific effects on tooth germ development in culture. Connect Tissue Res 2002. 43(2-3): 224-31.

[17] Tompkins K, Alvares K, George A, et al., Two related low molecular mass polypeptide isoforms of amelogenin have distinct activities in mouse tooth germ differentiation in vitro. J Bone Miner Res 2005. 20(2): 341-9.

[18] Tompkins, K., A. George, and A. Veis, Characterization of a mouse amelogenin [A-4]/M59 cell surface receptor. Bone 2006. 38(2): 172-180.

[19] Shapiro JL, Wen X, Okamoto CT, et al., Cellular uptake of amelogenin, and its localization to CD63, and Lamp1-positive vesicles. Cell Mol Life Sci 2007. 64(2): 244-56.

[20] Iacob, S. and A. Veis, Identification of the functional activity of the [A-4] amelogenin gene splice product in newborn mouse ameloblasts. Bone 2008. 42(6): 1072-9.

[21] Lacerda-Pinheiro S, Jegat N, Septier D, et al., Early in vivo and in vitro effects of amelogenin gene splice products on pulp cells. Eur J Oral Sci 2006. 114 Suppl 1: 232-8; discussion 254-6, 381-2.

[22] Boabaid F, Gibson CW, Kuehl MA et al., Leucine-rich amelogenin peptide: a candidate signaling molecule during cementogenesis. J Periodontol 2004. 75(8): 1126-36.
[23] Warotayanont R, Zhu D, Snead ML, et al., Leucine-rich amelogenin peptide induces osteogenesis in mouse embryonic stem cells. Biochem Biophys Res Commun 2008. 367(1): 1-6.
[24] Warotayanont R, Frenkel B, Snead ML, et al., Leucine-rich amelogenin peptide induces osteogenesis by activation of the Wnt pathway. Biochem Biophys Res Commun 2009. 387(3): 558-63.
[25] Matsuzawa, M., Sheu TJ, Lee YJ, et al., Putative signaling action of amelogenin utilizes the Wnt/beta-catenin pathway. J Periodontal Res 2009. 44(3): 289-96.
[26] Stupp SI and Braun PV Molecular manipulation of microstructures: biomaterials, ceramics, and semiconductors. Science 1997. 277(5330): 1242-8.
[27] Palmer LC, Newcomb CJ, Kaltz SR, et al., Biomimetic systems for hydroxyapatite mineralization inspired by bone and enamel. Chem Rev 2008. 108(11): 4754-83.
[28] Gong Y, Slee RB, Fukai N, et al., LDL receptor-related protein 5 (LRP5) affects bone accrual and eye development. Cell 2001. 107(4): 513-23.
[29] Ai M, Holmen SL, Van Hul W, et al., Reduced affinity to and inhibition by DKK1 form a common mechanism by which high bone mass-associated missense mutations in LRP5 affect canonical Wnt signaling. Mol Cell Biol 2005. 25(12): 4946-55.
[30] Boyden LM, Mao J, Belsky J, et al., High bone density due to a mutation in LDL-receptor-related protein 5. N Engl J Med 2002. 346(20):. 1513-21.
[31] Van Wesenbeeck L, Cleiren E, Gram J, et al., Six novel missense mutations in the LDL receptor-related protein 5 (LRP5) gene in different conditions with an increased bone density. Am J Hum Genet 2003. 72(3): 763-71.
[32] Kato M, patel MS, Levasseur R, et al., Cbfa1-independent decrease in osteoblast proliferation, osteopenia, and persistent embryonic eye vascularization in mice deficient in Lrp5, a Wnt coreceptor. J Cell Biol 2002. 157(2): 303-14.
[33] Babij P, Zhao W, Small C, et al., High bone mass in mice expressing a mutant LRP5 gene. J Bone Miner Res 2003. 18(6): 960-74.
[34] Li X, Zhang Y, Kang H, et al., Sclerostin binds to LRP5/6 and antagonizes canonical Wnt signaling. J Biol Chem 2005. 280(20): 19883-7.
[35] Bodine PV, Zhao W, Kharode YP, et al., The Wnt antagonist secreted frizzled-related protein-1 is a negative regulator of trabecular bone formation in adult mice. Mol Endocrinol 2004. 18(5): 1222-37.
[36] Lyngstadaas SP, Wohlfahrt JC, Brookes SJ, et al., Enamel matrix proteins; old molecules for new applications. Orthod Craniofac Res 2009. 12(3): 243-53.
[37] Evans, R.I., Invasive cervical resorption--a periodontist's perspective. Ann R Australas Coll Dent Surg 2000. 15: 327-30.

CHAPTER 17

Clinical Applications of an Enamel Matrix Protein Derivative in Regenerative Periodontal Therapy

Anton Sculean[1], Dieter D. Bosshardt[1] and Michel Brecx[2]

[1]Department of Periodontology, University of Bern, Bern, Switzerland and [2]Department of Conservative Dentistry and Periodontology, University of Tübingen, Tübingen, Germany

Abstract: The goal of regenerative periodontal therapy is the reconstitution of the lost periodontal structures (i.e. the new formation of root cementum, periodontal ligament and alveolar bone). Findings from basic research have pointed to the important role of an enamel matrix protein derivative (EMD) in periodontal wound healing. Histological results from acute and chronic animal models and from human case reports have provided evidence that treatment with EMD may indeed promote periodontal regeneration and positively influences wound healing in intrabony, class II furcation and recession type defects. Recent long-term randomized controlled clinical studies have demonstrated that the improvements obtained following surgery with EMD can be maintained on a long term basis. The aim of the present chapter is to provide an overwiev on the clinical applications for EMD in regenerative periodontal therapy.

Key Words: Enamel Matrix Derivative, Regenerative Periodontal Therapy, Periodontal Regeneration, Human Histology, Clinical Trials.

1. INTRODUCTION

The aims of periodontal therapy are to arrest and control the infection and, ultimately to regenerate the lost supporting apparatus of the tooth (i.e. root cementum, periodontal ligament and alveolar bone) [1].

One well established method to enhance periodontal regeneration is the use of an enamel matrix derivative (EMD). The rationale for the clinical use of EMD is the observation that enamel matrix proteins (EMPs) are deposited onto the surface of developing tooth roots prior to cementum formation [2-4].

Recent data indicate that EMD affects many different cell types including epithelial cells, periodontal ligament and gingival fibroblasts, and osteoblasts [5]. It has been shown that EMD has effects on cell attachment, spreading, and chemotaxis, cell proliferation and survival, expression of growth factors, cytokines, and extracellular matrix molecules, and on the expression of certain molecules which modulate bone remodeling [5].

A technique or a material must, however, fulfill the following criteria in order to be classified as "regeneration-promoting" [6]:

- In vitro studies, which confirm the action mechanism.
- Controlled histological animal studies, which demonstrate formation of new root cementum, periodontal ligament and alveolar bone (Figs. 1 and 2).
- Human biopsies, which show formation of root cementum, periodontal ligament and alveolar bone on a plaque-infected root surface.
- Controlled clinical studies, which prove a gain of clinical attachment and radiological new bone formation. In the following overview, the existing evidence regarding the clinical use of EMD is provided.

The aim of the present chapter is to provide an overwiev on the clinical applications for EMD in regenerative periodontal therapy, thus focusing on the evidence from human histologic studies and clinical trials.

***Correspondence Author:** Dr. Anton Sculean; Department of Periodontology, Dental School University of Bern, Freiburgstrasse 7, 3010 Bern, Switzerland; Tel: +41 (0)31 632 25 77; Fax: +41 (0)31 632 49 15; E-mail: anton.sculean@zmk.unibe.ch

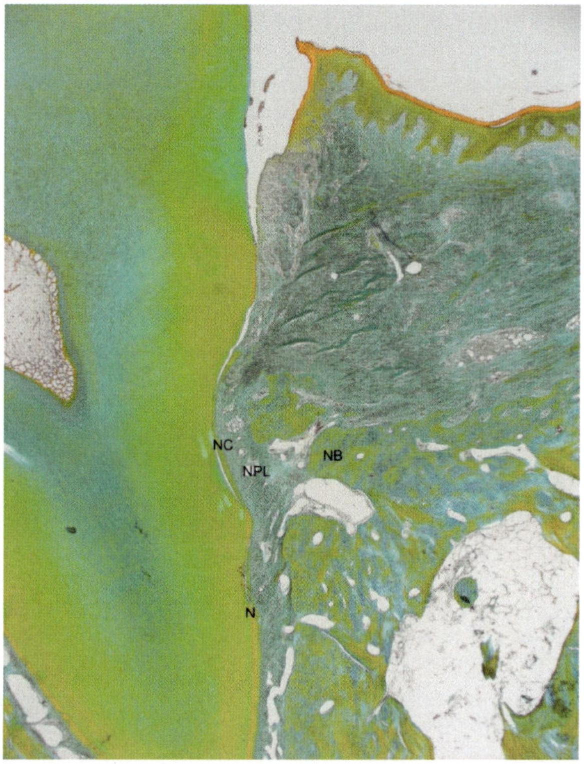

Figure 1: Representative photomicrograph of healing following treatment of a monkey intrabony defect with open flap debridement (OFD) and an enamel matrix derivative (EMD). New cementum (NC), new periodontal ligament (NPL) and new alveolar bone (NB) have formed coronal to the notch (N). Oxone-aldehyde-fuchsin-Halmi stain.

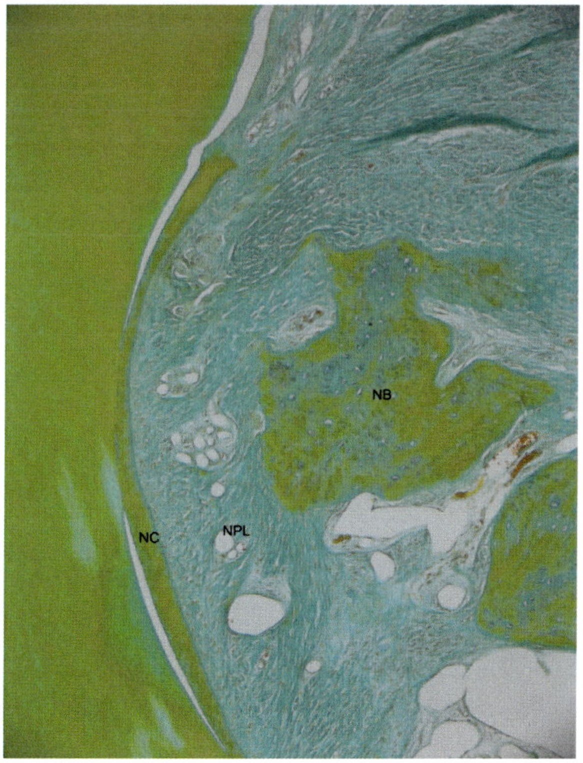

Figure 2: Higher magnification of the regenerated area shown in Fig. 1. Functionally oriented collagen fibers are inserting into the newly formed cementum (NC). NPL: new periodontal ligament, NB: new bone. Oxone-aldehyde-fuchsin-Halmi stain.

EVIDENCE FROM HUMAN HISTOLOGICAL STUDIES

Results of the first human-histological biopsy were published by Heijl [7]. A recession defect on a lower incisor was surgically created and treated with EMD. After a healing period of 4 months, the tooth as well as the surrounding soft and hard tissue was extracted and histologically evaluated. The histological investigation showed that a new layer of acellular root cementum covered 73% of the original defect depth. New alveolar bone has regenerated on 65% of the initial bone height. In another study Yukna and Mellonig [8] treated 10 intrabony periodontal defects in 8 patients with EMD. The histological analysis 6 months after the treatment has shown in 3 biopsies a complete periodontal regeneration (i.e. new formation of root cementum, periodontal ligament and alveolar bone), while in 3 further biopsies, the healing was characterized by a new connective tissue attachment (i.e. new cementum with inserting collagen fibers). 4 biopsies healed by a long junctional epithelium and without any signs of periodontal regeneration. In a comparative clinical and histological investigation the healing of intrabony periodontal defects was evaluated following treatment with EMD or Guided Tissue Regeneration (GTR) with a bioabsorbable barrier [9]. 6 months after therapy, the clinical attachment level (CAL) showed a mean gain of 3.2 ± 1.2 mm in the EMD group and of 3.6 ± 1.7 mm in the GTR group. The histological analysis showed that in both groups the healing was mainly characterized by periodontal regeneration [9]. The mean value of new cementum and periodontal ligament amounted to 2.6 ± 1.0 mm in the EMD group and to 2.1 ± 1.0 mm in the GTR group. The mean value of new alveolar bone was 0.9 ± 1.0 mm in the EMD group and of in the GTR group 2.1 ± 1.0 mm. A reparative healing by a long junctional epithelium occurred only in one biopsy from the EMD group. The results of the study have provided evidence that treatment with EMD promotes periodontal regeneration in humans and may lead to comparable clinical and histological results than the GTR therapy. These results were confirmed in subsequent reports by other authors, not only in intrabony but also in recession-type defects [10-15]. Subsequent immunohistological studies have shown that following surgery EMD remains up to 4 weeks on the root surface and, the wound healing and/or remodelling process can be followed for a period of up to 6 months after treatment with EMD therapy [16-18]. A subsequent human histologic study has attempted to characterize the tissues developing on the root surface at 2 to 6 weeks following treatment of intrabony defects with EMD [19, 20]. The results have shown that the newly formed tissues on the root surfaces were thick, collagenous, devoid of extrinsic fibers, and had an irregular surface contour. The presence of electron-dense, organic material in the collagenous matrix indicated at least partial mineralization. Embedded cells were numerous and the cells on the matrix surface were very large in size. It was concluded that following treatment with EMD, a bone-like tissue resembling cellular intrinsic fiber cementum may develop on the root surfaces, instead of acellular extrinsic fiber cementum. Furthermore, EMD may both induce de novo formation of a mineralized connective tissue on scaled root surfaces and stimulate matrix deposition on old native cementum.

The question whether periodontal regeneration may occur following non-surgical therapy and subsequent application of EMD is still difficult to be answered. In one study, sixteen patients, with one advanced intrabony defect were treated with: i) scaling and root planing with hand instruments and additional application of EMD, ii) scaling with an ultrasonic instrument and additional application of EMD, iii) scaling with an ultrasonic instrument alone [21]. At six months after surgery the clinical examination revealed a probing depth reduction and a gain of clinical attachment after all three treatment modalities. The histological evaluation, however, revealed that healing after all three treatment approaches was predominantly characterized by formation of a long junctional epithelium along the instrumented root surface and no predictable regeneration of attachment apparatus. On the other hand, a very recent study has demonstrated periodontal regeneration in 3 out of 4 intrabony defects treated with nonsurgical therapy and application of EMD [22].

Based on the available human histological evidence it may be concluded that the application of EMD may promote formation of new cementum, periodontal ligament and bone in intrabony and recession defects. A surgical access appears, however, to be preferable in order to better control the clinical procedure.

At present, there are no histologic data from human material evaluating the regenerative potential of EMD in furcation defects.

EVIDENCE ON THE EFFECT OF EMD ON EARLY WOUND HEALING

Several studies have attempted to evaluate the effect of EMD treatment on early wound healing [23-25]. In a double-masked, split-mouth, placebo-controlled, randomized study 28 patients with moderately advanced chronic periodontitis were scaled and root palned, and the soft tissue wall of the pocket was curetted to remove pocket epithelium and adjacent granulation tissue [23]. All experimental sites were carefully irrigated with saline. When the bleeding from the pocket had ceased, a 24% EDTA gel was applied in the sites and retained for 2 min. The sites were then thoroughly irrigated with saline to remove EDTA remnants. Subsequently, left and right quadrants were randomized to subgingival application of EMD (test) or vehicle (control). All sites were re-examined clinically after 1, 2 and 3 weeks. In addition, a visual analogue scale (VAS) was used to score the degree of post-treatment discomfort. The results indicated that EMD topically applied in instrumented sulci enhance the early healing of periodontal soft tissue wounds. Furthermore, at 1 week, the proportion of patients reporting a VAS score ≤ 20 was significantly higher for the EMD treated quadrants than for controls. Another study has evaluated by clinical means and as patient perception of post-operative events, the effect of EMD on the healing of soft-tissue wounds following periodontal surgery [25]. Patients scheduled for periodontal flap surgery were treated with either modified Widman flap and application of EMD (test) or with modified Widman flap alone (control). Clinical measurements were taken at four different points in time, at surgery, 1, 4 and 8 weeks after surgery. The results revealed that of all parameters evaluated, none showed a significant difference between the control and EMD groups, except for gingival swelling at the 1-week assessment where the EMD group exhibited a higher swelling score. It was concluded that the early wound healing of periodontal flap-surgeries in those sites treated with EMD is not different from control sites. Based on the available data, no definitive conclusions can be drawn to what extent the application of EMD may additionally enhance early wound healing following nonsurgical or surgical periodontal therapy.

EVIDENCE FROM CLINICAL STUDIES IN INTRABONY DEFECTS

Nonsurgical Periodontal Therapy

Two randomized, placebo controlled clinical studies have evaluated in intrabony defects the effects of EMD as adjunct to nonsurgical periodontal therapy [26, 27]. Both studies have failed to show a significant benefit of using EMD during nonsurgical periodontal therapy.

Surgical Periodontal Therapy

Side effects such as for example, incompatibility or allergic reactions even after repeated treatment with EMD have not yet been reported in any clinical trial [28-31]. A multi-center study evaluated the potential for sensitization to EMD in a subgroup of periodontal patients treated at least twice with at least 2 months between treatments [31]. Intrabony defects in 376 patients in 11 university-based postgraduate periodontics programs and five private practices were treated with open flap debridement, root conditioning with either citric acid pH = 1 or 24% EDTA followed by defect irrigation with sterile saline and application of EMD. The second test defect was treated in a similar manner at least 8 weeks after the first surgery. No clinical adverse reactions to multiple applications of EMD were noted. The results demonstrated a lack of clinical adverse reactions following 2 separate applications of EMD. Any subjective/objective adverse reactions experienced by the patient were typical complications following routine periodontal surgery and were not directly related to the use of EMD. Data from controlled clinical studies have demonstrated that treatment of intrabony defects with EMD results in a significant reduction of the probing depths and gain of clinical attachment. Moreover, it was shown that EMD attenuated the release of TNF-α and interleukin-8 in whole blood from healthy donors challenged by lipopolysaccharide or peptidoglycan, while the release of interleukin-10 was unchanged. EMD also produced a four-fold increase in the cAMP levels of peripheral blood mononuclear cell lysates, which in turn suggested that EMD has anti-inflammatory properties [31]. A randomized, placebo controlled multicenter-study examined the effectiveness of EMD in the split-mouth procedure in 33 patients [32]. The results after 36 months showed a mean CAL gain of 2.2 mm in the test group and of 1.7 mm in the control group (open flap debridement). The radiologically determined bone gain amounted to 2.6 mm in the test group, with a 66% fill of the bone defects. However, the control teeth did not show any bone gain. In another controlled clinical study Froum et al. [33], compared the treatment of deep intrabony defects by open flap surgery with and without EMD. In 23 patients with at least 2 intrabony defects each a total of 53 defects were treated with open flap surgery + EMD and 31 were treated only with open flap surgery alone. After a healing phase of 12 months the defects were again opened and the defect fill measured. The results showed that the treatment with open flap surgery + EMD resulted in a 3 x larger defect fill than the treatment with flap surgery alone (74% defect fill after flap surgery + EMD vs. 23% defect fill after flap surgery alone) [33]. In a further prospective, controlled clinical study a total of 40 patients were treated by surgical therapy with either EMD or GTR with a non-bioabsorbable or with 2 bioabsorbable barriers and compared to the open flap surgery (control) [34]. All 4 regenerative procedures were equally effective regarding probing depth (PD) reduction and CAL gain and, significantly better than the control treatment. A prospective, randomized, multi-center clinical study reported the treatment of intrabony defects with the papilla preservation technique with and without auxiliary application of EMD [35]. A total of 83 test and 83 control defects were treated. After 1 year the results showed significantly higher CAL gain in the test group than in the control group [35]. On the other hand, one randomized, double-masked, placebo-controlled clinical trial has failed to show significant differences in clinical and radiographic parameters following treatment of intrabony defects with open flap debridement and application of EMD or placebo [36]. Most data from controlled clinical studies, however, indicate that the additional application of EMD in the context of surgical therapy of deep intrabony periodontal defects may lead to significantly higher gains of clinical attachment and defect fill compared to open flap debridement [32-35, 37-42] (Table 1). Very recent data have also pointed to the potential advantage of EMD to be used in the context of minimally invasive surgical techniques, thus resulting in improved wound stability and less soft tissue recession and patient morbidity [43, 44]. Moreover, surgical treatment with EMD was also demonstrated to significantly improve supracrestal soft-tissue density compared to open flap debridement alone [45, 46]. In a recent study, supra-alveolar-type defects were randomly treated with open flap debridement (OFD) with and without EMD [46]. At one year after surgery, at sites ≥ 7 mm, the addition of EMD yielded statisticaly significant higher mean CAL gains compared to OFD (i.e. 2.72 mm vs. 0.78 mm, respectively). Although promising, these results need to be confirmed in large scale, multicenter controlled clinical trials.

Table 1: Controlled clinical studies comparing treatment of intrabony defects with Open Flap Debridement (OFD) with or without EMD.

Study	**Study design**	**Treatments**	**Mean PPD change (mm)**	**p value**	**Mean CAL change (mm)**	**p value**
Heijl et al. 199732	Split mouth	EMD OFD	3.3 2.6	<0.01	2.3 1.7	<0.01
Pontoriero et al. 199934	Split mouth	EMD OFD	4.4 3.5	<0.001	2.9 1.8	<0.001
Okuda et al. 200037	Split mouth	EMD OFD	3.00 2.22	<0.05	1.72 0.83	<0.05
Froum et al. 200133	Split mouth	EMD OFD	4.94 2.24	<0.0001	4.28 2.65	<0.0001
Silvestri et al. 200038	Parallel	EMD OFD	4.8 1.4	<0.01	4.5 1.2	<0.01
Sculean et al. 200139	Parallel	EMD OFD	4.1 3.7	n.s.	3.4 1.7	<0.05
Tonetti et al. 200235	Parallel	EMD OFD	3.9 3.3	0.02	3.1 2.5	<0.01
Zucchelli et al. 200240	Parallel	EMD OFD	5.1 4.5	<0.01	4.2 2.6	<0.01
Rösing et al. 200536	Split mouth	EMD OFD	4.17 4.39	n.s.	2.01 2.16	n.s.

The postoperative administration of amoxicillin and metronidazole or of a selective cyclo-oxygenase-2 inhibitor did not seem to additionally enhance the clinical results [47, 48]. Furthermore, two studies have suggested that the clinical outcomes in intrabony defects treated with EMD do not depend on the use of EDTA root conditioning [49, 50]. Comparative studies reported similar results after treatment of intrabony defects with EMD or GTR, whereby the type of the GTR barrier (non bioabsorbable or bioabsorbable) did not play a role [34, 38-41, 51, 52, 55, 56, 58, 60] (Table 2). Regarding the clinical relevance of using EMD or GTR, it should be pointed to the results of a prospective multicenter, randomized, controlled clinical trial compared the clinical outcomes of EMD versus GTR with a bioabsorbable membrane [52]. Seventy five patients with advanced chronic periodontitis were recruited in 7 centers in 3 countries. The surgical procedures included access for root instrumentation using the simplified papilla preservation flap and either the application of EMD or placement of a resorbable GTR membrane. The results of the trial have failed to demonstrate superiority of one treatment over the other. From a clinical point of view it is of interest to note that all cases treated with GTR presented at least one surgical complication, mostly membrane exposure, while only 6% of EMD treated sites displayed complications.

Findings from longitudinal studies have shown that the obtained clinical improvements with EMD can be maintained over a period of up to 10 years [53-60] (Figs. 3 and 4).

Table 2: Controlled clinical studies comparing treatment of intrabony defects with Open Flap Debridement (OFD) and EMD to OFD and GTR.

Study	Study design	Treatments	Mean PPD change (mm)	p value	Mean CAL change (mm)	p value
Sculean et al. 1999[51]	Split mouth	EMD GTR	3.8 4.0	n.s.	3.1 3.0	n.s.
Pontoriero et al. 1999[34]	Split mouth	EMD GTR	4.4 4.5	n.s.	2.9 3.1	n.s.
Silvestri et al. 2000[38]	Parallel	EMD GTR	4.8 5.9	n.s.	4.5 4.8	n.s.
Sculean et al. 2001[39]	Parallel	EMD GTR	4.1 4.2	n.s.	3.4 3.1	n.s.
Zucchelli et al. 2002[40]	Parallel	EMD GTR	5.1 6.5	<0.01	4.2 4.9	<0.01
Silvestri et al. 2003[41]	Parallel	EMD GTR	5.3 5.6	n.s.	4.1 4.3	n.s.
Sanz et al. 2004[52]	Parallel	EMD GTR	3.8 3.3	n.s.	3.1 2.5	n.s.

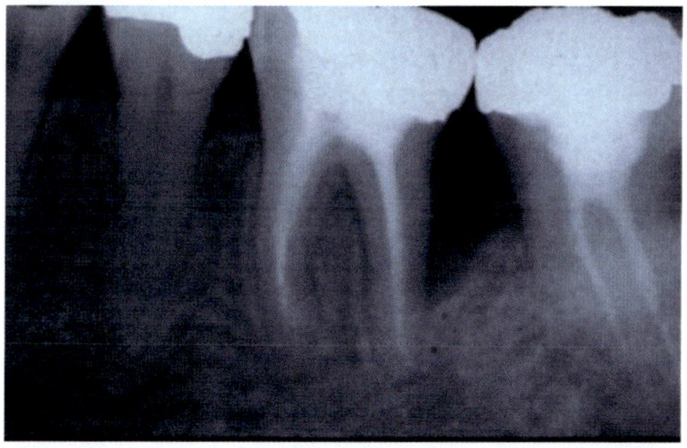

Figure 3: Intraoperative radiograph demonstrating a deep intrabony defect located at the distal aspect of a mandibular molar.

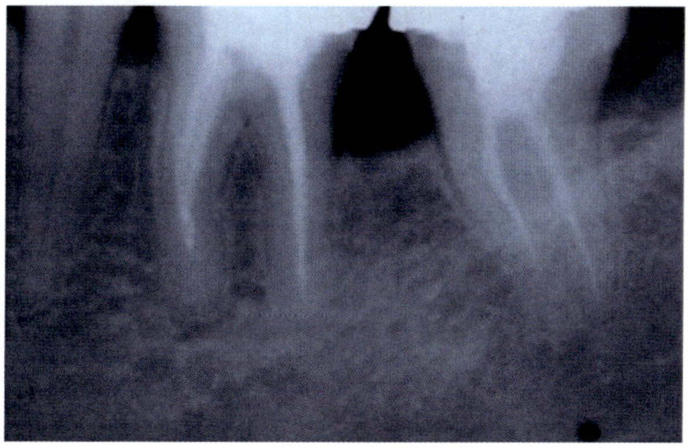

Figure 4: At ten years following regenerative surgery with OFD and EMD the intraoral radiograph revealed a complete fill of the intrabony defect.

Combination of EMD and Barrier Membranes or Grafting Materials

Experimental and clinical studies have indicated that the extent of the regeneration is determined by the available space under the mucoperiostal flap [1, 61, 62]. A collapse of the mucoperiostal flap may limit the area needed for the regeneration process and may thus affect the result of the therapy. In order to avoid these disadvantages, combination therapies between EMD and GTR and/or EMD and bone substitutes were tested. Observations from animal-histological and human-histological studies have demonstrated periodontal regeneration after treatment of intrabony defects with some of these combinations. In a prospective, controlled, clinical study the treatment of intrabony defects was evaluated following treatment with EMD, GTR, combination of EMD + GTR and open flap surgery [39]. The results have shown that all 3 regenerative procedures resulted in a significantly higher improvement of the clinical parameters compared to the conventional flap surgery; whereby the combination of EMD + GTR led to no additional improvement. Comparable results were also reported by others [63, 64]. A prospective, controlled split-mouth study has evaluated in 11 patients with a total of 12 pairs of intrabony defects the clinical response of EMD with or without a combination of a tertracycline-coated expanded polytetrafluoroethylene barrier membrane (e-PTFE) [64]. The results were evaluated at 6- and at 12 months following therapy. After 12 months, the mean CAL gain measured 1.28 ± 2.04 mm in the EMD group and 1.65 ± 1.29 mm in the EMD + GTR group, respectively. Except for more postoperative discomfort at the membrane treated sites, the results failed to reveal any significant differences between the 2 groups.

Several studies have evaluated the effect of a combination of EMD and various types of bone grafts/bone substitutes in the treatment of intrabony defects. Data from human histologic studies have provided evidence for regeneration of cementum, periodontal ligament and bone following a combination of EMD and a natural bone mineral or bioactive glass [65-67]. When the defects were filled with a bioactive glass alone, the healing occurred predominantly through formation of a long junction epithelium along the debrided root surface and connective tissue encapsulation of the graft particles [67].

Findings from controlled clinical studies seem to indicate that a combination of EMD and certain types of grafting materials such as autogenous bone, DFDBA, a natural bone mineral or a bioactive glass (BG) may additionally improve the hard and soft tissue parameters compared to treatment with EMD alone or to DFDBA alone [68-74]. Other studies have, however, failed to show statistically significant differences comparing the combination of EMD with either a beta tricalcium phosphate (β-TCP), a biphasic calcium phosphate (BCP) or BG with treatment using EMD alone [75-78].

Furthermore, clinical studies comparing various combinations of EMD and grafting materials to grafting materials alone are controversional (Table 3). While some studies have failed to shown an advantage of the combination approach others have found additional hard and soft tissue improvements following the combination approach [73, 79-81]. It may thus be speculated that the type of the bone graft/bone substitute and the volume and configuration of the defects are also important factors which might influence the clinical results. Furher, well designed controlled clinical studies are necessary in order to definitively elucidate the benefit of a combination therapy in relation to the single therapies.

Table 3: Controlled clinical studies comparing various combination modalities of EMD and either barrier membranes or grafting materials to the use of EMD alone.

Study	Study design	Treatments	Mean PPD change (mm)	p value	Mean CAL change (mm)	p value
Sculean et al. 200139	Parallel	EMD	4.1	n.s.	3.4	n.s.
		GTR	4.2	n.s.	3.1	n.s.
		EMD + GTR	4.3	n.s.	3.4	n.s.
		OFD	3.7	n.s.	1.7	<0.05
Minabe et al. 200263	Parallel	EMD + GTR	4.3	n.s.	3.0	n.s.
		EMD	3.8	n.s.	2.6	n.s.
		GTR	3.7	n.s.	2.8	n.s.
Sipos et al. 200564	Split mouth	EMD	2.86	n.s.	1.28	n.s.
		EMD + GTR	3.02	n.s.	1.65	n.s.
Lekovic et al.	Split mouth	EMD	1.91	<0.001	1.72	<0.001

200069		EMD + ABBM	3.43		3.13	
Velasquez-Plata et al. 200270	Split mouth	EMD	3.8	n.s.	2.9	n.s.
		EMD + ABBM	4.0	n.s.	3.4	n.s.
Zucchelli et al. 200371	Parallel	EMD	5.8	n.s.	5.8	<0.01
		EMD + ABBM	6.2	n.s.	4.9	
Gurinsky et al. 200472	Split mouth	EMD	4.0	n.s.	3.2	n.s.
		EMD + DFDBA	3.6	n.s.	3.0	n.s.
Guida et al. 200768	Parallel	EMD	5.6	n.s.	4.6	n.s.
		EMD + AB	5.1	n.s.	4.9	n.s.
Sculean et al. 200575	Parallel	EMD	4.5	n.s.	3.9	n.s.
		EMD + BG	4.2	n.s.	3.2	n.s.
Kuru et al. 200674	Split mouth	EMD	5.03	≤0.05	4.06	≤0.05
		EMD + BG	5.73		5.17	
Jepsen et al. 200878	Parallel	EMD	2.55	n.s.	1.83	n.s.
		EMD + BCP	1.93	n.s.	1.31	n.s.
Bokan et al. 200677	Parallel	EMD	3.9	n.s.	3.7	n.s.
		EMD + β-TCP	4.1	n.s.	4.0	n.s.
		OFD	3.8	n.s.	2.1	n.s.

EVIDENCE FROM CLINICAL STUDIES IN RECESSION DEFECTS

Human histological evidence for formation of cementum, periodontal ligament and bone was shown in several case reports following treatment of buccal recession defects with a coronally positioned flap and EMD alone or combined with a connective tissue graft [7, 13-15]. In two controlled clinical studies the treatment of buccal Miller class I and II gingival recessions with a coronally positioned flap and EMD or coronally positioned flap were examined using the split-mouth procedure [82, 83]. Over a short period of time (up to 1 year), the results did not show differences between the therapies in terms of root coverage. The additional application of EMD led, however, to statistically significantly higher formation of keratinized tissue than the coronally positioned flap technique alone [83]. A follow-up evaluation of this study has shown that over 2 years, complete root coverage could be maintained in 53% of the EMD group versus 23% in the control one [84]. A total of 47% of the treated recessions in the control group deteriorated again in second year after therapy compared to 22% in the EMD group indicating that EMD seems to provide better long-term results.

Similar results were obtained in a randomized controlled clinical study on 58 contralateral sites in 17 patients with > or = 2 mm of Miller Class I, II, and III buccal recessions treated with coronally positioned flap and EMD (test) or coronally positioned flap alone (control) [85]. At 6 months, there was a mean increase in keratinized tissue of 0.60 mm for the test sites and a mean decrease of 0.05 mm for the control sites. Test sites demonstrated better root coverage (i.e. 92.9% root coverage after 6 months) compared to the control sites (i.e. 66.8% root coverage after 6 months) [85]. These results were also corroborated by others [86]. Furthermore, a systematic review has recently demonstrated that the use of EMD in conjunction with a coronally advanced flap procedure, enhances the probability of obtaining complete root coverage in Miller Class I and II single gingival recessions [87].

In a controlled, clinical, split-mouth study involving 17 patients the therapy of buccal Miller class II recessions with a coronally positioned flap and EMD (test group) or with a coronally positioned flap and connective tissue graft (control) was compared [88]. The results have shown that 1 year after therapy the mean value of root coverage was 95.1% in the test group and 93.8% in the control group. A 100% root coverage was reached in 89.5% of the cases in the test group and in 79% of the cases in the control group. The additional histological evaluation of two biopsies showed that treatment of recession defects with a coronally positioned flap and EMD resulted in formation of root cementum, periodontal ligament and alveolar bone while treatment with a coronally positioned flap and a connective graft was characterized by a long junctional epithelium and even signs of root resorption [15]. Comparable results were also reported in a multicenter, controlled clinical trial comparing the clinical efficacy of a coronally advanced flap procedure with the additional use of EMD (test) to the coronally advanced flap procedure and subpedicle connective tissue graft (control) [89]. At 12 months the percent of root coverage in the test group was 71.7% ± 16.14

% and 87.0% ± 12.22% in the control one. The available data suggest that the use of EMD may enhance the outcome of root coverage procedures, but the additional application of a connective tissue graft seem to result in a higher increase of keratinized tissue [87-92]. It is interesting to note that most controlled clinical studies evaluating treatment of gingival recessions with coronally repositioned flaps and EMD reported stable clinical results after a longer time period (i.e. up to 2 years) and an increase in the with of keratinized tissue, thus indicating that EMD may have an effect upon proliferation and keratinization of gingival fibroblasts [84, 87, 91, 92] (Figs. 5 and 6).

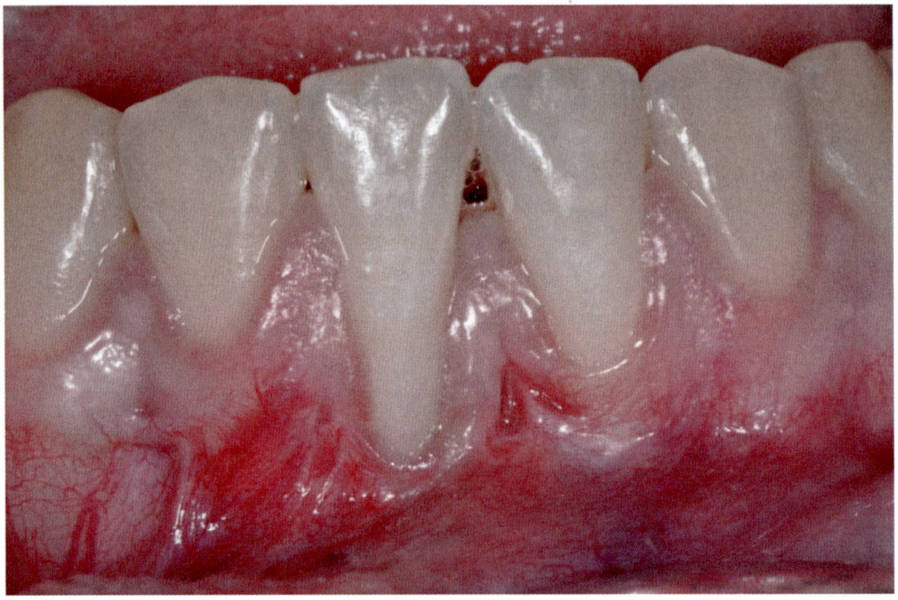

Figure 5: Deep gingival recession located at the vestibular aspect of the mandibular central incisors. Please note the scaring due to previous attempts to cover the recession.

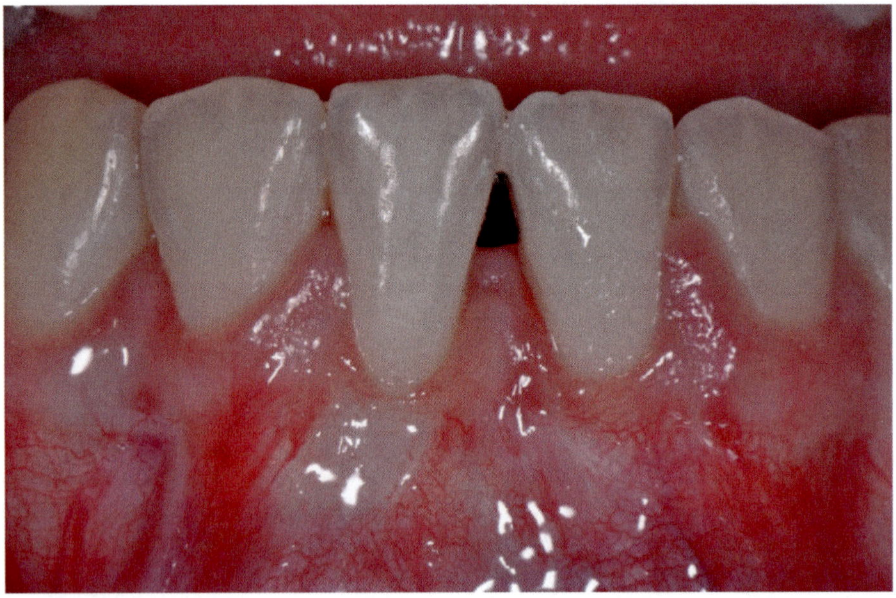

Figure 6: At six months following treatment with EMD and a connective tissue graft complete coverage of the recession are clearly visible. No scaring can any longer be distinguished.

EVIDENCE FROM CLINICAL STUDIES IN FURCATION DEFECTS

Data from controlled clinical studies evaluating the treatment of furcation defects by means of flap surgery with and without EMD are still limited. A multi-center, randomized, controlled, split-mouth, clinical study compared the treatment of mandibular class II furcation defects with EMD or GTR [93, 94]. A total of 44 patients with 90 comparable defects on contralateral molars were included. Defects were randomly assigned to treatment with EMD or GTR with a bioresorbable membrane. The results were evaluated at 8 and 14 months and included gingival margin levels, probing depths, bleeding on probing, vertical attachment levels, and vertical bone sounding from a stent at five buccal sites per tooth. Thc results have indicated that both treatment modalities led to significant clinical improvements. The median reduction of open horizontal furcation depth was 2.8 mm with the corresponding interquartile interval (1.5 mm, 3.5 mm) at test sites compared with 1.8 mm (1.0 mm, 2.8 mm) at control sites. The frequency of complete furcation closure was 8/45 (test) and 3/45 (control); partial closure, 27/45 in both groups; no change, 9/45 and 11/45, respectively. Deterioration was observed in 1/45 and 4/45 sites, respectively. The frequency of no pain or no swelling at 1 week post-surgery was 62% and 44%, respectively, at test sites and 12% and 6% at the control sites. It was concluded that there was a significantly greater reduction in horizontal furcation depth and a comparatively lower incidence of postoperative pain/swelling following EMD compared to GTR therapy. Recently, it was also shown that the use of EMD may also lead to clinical improvements in proximal class II furcation defects [95].

CONCLUSIONS

Based on the presented evidence the following conclusions can be drawn:

a. In intrabony defects, surgical periodontal therapy with EMD promotes periodontal regeneration and may lead to significantly higher clinical improvements than open flap debridement alone.

b. The results obtained following treatment with EMD are comparable to those following treatment with GTR and can be maintained over a long time period.

c. Treatment of intrabony defects with a combination of EMD + GTR does not seem to additionally improve the results compared to treatment with EMD alone or GTR alone.

d. The combination of EMD and certain types of grafting materials may result in additional improvements in the soft and hard tissue parameters compared to treatment with EMD alone. However, further studies are needed in order to definitively clarify the role of defect configuration and type of grafting material for the clinical outcomes.

e. Treatment of recession-type defects with coronally repositioned flaps and EMD may promote periodontal regeneration and may result in an increase in the width of keratinized tissue. The use of EMD in conjunction with a coronally advanced flap procedure, enhances the probability of obtaining complete root coverage in Miller Class I and II single gingival recessions and may provide better long-term results than coronally repositioned flaps alone.

f. Application of EMD may yield clinical improvements in mandibular and in maxillary proximal class II furcations. The clinical results are comparable to those obtained with GTR

REFERENCES

[1] Wikesjö UME and Selvig KA. Periodontal wound healing and regeneration. Periodontol 2000 1999; 19: 21-39.

[2] Hammarström L. Enamel matrix, cementum development and regeneration. J Clin Periodontol 1997; 24: 658-68.

[3] Slavkin HC and Boyde A. Cementum: An epithelial secretory product? J Dent Res 1975; 53: 157 (abstr. 409).

[4] Slavkin HC. Towards a cellular and molecular understanding of periodontics: Cementogenesis revisited. J Periodontol 1976; 47: 249-55.

[5] Bosshardt DD. Biological mediators and periodontal regeneration: a review of enamel matrix proteins at the cellular and molecular levels. J Clin Periodontol 2008,; 35 (Suppl. 8): 87-105.

[6] World Workshop in Periodontology. The American Academy of Periodontology. Ann Periodontol 1996; 1: 618-70.

[7] Heijl L. Periodontal regeneration with enamel matrix derivative in one human experimental defect. A case report. J Clin Periodontol 1997; 24: 693-6.

[8] Yukna RA and Mellonig J. Histologic evaluation of periodontal healing in humans following regenerative therapy with enamel matrix derivative. A 10-case series. J Periodontol 2000; 71: 752-9.

[9] Sculean A, Donos N, Windisch P, Gera I, Brecx M and Reich E. Healing of human intrabony defects following treatment with enamel matrix proteins or guided tissue regeneration. J Periodont Res 1999; 34: 310-22.

[10] Mellonig JT. Enamel matrix derivative for periodontal reconstructive surgery: technique and clinical and histologic case report. Int J Periodontics Restorative Dent 1999; 19: 9-19.

[11] Sculean A, Chiantella GC, Windisch P et al. Clinical and histologic evaluation of treatment of intrabony defects with an enamel matrix protein derivative (Emdogain®). Int J Periodont Rest Dent 2000; 20: 375-81.

[12] Mazjoub Z, Bobbo M, Atiyeh F, et al. Two patterns of histologic healing in an intrabony defect following treatment with an enamel matrix derivative: a human case report. Int J Periodontics Restorative Dent 2005; 25: 283-94.

[13] Rasperini G, Silvestri M, Schenk RK, et al. Clinical and histological evaluation of human gingival recession treated with a subepithelial connective tissue graft and enamel matrix derivative (Emdogain): a case report. Int J Periodontics Restorative Dent, 2000, 20: 269-75.

[14] Carnio J, Camargo PM, Kenney EB, et al. Histological evaluation of 4 cases of root coverage following a connective tissue graft combined with an enamel matrix derivative preparation. J Periodontol 2002, 73, 1534-43.

[15] McGuire MK and Cochran DL. Evaluation of human recession defects treated with coronally advanced flaps and either enamel matrix derivative or connective tissue. Part 2: Histological evaluation. J Periodontol 2003; 74: 1126-35.

[16] Sculean A, Windisch P, Keglevich T, et al. Presence of an enamel matrix protein derivative on human teeth following periodontal surgery. Clin Oral Invest 2002; 6: 183-7.

[17] Sculean A, Junker R, Donos N, et al. Immunohistochemical evaluation of matrix molecules associated with wound healing following treatment with an enamel matrix protein derivative in humans. Clin Oral Invest 2003; 7: 167-74.

[18] Sculean A, Berakdar M, Windisch P, et al. Immunohistochemical investigation on the pattern of vimentin expression in regenerated and intact monkey and human periodontal ligamemt. Arch Oral Biol 2003; 48: 77-86.

[19] Bosshardt DD, Sculean A, Windisch P, et al. Effects of enamel matrix proteins on tissue formation along the roots of human teeth. J Periodont Res 2005; 40: 158-67.

[20] Bosshardt DD, Sculean A, Donos N et al. Pattern of mineralization after periodontal tissue engineering with enamel matrix proteins. Eur J Oral Sci 2006; 114 (Suppl. 1): 225-31.

[21] Sculean A, Windisch P, Keglevich T and Gera I. Histologic evaluation of human intrabony defects following non-surgical periodontal therapy with and without application of an enamel matrix protein derivative. J Periodontol 2003; 74: 153-60.

[22] Mellonig JT, Valderrama P, Gregory HJ, et al. Clinical and histological evaluation of non-surgical periodontal therapy with an enamel matrix derivative: a report of four cases. J Periodontol 2009; 80: 1534-40.

[23] Wennström JL and Lindhe J. Some effects of enamel matrix proteins on wound healing in the dento-gingival region. J Clin Periodontol 2002; 29: 9-14.

[24] Hagenaars S, Louwerse PH, Timmerman MF, et al. Soft-tissue wound healing following periodontal surgery and Emdogain application. J Clin Periodontol 2004; 31: 850-6.

[25] Okuda K, Miyazaki A, Momose M, et al. Levels of tissue inhibitor of metalloproteinases-1 and matrix metalloproteinases-1 and –8 in gingival crevicular fluid following treatment with enamel matrix derivative (EMDOGAIN). J Periodont Res 2001; 36: 309-16.

[26] Gutierrez MA, Mellonig JT and Cochran DL. Evaluation of enamel matrix derivative as an adjunct to non-surgical periodontal therapy. J Clin Periodontol 2003; 30: 739-45.

[27] Mombelli A, Brochut P, Plagnat D, et al. Enamel matrix proteins and systemic antibiotics as adjuncts to non-surgical periodontal treatment: clinical effects. J Clin Periodontol 2005; 32: 225-30.

[28] Petinaki E, Nikolopoulos S and Castanas E. Low stimulation of peripheral lymphocytes, following in vitro application of Emdogain. J Clin Periodontol 1998; 25: 715-20.

[29] Nikolopoulos S, Petinaki E and Castanas E. Immunologic effects of Emdogain in humans: one-year results. Int J Periodont Rest Dent 2002; 22: 269-77.

[30] Zetterström O, Andersson C, Eriksson L, et al. Clinical safety of enamel matrix derivative (Emdogain®) in the treatment of periodontal defects. J Clin Periodontol 1997; 24: 697-704.

[31] Froum S, Weinberg M, Novak J, et al. A multicenter study evaluating the sensitization potential of enamel matrix derivative after treatment of two intrabony defects. J Periodontol 2004; 75: 1001-8.

[32] Heijl L, Heden G, Svardström G, et al. Enamel matrix derivative (Emdogain®) in the treatment of intrabony periodontal defects. J Clin Periodontol 1997; 24: 705-14.

[33] Froum SJ, Weinberg MA, Rosenberg E, et al. A comparative study utilizing open flap debridement with and without enamel matrix derivative in the treatment of periodontal intrabony defects: a 12-month re-entry study. J Periodontol 2001; 72: 25-34.

[34] Pontoriero R, Wennström J and Lindhe J. The use of barrier membranes and enamel matrix proteins in the treatment of angular bone defects. A prospective controlled clinical study. J Clin Periodontol 1999; 26: 833-40.

[35] Tonetti MS, Lang NP, Cortellini P, et al. Enamel matrix proteins in the regenerative therapy of deep intrabony defects. A multicenter randomized controlled clinical trial. J Clin Periodontol 2002; 29: 317-25.

[36] Rösing CK, Aass AM, Mavropoulos A, et al. Clinical and radiographic effects of enamel matrix derivative in the treatment of intrabony periodontal defects: a 12-month longitudinal placebo-controlled clinical trial in adult periodontitis patients. J Periodontol 2005; 76: 129-33.

[37] Okuda K, Momose M, Miyazaki A, et al. Enamel matrix derivative in the treatment of human intrabony osseous defects. J Periodontol 2000; 71: 1821-8.

[38] Silvestri M, Ricci G, Rasperini G, et al. Comparison of treatments of intrabony defects with enamel matrix derivative, guided tissue regeneration with a nonresorbable membrane and Widman modified flap. A pilot study. J Clin Periodontol 2000; 27: 603-10.

[39] Sculean A, Windisch P, Chiantella GC, et al. Treatment of intrabony defects with enamel matrix proteins and guided tissue regeneration. A prospective controlled clinical study. J Clin Periodontol 2001; 28: 397-403.

[40] Zucchelli G, Bernardi F, Montebugnoli L et al. Enamel matrix proteins and guided tissue regeneration with titanium-reinforced expanded polytetrafluoroethylene membranes in the treatment of intrabony defects: a comparative controlled clinical trial. J Periodontol 2002; 73: 3-12.

[41] Silvestri M, Sartori S, Rasperini G, et al. Comparison of intarbony defects treated with enamel matrix derivative versus guided tissue regeneration with a nonresorbable membrane. J Clin Periodontol 2003; 30: 386-93.

[42] Wachtel H, Schenk G, Bohm S, et al. Microsurgical access flap and enamel matrix derivative for the treatment of periodontal intrabony defects: a controlled clinical study. J Clin Periodontol 2003; 30: 496-504.

[43] Cortellini P and Tonetti MS. A minimally invasive surgical technique with an enamel matrix derivative in the regenerative treatment of intra-bony defects: a novel approach to limit morbidity. J Clin Periodontol 2007; 34: 87-93.

[44] Harrel SK, Wilson TG Jr and Nunn ME. Prospective assessment of the use of enamel matrix derivative with minimally invasive surgery: six year results. J Periodontol, 2010, (in press)

[45] Yilmaz S, Kuru B and Altuna-Kirac E. Enamel matrix proteins in the treatment of periodontal sites with horizontal type of bone loss. J Clin Periodontol 2003; 30: 197-206.

[46] Jentsch H and Purschwitz R. A clinical study evaluating the treatment of supra-alveolar-type defects with access flap surgery with and without an enamel matrix proetein derivative: a pilot study. J Clin Periodontol 2008; 35: 713-8.

[47] Sculean B, Blaes A, Arweiler N, et al. The effect of postsurgical antibiotics on the healing of intrabony defects following treatment with enamel matrix proteins. J Periodontol 2001; 72: 190-5.

[48] Sculean A, Berakdar M, Donos N, et al. The effect of postsurgical administration of a selective cyclo-oxygenase-2 inhibitor on the healing of intrabony defects following treatment with enamel matrix proteins. Clin Oral Invest 2003; 7: 108-12.

[49] Parashis AO, Tsiklakis K and Tatakis DN. EDTA gel root conditioning: lack of effect on clinical and radiographic outcomes of intrabony defcct treatment with enamel matrix derivative. J Periodontol 2006; 77: 103-10.

[50] Sculean A, Berakdar M, Willershausen B, et al. Effect of EDTA root conditioning on the healing of intrabony defects treated with an enamel matrix protein derivative. J Periodontol 2006; 77: 1167-72.

[51] Sculean A, Donos N, Blaes A, et al. Comparison of enamel matrix proteins and bioabsorbable membranes in the treatment of intrabony periodontal defects. A split-mouth study. J Periodontol 1999; 70: 255-62.

[52] Sanz M, Tonetti MS, Zabalegui I, et al. Treatment of intrabony defects with enamel matrix proteins or barrier membranes: results from a multicenter practice-based clinical trial. J Periodontol 2004; 75: 726-33.

[53] Francetti L, Del Fabro M, Basso M, et al. Enamel matrix proteins in the treatment of intra-bony defects. A prospective 24-month clinical trial. J Clin Periodontol 2004; 31: 52-9.

[54] Francetti L, Trombelli L, Lombardo G, et al. Evaluation of efficacy of enamel matrix derivative in the treatment of intrabony defects: a 24-month multicenter study. Int J Periodontics Restorative Dent 2005; 25: 461-73.

[55] Sculean A, Donos N, Miliauskaite A, et al. Treatment of intrabony defects with enamel matrix proteins or bioresorbable membranes. A four year follow up split-mouth study. J Periodontol 2001; 72: 1695-1701.

[56] Sculean A, Donos N, Schwarz F, et al. Five year results following treatment of intrabony defects with enamel matrix proteins and guided tissue regeneration. J Clin Periodontol 2004; 31: 545-9.

[57] Heden G and Wennström JL. Five-year follow-up of regenerative periodontal therapy with enamel matrix derivative at sites with angular bone defects. J Periodontol 2006; 77: 295-301.

[58] Sculean A, Schwarz F, Miliauskaite A, et al. Treatment of intrabony defects with an enamel matrix protein derivative or bioresorbable membrane: an 8-year follow-up split-mouth study. J Periodontol 2006; 77: 1879-86.

[59] Sculean A, Chiantella GC, Schwarz F, et al. Nine year results following treatment of intrabony periodontal defects with an enamel matrix protein derivative. Int J Periodontics Restorative Dent 2005; 27: 221-9.

[60] Sculean A, Kiss A, Miliauskaite A, et al. Ten-year results following treatment of intra-bony defects with enamel matrix proteins and guided tissue regeneration. J Clin Periodontol 2008; 35: 817-24.

[61] Polimeni G, Xiropaidis AV and Wikesjö UME. Biology and principles of periodontal wound healing/regeneration. Periodontol 2000 2006; 41: 30-47.

[62] Tonetti MS, Pini Prato G and Cortellini P. Factors affecting the healing response of intrabony defects following guided tissue regeneration and access flap surgery. J Clin Periodontol 1996; 23: 548-56.

[63] Minabe M, Kodama T, Kogou T, et al. A comparative study of combined treatment with a collagen membrane and enamel matrix proteins for the regeneration of intraosseous defects. Int J Periodontics Restorative Dent 2002; 22: 595-605.

[64] Sipos PM, Loos BG, Abbas F, et al. The combined use of enamel matrix proteins and a tetracycline-coated expanded polytetrafluoroethylene barrier membrane in the treatment of intra-osseous defects. J Clin Periodontol 2005; 32: 765-72.

[65] Sculean A, Windisch P, Keglevich T, et al. Clinical and histologic evaluation of human intrabony defects treated with an enamel matrix protein derivative combined with a bovine-derived xenograft. Int J Periodont Rest Dent 2003; 23: 47-55.

[66] Sculean A, Chiantella GC, Arweiler NB, et al. Five-year clinical and histologic results following treatment of human intrabony defects with an enamel matrix derivative combined with a natural bone mineral. Int J Periodont Rest Dent 2008; 28: 153-61.

[67] Sculean A, Windisch P, Keglevich T et al. Clinical and histological evaluation of an enamel matrix protein derivative combined with a bioactive glass for the treatment of intrabony periodontal defects in humans. Int J Periodont Rest Dent 2005; 25: 139-47.

[68] Guida L, Annunziata M, Belardo S, et al. Effect of autogenous cortical bone particulate in conjunction with enamel matrix derivative in the treatment of periodontal intraosseous defects. J Periodontol 2007; 78: 231-8.

[69] Lekovic V, Camargo PM, Weinlaender M, et al. A comparison between enamel matrix proteins used alone or in combination with bovine porous bone mineral in the treatment of intrabony periodontal defects in humans. J Periodontol 2000; 71: 1695-1701.

[70] Velasquez-Plata D, Scheyer ET and Mellonig JT. Clinical comparison of an enamel matrix derivative used alone or in combination with a bovine-derived xenograft for the treatment of periodontal osseous defects in humans. J Periodontol 2002; 73: 433-40.

[71] Zucchelli G, Amore C, Montebugnoli L et al. Enamel matrix proteins and bovine porous mineral in the treatment of intrabony defects: a comparative controlled clinical trial. J Periodontol 2003; 74: 1725-35.

[72] Gurinsky BS, Mills MP and Mellonig JT. Clinical evaluation of demineralized freeze-dried bone allograft and enamel matrix derivative versus enamel matrix derivative alone for the treatment of periodontal osseous defects in humans. J Periodontol 2004; 75, 1309-18.

[73] Hoidal J, Grimard BA, Mills MP, et al. Clinical evaluation of demineralized freeze-dried bone allograft with and without enamel matrix derivative for the treatment of periodontal osseous defects in humans. J Periodontol 2008; 79: 2273-80.

[74] Kuru B, Yilmaz S, Argin K, et al. Enamel matrix derivative alone or in combination with a bioactive glass in wide intrabony defects. Clin Oral Invest 2006; 10: 227-34.

[75] Sculean A, Pietruska M, Schwarz F, et al. Healing of human intrabony defects following regenerative periodontal therapy with an enamel matrix protein derivative alone or combined with a bioactive glass. A controlled clinical study. J Clin Periodontol 2005; 32: 111-7.

[76] Sculean A, Pietruska M, Arweiler NB, et al. Four year results of a prospective controlled clinical study evaluating healing of intrabony defects following treatment with an enamel matrix protein derivative alone or combined with a bioactive glass. J Clin Periodontol 2007; 34: 507-13.

[77] Bokan I, Bill JS and Schlagenhauf U. Primary flap closure combined with Emdogain® alone or Emdogain® and Cerasorb® in the treatment of intra-bony defects. J Clin Periodontol 2006; 33: 885–93.

[78] Jepsen S, Topoll H, Rengers H, et al. Clinical outcomes after treatment of intra-bony defects with an EMD/synthetic bone graft or EMD alone: a multicentre randomized controlled clinical trial. J Clin Periodontol 2008; 35: 420-8.

[79] Sculean A, Barbé G, Chiantella GC, et al. Clinical evaluation of an enamel matrix protein derivative combined with a bioactive glass for the treatment of intrabony periodontal defects in humans. J Periodontol 2002, 73: 401-8.

[80] Sculean A, Chiantella GC, Windisch P, et al. Clinical evaluation of an enamel matrix protein derivative (Emdogain®) combined with a bovine derived xenograft (Bio-Oss®) for the treatment of intrabony periodontal defects in humans. Int J Periodont Rest Dent 2002; 22: 259-67.

[81] Scheyer ET, Velasquez-Plata D, Brunsvold MA, et al. A clinical comparison of a bovine-derived xenograft used alone and in combination with enamel matrix derivative for the treatment of periodontal osseous defects in humans. J Periodontol 2002; 73: 423-32.

[82] Modica F, Del Pizzo M, Roccuzzo M, et al. Coronally advanced flap for the treatment of buccal gingival recessions with and without enamel matrix derivative. A split-mouth study. J Periodontol 2000; 71: 1693-8.

[83] Hägewald S, Spahr A, Rompola E, et al. Comparative study of Emdogain® and coronally advanced flap technique in the treatment of human gingival recessions. A prospective controlled clinical study. J Clin Periodontol 2002; 29: 35-41.

[84] Spahr A, Hägewald S, Tsoulfidou F, et al. Coverage of Miller class I and II recession defects using enamel matrix proteins versus coronally repositioned flap technique: a 2 year report. J Periodontol 2005; 76: 1871-80.

[85] Cueva MA, Boltchi FE, Hallmon WW, et al. A comparative study of coronally advanced flaps with and without the addition of enamel matrix derivative in the treatment of marginal tissue recession. J Periodontol 2004; 75: 949-56.

[86] Castellanos AT, de la Rosa MR, de la Garza M et al. Enamel matrix derivative and coronal flaps to cover marginal tissue recessions. J Periodontol 2006; 77: 7-14.

[87] Cairo F, Pagliaro U and Nieri M. Treatment of gingival recession with coronally advanced flap procedures: a systematic review. J Clin Periodontol 2008; 35 (Suppl. 8): 136-62.

[88] McGuire MK and Nunn M. Evaluation of human recession defects treated with coronally advanced flaps and either enamel matrix derivative or connective tissue. Part 1: Comparison of clinical parameters. J Periodontol 2003; 74: 1110-25.

[89] Nemcovsky CE, Artzi Z, Tal H, et al. A multicenter comparative study of two root coverage procedures: coronally advanced flap with addition of enamel matrix proteins and subpedicle connective tissue graft. J Periodontol 2004; 75: 600-7.

[90] Berlucchi I, Franchetti L, Del Fabro M, et al. Enamel matrix proteins (Emdogain) in combination with coronally advanced flap or subepithelial connective tissue graft in the treatment of shallow gingival recessions. Int J Periodont Rest Dent 2002; 22: 583-93.

[91] Del Pizzo M, Zucchelli G, Modica F, et al. Coronally advanced flap with or without enamel matrix derivative for root coverage: a 2 year study. J Clin Periodontol 2005; 32: 1181-7.

[92] Ofer M, Artzi Z, Sculean A, et al. Comparative study of 2 root coverage procedures: a 24-month follow-up multicenter study. J Periodontol 2006; 77: 195-202.

[93] Jepsen S, Heinz B, Jepsen K, et al. A randomized clinical trial comparing enamel matrix derivative and membrane treatment of buccal Class II furcation involvement in mandibular molars. Part I: study design and results for primary outcomes. J Periodontol 2004; 75: 1150-60.
[94] Meyle J, Gonzalez JR, Bodeker RH, et al. A randomized clinical trial comparing enamel matrix derivative and membrane treatment of buccal class II furcation involvement in mandibular molars. Part II: secondary outcomes. J Periodontol 2004; 75: 1188-95.
[95] Casarin RC, Del Peloso Ribeiro E, Nociti FH Jr, et al. A double-blind randomized clinical evaluation of enamel matrix derivative proteins for the treatment of proximal class II furcation involvements. J Clin Periodontol 2008; 35: 429-37.

Index

E

H

I

K

L

M

N

Made in the USA
Las Vegas, NV
15 April 2026

45339747R00148